T0384887

Helping the Hard-Core Smoker
A Clinician's Guide

•♈•

Helping the Hard-Core Smoker
A Clinician's Guide

•♈•

Edited by

Daniel F. Seidman
Columbia University
College of Physicians and Surgeons

Lirio S. Covey
New York State Psychiatric Institute
and
Columbia University

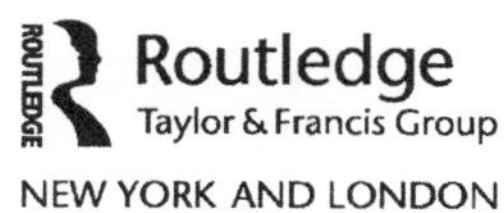

NEW YORK AND LONDON

First Published by
Lawrence Erlbaum Associates, Inc., Publishers
10 Industrial Avenue
Mahwah, NJ 07430

Transferred to Digital Printing 2009 by Routledge
270 Madison Ave, New York NY 10016
27 Church Road, Hove, East Sussex, BN3 2FA

Cover design by Kathryn Houghtaling Lacey

Library of Congress Cataloging-in-Publication Data

Helping the hard-core smoker : a clinician's guide / edited by Daniel F. Seidman, Lirio S. Covey

p. cm.

Includes bibliographical references and indexes.

ISBN 0-8058-2755-2 (cloth : alk. paper)

1. Tobacco habit—Treatment.. 2. Smoking cessation programs.

I. Seidman, Daniel F. II. Covey, Lirio S.

RC567.H45 1998

616.86'506—dc21

98-22971

CIP

Publisher's Note

The publisher has gone to great lengths to ensure the quality of this reprint but points out that some imperfections in the original may be apparent.

To our families

Susan, Lionel, and Ira Seidman
and
Michael, William, and Michael Lee Covey

Contents

Foreword

Joseph A. Califano, Jr.

In August 1975, on the beach at Gull Pond in Wellfleet, Massachussets, I asked my eleven-year-old son Joe III what he wanted for Christmas. "Your birthday is just after Christmas, so you never get a proper present," I said. "Let me know what you want and we'll get it in September."

"I want you to quit smoking," he responded immediately.

"Seriously, Joe, tell me what you want for your birthday."

"Seriously, Dad," he shot back, "I want you to quit smoking."

With that formidable task ahead, I returned to Washington on Labor Day.

Like the subjects of this book, I was a hard-core smoker. I had begun smoking in 1945 shortly before my 14th birthday. By the time I got to Harvard Law School in 1952, I was up to a pack a day, and I hit a whopping four packs daily from 1965 to 1969 while working as Lyndon Johnson's special assistant for domestic affairs.

In 1966, when I recommended to President Johnson that he send to Congress legislation to ban cigarette advertising from television, he looked at the cigarette between the fingers of my right hand and said, "When you stop, I'll send that legislation forward." Already at war with the Southern states over civil rights, his top national priority, LBJ had no intention of opening a second front in tobacco in states like North Carolina, Kentucky, and Virginia. He knew that by setting that condition on my proposal, he had tabled the issue for the duration of his presidency.

Lyndon Johnson himself had been a chain smoker until his massive heart attack in 1954. Though he quit smoking after that, on most days at the White House he would say, "The day I leave here, I'm going to light up a cigarette." Indeed he did—on the flight back to Texas on the afternoon of January 20, 1969, shortly after Richard Nixon was sworn in as president. He died of a heart attack 4 years later.

I did not seriously try to quit smoking while serving in the Johnson White House. On returning to law practice, I settled into a two-pack-a-day habit.

In 1975, faced with my son Joe's request, I sought help in quitting. My friend, Washington Post editor Ben Bradlee, and my law partner Vincent Fuller (who later represented John Hinkley, Jr., the disturbed young man who attempted to assassinate President Ronald Reagan) were enrolled in a smoking-cessation program. Bradlee had been told by his wife-to-be, Sally Quinn, that he had to quit if he wanted to continue their relationship. Fuller had been told by his doctor that he had the early symptoms of emphysema, and it was either quit smoking or prepare for disability and premature death.

I entered that smoking cessation program uncertain of my ability to quit. I followed the steps of the program, from switching from my chosen brand of cigarettes to another, to keeping my cigarette butts in a big jar on my bedroom dresser. On October 27, 1975, just before midnight, I took my last puff on a cigarette.

The quitting process was not easy, but it was successful. I was among the fortunate few life-long smokers who are able to quit on the first try.

When I became Secretary of Health, Education, and Welfare in January 1977, I had no intention of mounting an aggressive antismoking campaign. President Jimmy Carter and I were determined to focus the nation's attention on health promotion and disease prevention. As I interviewed more than 100 physicians for various posts in the department, and talked to many more already in the Public Health Service, I would ask them about health promotion and disease prevention. Without exception, the response was the same refrain: "You can't have a serious health promotion and disease prevention program unless you go after smoking."

We then conducted a survey that revealed two stunning facts: 90% of smokers were hooked before they reached age 21, and most smokers had tried to quit within the last year (they may not have made it out of bed in the morning without lighting up, but at least they went to sleep determined to stop smoking the next day). These findings spurred my decision to mount the antismoking campaign in January 1978, with an energetic effort aimed at reminding smokers of all the dangers of their habit in order to encourage them to hold fast to their determination to quit.

That program sparked the rapid decline in the social acceptability of smoking. As a result, hundreds of thousands of smokers broke their addiction. But oh, how many millions more would have stopped if this book had been available then!

Helping The Hard-Core Smoker: A Clinician's Guide belongs on the desk of every physician, psychiatrist, nurse practitioner, dentist, psychologist, elementary and secondary school teacher, and drug and alcohol counselor in the nation. The chapters are chock full of practical ideas on how to get smokers from early teens to late sixties to quit—and stay smoke-free permanently. They offer telling insights into the many obstacles faced by the smoker trying to quit, and into the mix of psychological, emotional, genetic, and environmental factors that contribute to nicotine dependence. This book contains workable techniques for targeting women, whose reasons for continuing to smoke—particularly weight control—may be quite distinct from those of men, and for intervening with older smokers (those over 49), who may not realize the extent to which they can improve the quality of their lives if they break the habit.

Of particular importance, in view of the alarming increases in teen smoking, is the piece by Gil Botvin and Jennifer Epstein. Its analysis of why teens start and continue to smoke, and its emphasis on the importance of *comprehensive* school programs are invaluable to school boards, administrators and teachers, and parents committed to stemming this increase.

At The National Center on Addiction and Substance Abuse at Columbia University, we are testing a program to help women on welfare shake their substance abuse and addiction. We have found Michelle Drayton-Martin et al's chapter on implementation of a prenatal smoking cessation program in three inner city communities a priceless source of invaluable ideas.

The essays in this book present a wide range of treatment options for nicotine dependence, from nicotine and nonnicotine medications to short-term individual psychotherapy, group therapy, and hypnosis, as well as techniques for preventing relapse among former smokers. The potential efficacy of these treatments will provide hope to the practitioner attempting to help the hard-core smoker quit.

Among the most critical points made in this collection of pieces is the largely untapped potential of physicians and dentists to promote smoking cessation, as underscored in the last two chapters. As Glynn et al's essay notes, even a brief intervention by a physician or dentist can make the difference for an individual trying to quit.

Any practitioner looking for help to encourage smokers to stop, and practical suggestions to provide that help could find no better resource than this extraordinary collection of essays. For those who harbor any doubts about the economic, social, and public health benefits in getting the hard-core smokers to quit, the afterword by Dr. Cheryl Healton provides a powerful conclusion to this work.

My son Joe's gift to me was to get me to quit smoking more than 20 years ago. He is now an otolaryngologist focused on cancer research and surgery. He often bemoans the failure of his patients to quit smoking. This book will give him a sense of hope borne of the fact that some of our nation's finest minds in this field have put it all together to increase the effectiveness of those on the front lines in getting the hard-core smoker to quit. That is the gift that Daniel Seidman and Lirio Covey have given our nation and its 50 million remaining smokers, with their tenacious and hard work in assembling and editing this extraordinary collection of essays.

Preface

Our work on this volume represents the combined experience of more than two decades of research and clinical practice in the area of smoking cessation. In 1987, Alexander Glassman, as Chief of its Department of Clinical Psychopharmacology, was developing a smoking cessation research unit at the New York Psychiatric Institute (NYSPI) and a smoking cessation treatment service at the Columbia Presbyterian Medical Center (CPMC). July 1 of that year marked the first employment day for both Lirio Covey as researcher-clinician at NYSPI, and Daniel Seidman as the clinical psychologist for the CPMC smoking cessation service. For Covey, the new challenge marked an integration of previous epidemiological research activities, with Ernst Wynder at the American Health Foundation, which had made clear the abundance of health reasons for avoiding or terminating tobacco use, and an academic background in psychology and psychiatric research. For Seidman, his work with smokers at the CPMC Smoking Cessation Service coincided with other work in the Department of Psychiatry with cocaine, alcohol, and other substance abusers, an experience that provided him with a particular perspective in working with the problems of cigarette smokers.

A result of this work since the 1980s has been, for both of us, an intimate familiarity with the subject of this volume: smokers who have made numerous attempts to stop smoking, but have failed. Additionally, that work enabled us to develop ideas and strategies for helping these patients not only to stop smoking but also to relinquish attitudes and behaviors that accompanied and often sustained the need to continue to smoke, and then move on to productive and satisfying nonsmoking patterns of behavior, thinking, and feeling.

During this period, we were frequently invited by various medical and health care organizations to give lectures and provide consultation in their efforts to assist smokers. The educational flow in these contacts was, in fact, in both directions. To our gain, these experiences indicated to us a widespread lack of recognition of the special difficulties of the highly addicted smoker as well as the need for disseminating the knowledge that we had gained about how best to help those smokers. This background motivated the preparation of this book.

Recent data on the prevalence of cigarette smoking among adolescents constitute another important purpose for this book. Instead of continuing to decline, as would be expected from the historical trend, the rate of cigarette smoking among teenagers in the United States has increased. This is an ominous statistic. Although the causes of the increased prevalence of smoking among young persons are yet to be determined, and society's ability to control them may be in doubt, what is quite certain is that many of those teenaged smokers will become tomorrow's highly addicted adult smokers. Like the generation before them, those hard-core smokers of the future will be at high risk for a significant number of smoking-related illnesses. Although societal efforts had not sufficed to prevent them from beginning to smoke, perhaps timely and well-placed interventions will help them to stop smoking.

Among the central beliefs to grow out of our work were, first of all, that no single personal or demographic trait—neither age, sex, nor medical or psychiatric history, characterizes the hard-core smoker; and secondly, that no single type of treatment modality will work for all smokers. Nevertheless, some smoker subgroups do carry particular areas of vulnerability and require special care. These include women, low-income groups, adolescents, and the elderly. Issues relating to those groups of smokers, as well as an array of psychological and pharmacological treatments that have been employed to help them quit, are discussed in Part III of this volume.

We have designed this book for professionals who are in a position to help today's difficult-to-treat smokers: clinicians in the field of mental health; physicians, dentists, nurses, pharmacists, and other health care professionals; human-resource and employee-assistance program corporate staff; teachers and guidance counselors; and clergy.

We are grateful to our colleagues who contributed chapters and gave generously of both their time and expertise toward the completion of this book.

We are also grateful to Alexander H. Glassman, Chief of Clinical Psychopharmacology at the New York State Psychiatric Institute and Columbia University, and Donald S. Kornfeld, Director of the Behavioral Medicine program at Columbia University for the opportunity to develop the perspectives we have put forth in this work. We also thank our colleagues at the New York State Psychiatric Institute: Elmer Struening, Fay Stetner, Janel Carino, and Sally Woodring; and our colleagues in the Behavioral Medicine Program: Kenneth Frank, Ethan Gorenstein, Kenneth Gorfinkle, Kenneth Greenspan, and Richard Sloan, for creating the intellectually challenging and supportive environment in which this book took shape. Finally, we are grateful to our patients whose hard work and perserverance helped to educate us about nicotine dependence.

Despite the enormous amount of research on the problem of smoking cessation, the success rates of hard-core smokers have remained low. We hope that the concepts and treatment approaches presented in this guide will lead to improved services for hard-core smokers. We also hope that this volume will stimulate further thinking and research on how best to help smokers who continue to struggle with their addiction.

—Lirio S. Covey
—Daniel F. Seidman

Part I

Background Conceptual Issues

CHAPTER ONE

Biological and Clinical Perspectives on Nicotine Addiction

Daniel F. Seidman
Jeffrey Rosecan
Lorna Role
Columbia University

Although smoking cigarettes continues to be portrayed as glamorous in advertisements and to attract a new generation of smokers, it has undergone a transformation in public awareness from bad habit to drug addiction. The health consequences of smoking have also been well established and publicized. This chapter provides a foundation for understanding nicotine addiction by examining two different approaches to the same phenomenon. One approach looks at nicotine addiction from the perspective of the cell, and the other from the perspective of the whole person. One approach examines nicotine addiction viewed from recent developments in neuroanatomy and neurophysiology. In the other approach, cigarette smoking is examined as a clinical disorder.

Promising patients to address their smoking addictions "later," or admonishing them to "just stop smoking," can mean missed opportunities (Fiore, Epps, & Manley, 1994). This applies not only to helping patients with their cigarette addiction, and to teaching new clinicians about effective interventions, but also to a lost opportunity to deepen the relationship between patient and doctor, dentist, or other health care professional.

Although some smokers can and do quit on their own, increasingly, many others are in need of clinical assistance. This is especially the case for the hard-core smoker.

In this chapter we define *hard-core smokers*, and distinguish between the habit of smoking and nicotine addiction. We also compare the rates of addiction and relapse in smokers with those of people addicted to other drugs and alcohol.

We then review recent developments in basic research science to provide the practicing clinician with new insight into the underlying biological foundation of nicotine addiction. Finally, we develop a clinical perspective that views nicotine addiction as a complex interaction among three factors: (a) the brain pathways that are altered by smoking tobacco, and the impact of smoking the drug nicotine on mood, perception, arousal, and attention; (b) the psychological adjustment of the individual and the use of smoking as a "psychological tool"; and (c) the role of the sociocultural context in the initiation, maintenance, and relapse back to smoking behavior. This clinical perspective on nicotine addiction concludes with a brief review of four practical criteria for diagnosing cigarette smoking as an addictive disorder.

DEFINING HARD-CORE SMOKERS

The first group of smokers defined here as *hard core* are smokers who are medically ill but who continue to smoke. The literature contains a number of studies of cancer patients who continued to smoke at high rates even after diagnosis and treatment (Davidson & Duffy, 1982; Spitz, Fueger, Chamberlain, Goepfert, & Newell, 1990). Several studies also report high rates of continued smoking after myocardial infarction (Havik & Maeland, 1988; Taylor, Houston-Miller, Killen, & DeBusk, 1990).

The second group of smokers we define as hard core are those who score greater than 7 on the Fagerstrom Test for Nicotine Dependence (Fagerstrom & Schneider, 1989). According to this test, smokers high in nicotine dependence often smoke more than 20 cigarettes per day and begin smoking within 5 min of awakening in the morning. Highly nicotine-dependent smokers also report severe symptoms of nicotine withdrawal (U.S. Department of Health and Human Services, 1996).

Finally, the third group we define as hard-core smokers are those with comorbid psychological or psychiatric conditions, which are associated with increased risks of becoming addicted to, and difficulties in cessation from, cigarette smoking (see chap. 2, this volume). This group of smokers includes those depressed smokers referred to in the 1990 *JAMA* editorial "Blue Mood, Blackened Lungs." This editorial concluded that "about 20% of smokers have high depressive symptom scores, this means that depression may be a contributing factor to the smoking of more than 10 million Americans, who are 40% less likely to quit smoking than are nondepressed smokers" (Glass, 1990, p. 1584).

HABIT VERSUS ADDICTION

Cigarette smoking often appears to be only a habit—an automatic behavior pattern influenced primarily by learning and reinforcement—because it is a repetitive behavior, it is learned, and in many smokers it tends to increase under stress. It is used as a tension reducer in anxiety-provoking situations. It is also pleasurable for many people, and this pleasure is reinforced when smoking accompanies activities such as a meal, coffee, or sex. The constant repetition of smoking behavior many times per day involves tremendous habit strength and conditioning and can become an automatic part of life, a ritual. In fact, smoking behavior is so "overlearned" that smokers often light up a cigarette and let it burn down in an ashtray without even realizing it.

Gum chewing also fits the definition of a habit: It is an automatic behavior pattern that is learned, and can be used to reduce tension or for pleasure. People are aware of unwrapping a piece of gum and putting it in their mouths, but tend to forget that they are chewing it until the flavor runs out. People can chew gum for years without thinking twice about it, and aside from minor dental problems suffer no real adverse consequences.

There are, however, important reasons why we feel cigarette smoking is much more than a habit like chewing gum. One principal reason is the presence of nicotine withdrawal after stopping:

> The misery of abstinence has been far greater than I ever imagined . . . suddenly there came a severe cardiac misery, greater than I ever had while smoking. The most violent arrythmia, constant tension, pressure, burning in the heart region, shooting pains down my left arm . . . and with it a feeling of depression which took the form of visions of death. (quoted in Masson, 1985, p. 67)

This unfortunate individual is Dr. Sigmund Freud, founder of modern psychiatry and psychoanalysis, after trying unsuccessfully to stop smoking his famous cigar for a few weeks in 1894. It is, to our knowledge, the earliest description of the nicotine withdrawal syndrome.

A defined withdrawal syndrome establishes a biological basis for addiction. In contrast to what happens when an addicted smoker stops smoking, there is no withdrawal syndrome from stopping the habit of chewing gum. The withdrawal syndrome is thus one of the hallmarks of an addiction, whether it be to alcohol ("the DTs"), heroin ("cold turkey"), cocaine ("the crash"), or nicotine. The common symptoms associated with nicotine withdrawal are:

- Dysphoric or depressed mood
- Insomnia
- Irritability, frustration, or anger
- Anxiety
- Difficulty concentrating
- Restlessness

- Decreased heart rate
- Increased appetite or weight gain (*DSM–IV*, APA, 1994)

Although the medical and scientific community would prefer not to use the term *addiction*, the term is widely used to imply a severe drug dependence. The legitimacy of viewing cigarette smoking as an addiction has been increasingly accepted (U.S. Department of Health and Human Services, 1988) and with that acceptance, its comparison to heroin, cocaine, and alcohol addiction has also grown.

RATES OF ADDICTION AND RELAPSE

How addicting is smoking nicotine? There are a variety of ways to measure addiction. One is the *graduation rate* from recreational, casual, or social use of a substance to daily, compulsive use or abuse of a substance. The graduation rate is a measure of the incidence of addictive use or abuse of a substance, versus its experimental or recreational use.

For nicotine, the graduation rate from experimental or recreational use to daily use for 20-year-olds who are still smoking is 95% (APA, 1994). Further, out of 10 people who become smokers, 9 smoke more than five cigarettes a day (Henningfield, Cohen, & Slade, 1991). The 10% or less of smokers who smoke five or fewer cigarettes per day have been called "chippers." The term, borrowed from some opiate addicts, refers to light use without becoming addicted (Shiffman, 1989). Seventy-five percent of smokers meet diagnostic criteria for nicotine dependence (see chap. 2, this volume).

For nasal cocaine use, the rate of progression to dependence (i.e., graduation rate) has been estimated at 25% of regular users (Jaffe, 1990). Although difficult to estimate precisely, the graduation rate to compulsive use for crack smoking is undoubtedly much higher. This is because the addiction to crack can be instantaneous on the first try, or a matter of weeks or months, compared with a pattern of escalating use over several years in cigarette, heroin, and alcohol addiction.

For narcotics (heroin and opium), the graduation rate to addiction can be circumstantial (i.e., dependent on social circumstances, e.g., combat service). A study by Robins, Helzer, and Davis (1975), using U.S. army enlistees, found only 14% of those highly addicted to narcotics in Vietnam to be still addicted 10 months after returning to the United States.

Finally, for alcohol, the graduation rate to dependence is conservatively estimated as 5–10% for adult men, and approximately one third of that for adult women (Schuckit, 1989).

A second way to measure addiction is by how difficult it is to stay away from a substance. In one study (Blumberg et al., 1974) polysubstance abusers were asked to compare their need on a 1 (no need) to 4 (need a lot) scale. The results showed the following ratings: tobacco (3.3), heroin (2.8), cocaine (1.5), and alcohol (1.3). In a second study of patients in treatment for drug and alcohol abuse (Kozlowski et al., 1989), 74% of these patients reported that giving up cigarettes was at least as difficult as giving up their primary problem substance. Over half, or 57%, of this patient sample stated that giving up cigarettes would be *more* difficult than giving up the drug that originally brought them to treatment.

Further, it turns out that heroin, alcohol, and nicotine addiction (smoking cessation) programs have similar outcome rates or rates of success and failure (Hunt, Barnett, & Branch, 1971). Hunt and colleagues, writing in 1971, found relapse rates in addiction programs of 60–65% to be common in the first 3 months of treatment, 70–80% at 1 year. Over 20 years later, Hurt and colleagues (1992) reported a 1-year abstinence rate of 29% from an in-patient service for difficult-to-help smokers. This outcome is comparable to many good addiction treatment programs.

This means, however, that 70–80% of patients go on smoking, drinking, and taking heroin after treatment, despite the problems these drugs cause or may cause in their lives. Smoking is an addiction of major magnitude. We now discuss how the biological processes underlying cigarette addiction contribute to its refractory clinical presentation.

NICOTINE ADDICTION: BRAIN AND BEHAVIOR

Biological Perspectives

A biologically based approach to understanding the roots of tobacco addiction comes from the work of basic scientists studying the interactions of nicotine with various brain structures. From their work, we glean important insights into the effects of smoking on nerve cells within the "reward systems" of the brain. This perspective evolves from studies of the primary addictive substance in cigarettes: nicotine (Corrigall & Coen, 1989; Dani & Heinemann, 1996; Stolerman & Shoaib, 1991).

Recognizing the versatility and comprehensiveness of the many brain pathways affected by smoking underscores the biological basis of smoking as an addictive disorder. This can help counter the smoker's view of cigarette use as merely a "bad habit" they will eventually be able to control. It can also help smokers to understand why quitting often requires clinical intervention, and why, once they are addicted, they "can't just take one" cigarette. One cigarette will stimulate an addictive reward system that it then won't be able to satisfy.

Compelling evidence has accrued implicating nicotine as the active compound in the behavioral, cognitive, and addictive effects of cigarette smoking. Nicotine by itself, in the absence of any other tobacco-derived products, elicits drug-seeking behavior. Animal studies demonstrate that nicotine per se can increase locomotor activity and potently reinforce self-administration and place-preference behaviors in ways similar to other substances of abuse (Adikofer & Thurau, 1991; Goldberg & Henningfield, 1988; Stolerman & Shoaib, 1991). The mechanisms underlying nicotine addiction are far from understood in their entirety. Nevertheless, the physical localization of nicotinic receptors in the brain and the demonstrated effects of nicotine on neuronal activity underscore the importance of this nicotine research for understanding the physiological basis of nicotine addiction.

Basic research efforts on nicotine have already elucidated fundamental aspects of disorders such as schizophrenia, Alzheimer's, and Parkinson's, and suggest that nicotine-related drugs may have therapeutic potential for treating the symptoms of these disorders, as well as for smoking cessation. As such, the findings from basic research efforts on the physiology of nicotine, although often less familiar to the clinician, provide essential background information for modern health care practitioners whose patient populations include smokers. In view of the (unexpected) discovery of the potential therapeutic value of nicotine in diseases as prevalent and devastating as Alzheimer's, a fundamental understanding of the physiology of nicotine is essential to the informed physician. For these reasons, we present a brief primer on the highlights of recent research into nicotine's effects on the brain.

Nicotine functionally mimics *acetylcholine*, an endogenous component of neural tissue that serves as a neurotransmitter in specific regions of the brain. Like acetylcholine, nicotine can excite individual neurons in the brain by virtue of its ability to interact with a particular set of transmitter recognition sites, which were dubbed *nicotinic receptors* in the late 1800s (!) by one of the grandfathers of neurobiology, J. Langley (Langley & Anderson, 1892). More than a century of study of nicotinic receptors has yielded considerable insight into the molecular and biophysical details of their function. The most essential elements are:

1. The effects of nicotine are mediated by the direct activation of nicotinic receptor sites in the brain.

2. Nicotinic receptors are expressed in specific regions of the brain and in particular groups of neurons within these regions. Of special interest in this regard is the high level of expression of nicotinic receptors in the "reward" or "reinforcement" centers of the brain: that is, neurons of the mesolimbic system, as well as neurons within and projecting to the accumbens, amygdala, and hippocampus.

3. Individual neurons can express more than one subtype of nicotinic receptors (of which there are many; see Role & Berg, 1996, for a recent review).

4. Nicotinic receptors can be both on the neuronal cell body and on neuronal synaptic terminals. Furthermore, distinct subtypes of nicotinic receptors can be selectively localized to either the cell body or terminals of an individual neuron.

It is important to note that depending on both the type of nicotinic receptor and the cellular localization (i.e., where on the neuron the receptors are expressed) nicotine can have dramatically different physiological effects.

Possibly the most important findings relative to how nicotine works in the brain have emerged from cellular physiology studies (for reviews see McGehee & Role, 1995, 1996; Role & Berg, 1996; Wonnacott, 1997). The "classical" notion of where nicotinic receptors are located and how nicotine changes neuronal excitability is illustrated in Fig. 1.1A. Here, the nicotinic receptors are located on the postsynaptic neuron. The release of the natural transmitter, acetylcholine, from a presynaptic neuron (a *cholinergic* neuron, which is one that is capable of synthesizing and releasing acetylcholine from its synaptic terminals) results in the direct activation of the postsynaptic neuron. This activation is initiated by the interaction of acetylcholine with nicotinic receptors on the surface of the postsynaptic neurons that both bind the neurotransmitter and, once bound, open a "channel" or membrane pore through which positively charged ions flow into the cell. The result of this current influx is physiologically manifest as an increase in excitability, that is, an increase in the number and frequency of action potentials fired.

The increase in current flow and the consequent increase in neuronal excitability can also be achieved by exposure of a neuron to exogenous nicotine if (and only if) the neuron expresses nicotinic receptors (e.g., Fig. 1.1A). A prime example of a place in the nervous system where this can happen is in the peripheral autonomic ganglia. In this case, acetylcholine is released from a presynaptic neuron and postsynaptic nicotinic receptors directly mediate synaptic transmission (see Fig. 1.1A). In the central nervous system (CNS), however, researchers have demonstrated that the receptors that bind acetylcholine and nicotine are localized on the presynaptic terminals, as well as on neuronal cell bodies. Furthermore, electrophysiological studies have revealed that, although direct nicotinic transmission does occur within specific regions of the CNS, documented examples of synapses like the one illustrated in Fig. 1.1A are relatively scarce (for reviews see Role & Berg, 1996; Wonnacott, 1997).

Another mechanism by which acetylcholine and nicotine can alter the excitability of neurons, illustrated in Fig. 1.1B, may account for the widespread effects of nicotine in the CNS. Recent work demonstrates that nicotinic

A. Post-synaptic actions of ACh and nicotine

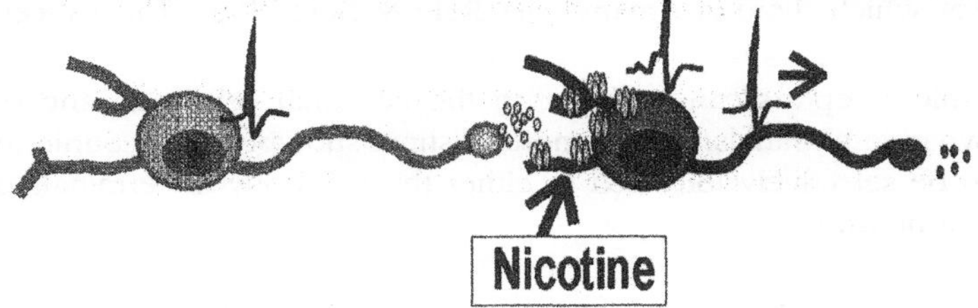

B. Pre-synaptic actions of ACh and nicotine

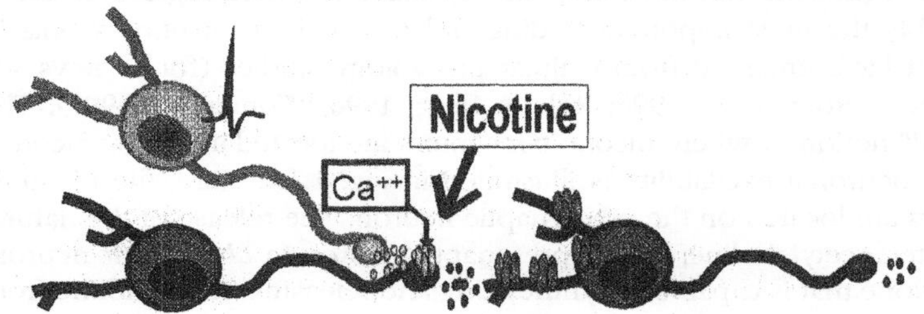

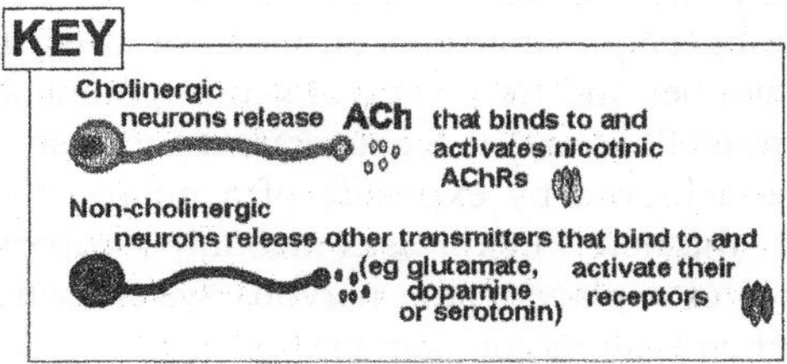

FIG. 1.1

receptors can be targeted or shipped from the cell body to the presynaptic neuronal axon terminals—the site of transmitter release from neurons (Fig. 1.1B). When either acetylcholine or nicotine binds to these nicotinic receptors, the receptor channel opens and positive ions flow into the synaptic terminal. However, because the volume of a synaptic terminal is so small, the net effect of the current influx on the local concentration of calcium and other cations is huge. The net effect of the activation of even a few such strategically localized receptors will dramatically increase the amount of transmitter released from the synaptic terminal.

Neuronal nicotinic receptors are particularly well suited to enhancing transmitter release because the ion pore they comprise is highly permeable to calcium. Activating presynaptic nicotinic receptors—whether by the endogenous transmitter (acetylcholine) or by exogenously administered nicotine—causes calcium influx, which in turn increases the release of the stored neurotransmitter. It is particularly important to note that nicotine-induced facilitation of transmitter release can and does occur at synapses mediated by the full gamut of known transmitters. The result is that nicotine can enhance the release of dopamine (from meso-limbic projections to nucleus accumbens), norepinephrine (from nigral neurons projecting to ventral striatum), and facilitates synaptic transmission at gamma-aminobutyric acid (GABA), glutamate, and serotonin synapses within the interpeduncular nucleus, prefrontal cortex, and hippocampus (for reviews see McGehee & Role, 1996; Role & Berg, 1996; Wonnacott, 1997).

Because nicotinic receptors are present on synaptic terminals containing different neurotransmitters, the effect of nicotine administration will be a combination of the effects of each of the transmitters whose release is potentiated by nicotine. In addition, the extent to which nicotine increases neurotransmitter release from a particular synaptic terminal will depend on the specific subtype of nicotinic receptor that is expressed on that synaptic terminal. For example, it is known that a particular type of nicotinic receptor is on terminals that contain and release glutamate in several brain areas (including the habenula and hippocampus). This receptor subtype is characterized by a particularly high permeability to calcium, and more robust activation by nicotine than by acetylcholine. Nicotine potently increases the release of glutamate from these neurons, increasing synaptic transmission and excitability within these brain regions. The current notion is that the ability of nicotine to enhance excitability within hippocampus, habenula, and prefrontal cortex may be responsible for enhanced perception, arousal, and attention associated with nicotine self-administration.

In another example, certain forms of depression are commonly associated with altered serotonin metabolism. Thus, drugs that enhance serotonin function (e.g., blocking the inactivation of serotonin by the serotonin transporter, as is the case with Prozac-like drugs) improve mood. Nicotine elevates mood by increasing serotinergic transmission through the release of serotonin. The type of nicotinic receptor present on serotonin-containing terminals is different from those on glutamate-releasing terminals within the hippocampus. At present, it is not known how nicotine may be involved in the reported anxiolytic effects of smoking. The perceived relief from anxiety reported by smokers may be a function of the ability of nicotine to enhance attention (Kassel & Shiffman, 1997). A capacity to decrease disruptive attention deficits by smoking, as can be seen in schizophrenics, may be a factor in directly mediating smokers' anxiety, and in helping them to reduce it.

The convergence of neuroanatomical and neurophysiological studies just summarized suggests that nicotine potently increases the excitability of neurons involved in reinforcement and reward (Fig. 1.2). Studies of the cellular mechanisms of nicotine action reveal that nicotine enhances synaptic transmission in areas involved in (a) appetitive and addictive behaviors (such as the nucleus accumbens), and in (b) areas implicated in alertness, arousal, working memory, and short-term memory consolidation (e.g., prefrontal cortex, habenula, hippocampus).

The effects of nicotine in these regions are likely to involve both pre- and postsynaptic nicotinic receptor activation (Fig. 1.2). In view of numerous reports from smokers that among the perceived benefits of smoking is improved cognitive performance (i.e., better concentration, focus, memory), these functions of nicotine are of particular interest in potential drug design protocols. Distinctions between the nicotinic receptor subtypes subserving addictive effects of nicotine, compared with those involved in enhanced

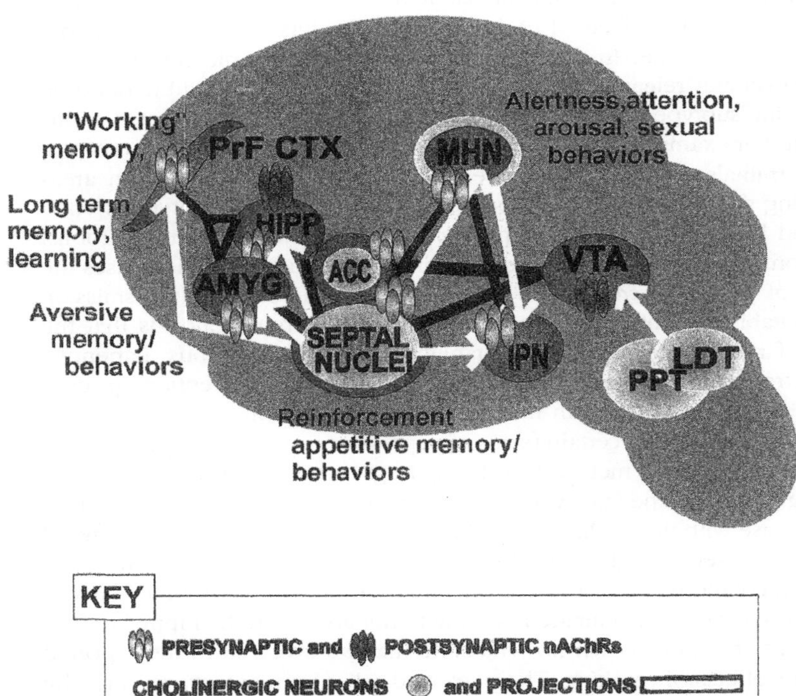

FIG. 1.2

memory and alertness, could permit the design of drugs that selectively target particular functional effects of nicotine. Recent studies indicate that this is indeed the case: The subunit composition of the presynaptic nicotine receptors in nucleus accumbens, ventral striatum, and prefrontal cortex appears to be strikingly different from the composition of those in hippocampus and habenula.

The potential therapeutic value of "functionally targeted" versions of nicotine extends beyond smoking cessation. Nicotine and nicotine analogs have been strongly implicated in the amelioration of several cognitive and behavioral disorders, most notably improving performance on memory tasks in patients with Alzheimer's, and reducing tics and increasing concentration span in Tourette's syndrome patients (see Perkins et al., 1996, for review). Perhaps most intriguing are recent studies by Freedman and his colleagues. These investigators have shed new light on why patients with schizophrenia are typically heavy smokers. They demonstrate strong genetic concordance of schizophrenia and a mutation in a nicotinic receptor subunit gene ($\alpha 7$) that is expressed in many limbic areas, including hippocampus, and is thought to comprise presynaptic nicotine acetylcholine receptors (nAChRs) that control glutamate release (Freedman et al., 1997; Gray, Rajan, Radcliffe, Yakehiro, & Dani, 1996; McGehee, Heath, Gelber, Devay, & Role, 1995). The $\alpha 7$ nicotine receptor subunit may be involved in higher order aspects of auditory processing—a mechanism referred to as *auditory gating*—that allows individuals to screen out irrelevant or repeated auditory stimuli. Patients with schizophrenia typically have significant problems with filtering auditory stimuli, and nicotine administration restores a more normal pattern of excitability in brain regions involved in auditory gating. The precise role of $\alpha 7$ in auditory gating and its relationship (if any) to other symptoms of schizophrenia are not yet known, but this promises to evolve as a particularly exciting area of research.

The key to nicotine's addictive effects may well be in the pattern of delivery of the exogenous drug, as opposed to the endogenous transmitter. The activity of endogenous cholinergic inputs, and hence the extent of acetylcholine-mediated synaptic facilitation via presynaptic receptors, is regulated closely in a drug-free brain. Under circumstances where enhanced transmission is appropriate, acetylcholine is released in the vicinity of nicotine-receptor–studded terminals, the receptors are activated, there is increased calcium influx into the terminal and hence increased release of neurotransmitter (Fig. 1.1B). In contrast, the chronic administration of nicotine, achieved by relatively brief but frequent periods of smoking, produces two important changes in the brain milieu. With each bolus of nicotine administered (i.e., each cigarette puff), peak arterial values can be as much as 0.5 μM (see Dani & Heinemann, 1996, for review). This represents the peak or upper limit of nicotine concentrations reached in smoking, after which they decline. These concentrations of nicotine are lower when compared to acetylcholine (ACh), but are more persistent in producing a stimulant effect.

Furthermore, because of the chemical stability of nicotine compared with acetylcholine, the steady state levels of nicotine in the brain can reach 0.5 μM (breakdown of nicotine occurs over several hours, whereas acetylcholine is hydrolized within milliseconds of its release). This pattern of nicotine administration results in both transient activation and long-term inactivation (or desensitization) of an increasing percentage of the nicotine receptors (see Dani & Heinemann, 1996, for detailed discussion of this issue). The net effects of chronic nicotine administration will then be an "average" of the nicotine-induced increases in transmitter release (due to nicotine's interaction with receptors not yet desensitized) and the nicotine-induced block of the effects of endogenous acetylcholine input (due to the progressive desensitization of nicotine receptors). The desensitization of nicotine receptors with continued exposure is consistent with the reported need to increase the drug dose to elicit a response, and with the classic smokers' experience that the first cigarette of the day is the "best." The latter phenomenon likely results from the recovery of receptors from their inactivated state during overnight nicotine deprivation.

In summary, recent animal and cellular physiology experiments provide an increasingly clear view of where and how nicotine acts in the brain. The brain regions, receptors, and mechanisms of nicotine-induced changes in neuronal excitability have been elucidated. Additional molecular dissection of the pathways and the receptors involved may well help with the development of novel, highly selective antismoking treatments, and may further elucidate other therapeutic potentials of nicotine receptor activation in the CNS. We now discuss how these underlying biological processes contribute, along with other factors, to nicotine addiction as a clinical disorder.

Clinical Perspectives on Nicotine Addiction

Nicotine addiction, like cocaine and other drug addictions, can be conceptualized as a triangle showing the complex interaction among three factors: the individual, the environment, and the drug itself (see Fig. 1.3; Spitz & Rosecan, 1987, pp. 13–15). All three factors are important, but depending on the situation, one factor outweighs the others.

Social Environment. Let's begin with *messages in the social environment.* These include easy access, low prices, no legal consequences, and successful marketing (Henningfield et al., 1991). Imagine for a moment a heroin addict trying to quit but living with another addict, or finding people injecting heroin in designated areas at work, in bathroom stalls, or on the

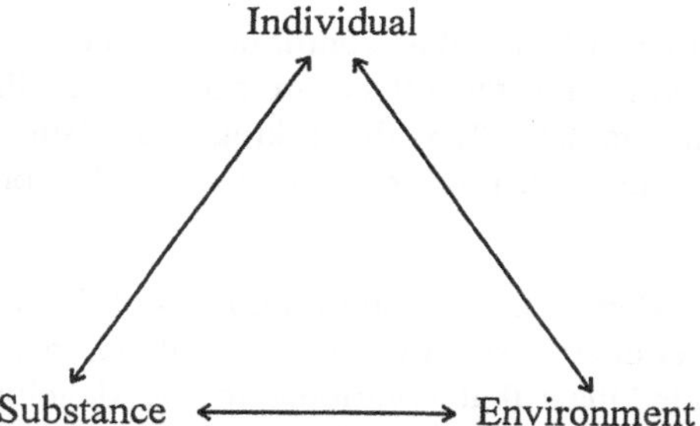

FIG. 1.3. Factors involved in the development of an addiction.

sidewalk in front of the building. We would all think it highly unlikely that the heroin addict would make it under these circumstances. And yet, smokers trying to quit face this every day.

On the other hand, the social environment is changing, due in part to the publicity surrounding environmental or "passive" tobacco smoke. There is a cartoon of a man sitting in the smoking section of a restaurant by the exit with the garbage cans and a sign above him says, "If you must smoke, please do not exhale." Another cartoon pictures a king, across the moat, stealing a smoke outside his castle.

Part of what makes smoking nicotine so prevalent is its social availability and acceptability. It is therefore important when evaluating smokers who want to quit to know whether they will be exposed to smoking at work or at home. Anyone working in this field or trying to quit smoking knows what a powerful trigger a cigarette-smoking spouse, boss, or coworker can be.

Substance: Smoking Tobacco. In addition to the contribution of the social environment to nicotine dependence, there is the drug experience itself of smoking tobacco. This includes its daily pattern of use and its pharmacological action (as discussed in the previous section). Is a smoker who smokes 20 or 30 cigarettes (or has 200–300 nicotine hits per day) as addicted as a heroin addict who uses heroin two times a day? Not only do smokers use their drug more often than heroin addicts, but the smoker's 7-sec "hit" is faster than the heroin user's.

Part of what makes it so difficult to stop smoking is the associations that develop between a smoker's extensive daily pattern of use and an equally long list of physical, situational, and emotional cues to smoke. When the smoker tries to quit, these cues continue to be prompts to smoke. Clinically, the three most common sources of relapse are drinking alcohol, socializing with smokers, and experiencing emotional discomfort.

Another pharmacological factor that contributes to the development of nicotine addiction is that its negative effects are not as immediate and overt (and do not interfere as dramatically with working and relationships) as the negative effects from other addicting drugs such as alcohol or cocaine.

The Individual Smoker. In addition to the roles of the social environment and the drug experience of smoking cigarettes, there are also important differences among individuals that contribute to the development of an addiction to cigarettes. What are the individual factors that contribute to people continuing a behavior that they know could kill them? Why do some people quit with relative ease, and some have difficulty but quit for good anyway, whereas some people never feel right without their cigarettes and still others can't even quit for 24 hours?

Many people blame themselves for a lack of "willpower" when they can't quit. Recent evidence suggests, though, that when it comes to quitting smoking, for some people willpower is not the issue. They have special problems, such as depression or anxiety, that are associated with smoking, and difficulties in quitting (see chap. 2, this volume). Clinicians will recognize the kind of smoker who gets that "sinking feeling" without cigarettes, who reports being "let down" or just "not happy" when not smoking. This may be part of the sense of loss or the adjustment process often associated with the transition to not smoking. However, some refractory smokers do suffer from the association between cigarette smoking and clinical depression, making it harder for them to stop and stay stopped. We treated a woman who took 12 years to quit smoking. She traveled all over the country going to smoking cessation programs and would quit but never felt quite right. After a few months of grim determination, and a morbid daily existence without letup, she would return to smoking and her depression would lift.

After a similarly unproductive period of abstinence in our program, this woman was treated with an antidepressant medication. Interestingly, her craving to smoke then diminished the way, for instance, we usually expect a smoker's craving to diminish over a period of abstinence. Despite multiple problems, this woman, who also had emphysema and was a recovering alcoholic, has now been cigarette free for over 2 years.

The tendency to use drugs to medicate painful emotions is the basis of a very influential theory developed by Edward Khantzian (1985) called the *Self-medication hypothesis of addictive disorders.* Khantzian viewed the choice of a drug "as an interaction between the pharmacological action of the drug and the dominant painful feelings" of the individual. For example, he viewed opiate addicts as medicating the disorganizing effects of "rage and aggression," and cocaine addicts as medicating the distress of "depression, hypomania and hyperactivity."

Where would cigarette smoking fit into Khantzian's picture? The British smoking researchers Heather Ashton and Rob Stepney (1982) described a model of smoking as a "psychological tool." In a research review, as early as 1982, they wrote:

> The evidence indicating more intensive smoking under short-term increases in anxiety is complemented by a number of non-laboratory studies which have shown that smoking is associated with longer-term stressful life events and high levels of personal anger and anxiety. (1982, p. 111)

Pomerleau and Pomerleau (1984) also reported numerous ways smokers turn to smoking as a psychological tool. They listed the following: to increase concentration, memory recall, psychomotor performance, alertness and arousal, pain endurance, and pleasure, and to decrease anxiety/tension, body weight, and hunger. Cigarette smoking has also been shown to help smokers perform better on certain kinds of tasks, including those described as boring or monotonous (Wesnes & Warburton, 1983).

Paradoxical Effects of Smoking. Many smoking researchers have described paradoxical or biphasic effects of smoking (Nesbitt, 1973; Pomerleau & Pomerleau, 1984). This refers to the use of cigarettes for stimulation and alertness at some times, and for their tranquilizing and relaxing effects at other times. Although the emotional effect is subtle and fleeting, cigarettes seem to provide a combination of the calming effects of heroin and the stimulating effects of cocaine. Ashton and Stepney (1982) suggested that these bidirectional responses were a function of nicotine dosing based on the smoker's individual smoking style and circumstances of the moment. For example, according to this view, by taking deep drags a smoker can obtain high levels of nicotine, which are sedating. In contrast, by taking short quick puffs a smoker can give the nervous system a stimulating start-up (Ashton & Stepney, 1982; Pomerleau & Pomerleau, 1984). Only more recently, with the discovery of neurophysiological mechanisms at the cellular level, have these observations been more clearly elucidated. Current evidence suggests, however, that nicotine is not titrated by the smoker, but that the smoker first achieves and then retains a relatively steady state of nicotine level. The varying subjective responses to smoking therefore depend not on changes in nicotine dose delivery, but on a different and more complex set of biological interactions, as discussed previously. In this view, the psychological effects of cigarette smoking may be better described as *diverse* rather than as *paradoxical.*

The use of cigarette smoking as a psychological tool for dealing with anger, anxiety, stress, boredom, pain, tension, and the need to concentrate may help explain its association with psychiatric disorders such as depression and anxiety. Individuals with psychiatric conditions, and those with less severe psychological problems, may use cigarette smoking as a tool to help them cope with, and self-medicate, the ongoing psychological distress in their lives.

From a clinical perspective, understanding smoking as a psychological tool presents important advantages. This is especially the case when the clinician is faced with behavior that smokers themselves regard as self-destructive, "crazy," and, at times, bewilderingly irrational. The model of smoking as psychological tool helps smokers to see their smoking as an important, although limited, way in which they have learned to cope with their lives. This applies both when they have needed to be alert to perform some task, and when they have sought to reduce the pain associated with a negative emotional state. Viewing smoking as a psychological tool can also help clinicians counter their own, sometimes negative, responses to smokers' "out-of-control" behavior. Together, clinician and patient can then focus on developing new psychological tools as an alternative to smoking and its unwanted negative consequences.

Practical Criteria

In diagnosing addictive disorders, four main criteria, important for clinicians to recognize, are generally present:

1. Preoccupation
2. Continued use despite adverse consequences
3. Loss of control
4. Denial

Preoccupation

The smoker spends much of his or her time thinking about smoking—how many cigarettes there are left in the pack, how many packs are left, what time the store closes if he or she should run out, and so on. As is the case with other drugs like cocaine or heroin, the preoccupation centers around assuring a steady supply. The preoccupation can also fit the definition of an obsession, according to *DSM–IV* (APA, 1994), if it is not wanted and causes the person "marked anxiety or distress."

Closely related to preoccupation and obsession is compulsion, which is defined as a pressure to act—in this case to smoke nicotine—which the person recognizes is excessive. Compulsions are the behavioral expression of preoccupation or obsession. This compulsion to smoke is present even after the addict has stopped smoking (which differentiates it from loss of control; see later section). However, it is intensified in the active smoker. In the Smoking Cessation Program at our hospital, we commonly hear comments like, "I had to drive 10 miles out of my way to buy cigarettes at the 7–11 because my usual late-night cigarette machine was empty," or, "When no one was looking I picked up a butt on the street because I ran out." The person feels driven to act to reduce the distress associated with his or her preoccupation with smoking.

Continued Use

Smokers as a group continue their smoking despite knowledge of adverse medical consequences. We commonly see this behavior in alcoholics and other addicts, where the alcoholic continues to drink for years after being told he or she has liver cirrhosis. The alcoholic tries to stop drinking but cannot. This continued use despite adverse consequences is not found with behaviors that are merely bad habits. It is an important clinical criteria for diagnosing an addiction. Many continue to smoke despite medical problems associated with smoking that have been identified by their physicians. Others have had the personal risks pointedly explained to them not only by physicians, but also by concerned family and friends. Since the first Surgeon General's report in 1964 linking cigarette smoking with lung cancer, there has also been widespread publicity regarding the medical risks of smoking. The typical smoker we treat comes to our program at the insistence of the doctor, spouse, children, and sometimes through the suggestion of the employer. Often the smoker has just learned from the doctor that he or she has lung disease (emphysema, bronchitis, a lung tumor that might be cancerous) or heart disease (high blood pressure, angina or chest pain, myocardial infarction, or heart attack), and that stopping smoking is a matter of life or death.

Case Example. Harold[1] is a 65 year-old retired engineer who was referred to our program by his surgeon after a routine chest x-ray showed the presence of a mass lesion. Harold had smoked three packs of cigarettes a day for 40 years, but aside from bronchitis, which became severe in the winters, he has been in fairly good health. A biopsy of the lesion proved it to be a cancerous tumor, and Harold was advised to stop smoking immediately and was scheduled for surgery in one week. Harold was understandably terrified and was able to throw out all of his cigarettes and stop. He had a lung removed, yet within days after leaving the hospital began to smoke again. Within weeks, he was again smoking three packs a day.

Harold desperately wanted to stop smoking, but could not. After interviewing Harold, we started him on antidepressant medication, nicotine patches, and put him in one of our stop-smoking groups. Within 3 weeks on this comprehensive regimen he stopped smoking and was cigarette free for over 6 months when we last saw him.

---

[1]All clinical examples are carefully disguised.

Loss of Control

Loss of control is the third cardinal feature of addictions and can be defined as the inability to stop smoking once the smoker takes even one cigarette. It is difficult to understand why some smokers appear to stop relatively easily using willpower alone, whereas many others are unable to control their smoking at all without a great deal of intervention and support. One reason is that loss of control may not be apparent until a period of time has passed.

The concept of developing an addiction over time is an attempt to explain why some smokers can quit using willpower on their own or with less intensive interventions such as hypnosis, acupuncture, or a behavioral program without medications. These smokers are stopping earlier in the development of their smoking addiction. If they tried to stop again a few years after smoking continuously, willpower or less intensive approaches alone may not work. Most smokers in our program are considered refractory because over 85% of them have already failed at another smoking cessation program or with prior professional help. Cigarette smoking, as a developmental process, can lead to *tolerance* (or the need for more cigarettes to achieve the same effect) or *desensitization* (inactivation of the pharmacological effects of smoking). Smokers often need help to stop trying to control their "bad habit" through willpower. When they realize they have lost control due to the addictive nature of cigarette smoking, they may stop blaming themselves for their inability to stop and accept the need for a more intensive treatment option.

Denial

Denial, the fourth cardinal symptom of addiction, is the catalyst for the other three. For smokers, denial is especially important (see chap. 12, this volume). This is because, compared to other addictions, the medical consequences of smoking are, as one patient put it, "so far in the future that I can't worry about it now. I could be struck by lightning before cigarettes get me." The psychological disconnection between addictive behavior and its unpleasant consequences is an important hallmark of denial.

A study by Chapman, Leng Wong, and Smith (1993) found smokers were significantly more likely than ex-smokers to have "self-exempting beliefs." These include, for example, that "most lung cancer is caused by air pollution," that "most people smoke," and that "it's safe to smoke low-tar cigarettes." Smokers, like alcoholics and other drug addicts, are masters of rationalization. Examples include, "I can stop whenever I like (I've done it many times)," "I only smoke low tar cigarettes, and I don't inhale much anyway," and "I only smoke because my wife smokes." Rationalization serves to minimize problems and to overlook their seriousness. Although smokers as a group generally know the medical risks of tobacco, it is their selective denial of this knowledge which is diagnostic of the addiction.

SUMMARY

In this chapter we have shown that the behavior of cigarette smoking fits the definition of a drug addiction: There is a clearly defined withdrawal syndrome, it fits the clinical criteria for addiction, and it is definitely addicting when compared to other chemicals such as alcohol, heroin, and cocaine.

Recent developments in basic science research in the field of nicotine receptors suggest that where nicotine acts in the brain, how it affects receptors, and the mechanisms by which these changes affect neuron excitability will elucidate the biological underpinnings of disorders previously defined primarily by clinical evaluation. Understanding these mechanisms also makes the pathways in question vulnerable to pharmacological intervention, which in turn will give the clinician more carefully calibrated tools with which to help patients.

A careful clinical evaluation of all three aspects of an addiction (i.e., the use of the substance itself, the role of the environment, and the psychological adjustment of the individual) is the first step in helping smokers to prepare to quit. Clinicians' understanding of cigarette smoking as an addiction with a strong physiological basis can help them to help smokers stop blaming themselves for their "bad habit" and "lack of willpower," and instead to focus on how to make best use of the currently available medical and psychological treatment options. It is our hope that the synergy of understanding both biological and clinical perspectives on nicotine addiction will soon lead to widespread improvements in patient care.

REFERENCES

Adikofer, F., & Thurau, K. (Eds.). (1991). *Effects of nicotine in biological systems* (pp. 285–294). Basel: Birkhauser Verlag.

American Psychiatric Association. (1994). *Diagnostic and statistical manual of mental disorders* (4th ed.). Washington, DC: American Psychiatric Association.

Ashton, H., & Stepney, R. (1982). Smoking as a psychological tool. In H. Ashton & R. Stepney (Eds.), *Smoking: Psychology and pharmacology* (pp. 91–119). London: Tavistock.

Blumberg, H., Cohen, S., Dronfield, B., Mordecai, E., Roberts, J., & Hawks, D. (1974). British opiate users I. People approaching London drug treatment centers. *International Journal of Addiction, 9,* 1–23.

Chapman, S., Leng Wong, W., & Smith, W. (1993). Self-exempting beliefs about smoking and health: Differences between smokers and ex-smokers. *American Journal of Public Health, 83,* 215–219.

Corrigall, W. A., & Coen, K. M. (1989). Nicotine maintains robust self-administration in rats on a limited access schedule. *Psychopharmacology, 99,* 473–478.

Dani, J. A., & Heinemann, S. (1996). Molecular and cellular aspects of nicotine abuse. *Neuron, 16,* 905–908.

Davidson, G., & Duffy, M. (1982). Smoking habits of long-term survivors of surgery for lung cancer. *Thorax, 37,* 331–333.

Fagerstrom, K. O., & Schneider, N. G. (1989). Measuring nicotine dependence: A review of the Fagerstrom Tolerance Questionnaire. *J. Behav. Med., 12,* 159–182.

Fiore, M. C., Epps, R. P., & Manley, M. W. (1994). Missed opportunities: Teaching medical students about tobacco cessation and prevention. *JAMA, 271*(8), 624–626.

Freedman, R., Coon, H., Myles-Worsley, M., Orr-Urtreger, A., Olincy, A., Davis, A., Polymeropoulos, M., Holik, J., Hopkins, J., Hoff, M., Rosenthal, J., Waldo, M. C., Reimherr, F., Wender, P., Yaw, J., Young, D. A., Breese, C. R., Adams, C., Patterson, D., Adler L. E., Kruglyak, L., Leonard, S., & Byerley, W. (1997). Linkage of a neurophysiological deficit in schizophrenia to a chromosome 15. *Proceedings of the National Academy of Science, USA, 94*(2), 587–592.

Glass, R. (1990). Blue mood, blackened lungs, depression and smoking. *JAMA, 264*(12), 1583–1584.

Goldberg, S. R., & Henningfield, J. E. (1988). Reinforcing effects of nicotine in humans and experimental animals responding under intermittent schedules of intravenous drug injection. *Pharmacology, Biochemistry, Behavior, 30,* 227–234.

Gray, R., Rajan, A. S., Radcliffe, K. A., Yakehiro, M., & Dani, J. A. (1996). Hippocampal synaptic transmission enhanced by low concentrations of nicotine. *Nature, 383*(6602), 713–716.

Havik, O. E., & Maeland, J. G. (1988). Changes in smoking behavior after myocardial infarction. *Health-Psychology, 7*(5), 403–420.

Henningfield, J. E., Cohen, C., & Slade, J. (1991). Is nicotine more addictive than cocaine? *British Journal of Addiction, 86,* 565–569.

Hunt, W. A., Barnett, W., & Branch, L. G. (1971). Relapse rates in addiction programs. *Journal of Clinical Psychology, 27,* 455–456.

Hurt, R., Dale, L., Offord, K., Bruce, B., McClain, F., & Eberman, K. (1992). Inpatient treatment of severe nicotine dependence. *Mayo Clinic Proceedings, 67,* 823–828.

Jaffe, J. (1990). Drug addiction and drug abuse. In G. Gilman, T. W. Rall, A. S. Nies, & P. Taylor (Eds.), *Goodman and Gilman's the pharmacological basis of therapeutics* (8th ed., pp. 522–573). New York: Pergamon.

Kassel, J. D., & Shiffman, S. M. (1997). Attentional mediation of cigarette smoking's effect on anxiety. *Health Psychology, 16*(4), 359–368.

Khantzian, E. (1985). The self-medication hypothesis of addictive disorders: Focus on heroin and cocaine dependence. *American Journal of Psychiatry, 142,* 1259–1264.

Kozlowski, L. T., Wilkinson, A., Skinner, W., Kent, C., Franklin, T., & Pope, M. (1989). Comparing tobacco cigarette dependence with other drug dependencies. *JAMA, 261*(6), 898–901.

Langley, J. N., & Anderson, H. K. (1892). The actions of nicotine on the ciliary ganglion and on endings of the third cranial nerve. *Journal of Physiology (London), 13,* 460–468.

Masson, J. (Ed.). (1985). *The complete letters of Sigmund Freud to Wilhelm Fliess 1887–1904.* Cambridge, MA: Harvard University Press.

McGehee, D. S., & Role, L. W. (1995). Physiological diversity of nicotinic acetylcholine receptors expressed by vertebrate neurons. *Annual Review of Physiology, 57,* 521–546.

McGehee, D., & Role, L. (1996). Presynaptic ionotropic receptors. *Current Opinions in Neurobiology, 6,* 342–349.

McGehee, D., Heath, M., Gelber, S., Devay, P., & Role, L. W. (1995). Nicotine enhancement of fast excitatory synaptic transmission in CNS by presynaptic receptors. *Science, 269,* 1692–1697.

Nesbitt, P. (1973). Smoking, physiological arousal, and emotional response. *Journal of Personality and Social Psychology, 25*(1), 137–144.

Perkins, K. A., Benowitz, N., Henningfield, J., Newhouse, P., Pomerleau, O. F., & Swan, G. (1996). Society for Research on Nicotine and Tobacco (Proceedings). *Addiction, 91*(1), 129–144.

Pomerleau, O. F., & Pomerleau, C. (1984). Neuroregulators and the reinforcement of smoking: Towards a biobehavioral explanation. *Neuroscience & Biobehavioral Reviews, 8,* 503–513.

Robins, L. N., Helzer, J. E., & Davis, D. (1975). Narcotic use in Southeast Asia and afterward. *Archives of General Psychiatry, 32,* 955–961.

Role, L. W., & Berg, D. K. (1996). Nicotinic receptors in the development and modulation of CNS synapses. *Neuron, 16,* 1077–1085.

Schuckit, M. A. (1989). *Drug and alcohol abuse. A clinical guide to diagnosis and treatment.* New York and London: Plenum Medical Book Company.

Shiffman, S. M. (1989). Tobacco "chippers"—Individual differences in tobacco dependence. *Psychopharmacology, 97,* 539–547.

Spitz, H., & Rosecan, J. (1987). *Cocaine abuse: New directions in treatment and research.* New York: Brunner/Mazel.

Spitz, M. R., Fueger, J. J., Chamberlain, R. M., Goepfert, H., & Newell, G. R. (1990). Cigarette smoking patterns in patients after treatment of upper aerodigestive tract cancers. *Journal of Cancer Education, 5*(2), 109–113.

Stolerman, I. P., & Shoaib, M. (1991). The neurobiology of tobacco addiction. *Trends in Pharmacological Science, 12,* 466–473.

Taylor, C. B., Houston-Miller, N., Killen, J. D., & DeBusk, R. F. (1990). Smoking cessation after acute myocardial infarction: Effects of a nurse-managed intervention. *Annals of Internal Medicine, 113*(2), 118–123.

U.S. Department of Health and Human Services. (1988). *The health consequences of smoking: Nicotine addiction. A report of the Surgeon General, 1988* (DHHS Publication No. [CDC] 88-8406). Rockville, MD: U.S. Department of Health and Human Services, Public Health Service, Centers for Disease Control, Center for Health Promotion and Education, Office on Smoking and Health.

U.S. Department of Health and Human Services. (1996). *Clinical practice guideline: Smoking cessation* (AHCPR Publication No. 96-0692). Rockville, MD: Author.

Wesnes, K., & Warburton, D. M. (1983). Smoking, nicotine, and human performance. *Pharmacology & Therapeutics, 21,* 189–208.

Wonnacott, S. (1997). Presynaptic nicotinic ACh receptors. *Trends in Neuroscience, 20*(2), 92–98.

Rose, J. E., [illegible] & [illegible] (1987). [illegible] and [illegible] *Archives of General Psychiatry, 44*, [illegible]

Rose, J. E., & [illegible] (1990). [illegible] in the [illegible] and [illegible] of [illegible] *Pharmacology Biochemistry and Behavior*, [illegible]

Spitz, M. R., [illegible] [illegible], & [illegible] (1998). [illegible] in [illegible] after [illegible] of [illegible] *Journal of the National Cancer Institute, 90*, 100–11[illegible]

Tiffany, S. T., Drobes, D. J., & [illegible] [illegible] [illegible] [illegible] [illegible] *Psychopharmacology*, [illegible] 1[illegible]

[illegible], & Wahlgren, D. R. (19[illegible]). [illegible] *[illegible] 21*, [illegible]

[illegible], S. (1987). Prescription [illegible] [illegible] 1–9.

Part II

Developments in Clinical Research

CHAPTER TWO

Nicotine Dependence and Its Associations With Psychiatric Disorders: Research Evidence and Treatment Implications

Lirio S. Covey
New York State Psychiatric Institute, and Columbia University

As recently as 30 years ago, when smoking was socially acceptable for men and in many circles for women as well, it would have been difficult to demonstrate a relationship between the regular use of tobacco and a psychiatric condition. However, in the past 10 years, as many smokers quit smoking or attempted to do so in response to the negative information about the health consequences of smoking, considerable scientific evidence emerged pointing to dramatic differences in the rates of smoking according to the presence of a psychiatric history. The earliest report linking psychiatric diagnoses and smoking appeared in 1986, when a group of psychiatric researchers in Minnesota observed a higher prevalence of smoking among patients in a mental health clinic who suffered from major depression, anxiety, or schizophrenia, when compared with representative individuals drawn from the community (Hughes, Hatsukami, Mitchell, & Dahlgren, 1986). Numerous studies since then have pointed to a greater propensity of persons with those disorders as well as those with alcoholism to become cigarette smokers, to smoke more heavily, and to have greater difficulties when stopping when compared with nonaffected individuals.

In this chapter, I describe addiction to nicotine, also known as nicotine dependence, and review the evidence concerning its association with the psychiatric conditions that appear to have the strongest associations with cigarette smoking: major depression, alcoholism, anxiety disorders, and schizophrenia. The limited evidence on the association between attention deficit hyperactivity disorder and cigarette smoking is also reviewed. Based on empirical evidence and a history of clinical work predominantly among smokers with a history of depressive illness, I then discuss treatment considerations involving pharmacological and psychological interventions.

NICOTINE DEPENDENCE

Nicotine, the main pharmacologic agent in cigarettes, has been shown to be a powerfully addicting drug (U.S. Department of Health and Human Services, 1988). Yet for a long time, cigarette smoking was perceived as being just a "habit," in part because of the absence of debilitating intoxicating symptoms or the marked social and occupational impairments associated with the use of other addictive drugs such as alcohol or heroin. However, individuals who have been dually addicted to heroin and nicotine or to alcohol and nicotine are likely to describe abstaining from nicotine as the more difficult task (Kozlowski, Skinner, & Kent, 1989). This increased difficulty flows, in part, from the fact that cigarette smoking, much more than other addictive substances, is so pervasively intermingled with the smoker's day-to-day activities and behaviors.

The term *nicotine dependence* entered diagnostic terminology in the third edition of the American Psychiatric Association's *Diagnostic Statistical Manual of Mental Disorders* (*DSM–III*) with the designation *tobacco dependence* (APA, 1980). In the later editions, *DSM–III–R* (APA, 1987) and *DSM–IV* (APA, 1994), the term was changed to *nicotine dependence* in acknowledgment of the abundant scientific evidence concerning the addictive quality of nicotine (U.S. Department of Health and Human Services, 1988). In each of those diagnostic systems (as well as in the International Classification of Diseases published by the World Health Organization), dependence on nicotine (or tobacco) is classed among the disorders of dependence to addictive substances, along with alcohol, cocaine, opiates, amphetamines, and marijuana. The same set of symptoms is used as criteria for defining all the substance dependence disorders. *DSM–IV* (APA, 1994) lists the following the criteria for substance dependence:

1. Tolerance—a need for markedly increased amounts of the substance or markedly diminished effect with continued use of the same amount of the substance.
2. Characteristic withdrawal symptoms (including depressed mood, insomnia, irritability, anxiety, difficulty concentrating, restlessness, decreased heart rate, and increased appetite).
3. Taking the substance in larger amounts or over a longer period than intended.

4. Persistent desire or unsuccessful efforts to cut down or control substance use.
5. A great deal of time is spent in activities necessary to obtain the substance.
6. Important social, occupational, or recreational activities are given up or reduced because of substance use.
7. The substance use is continued despite knowledge of having a persistent or recurrent physical or psychological problem that is likely to have been caused or exacerbated by the substance.

According to the *DSM–IV*, smokers who meet three or more of these criteria when applied to nicotine are considered nicotine dependent. Epidemiological studies have shown that about 75% of all smokers meet those criteria (Anthony, Warner, & Kessler, 1995). Furthermore, the more criteria are met, the higher the likelihood that nicotine dependence occurs with a psychiatric condition (Breslau, Kilbey, & Andreski, 1991).

Measurements of Nicotine Dependence

For a long time, the most widely used instrument for measuring nicotine dependence was the Fagerström Tolerance Questionnaire (FTQ, Fagerström, 1978) whose eight items, shown in Table 2.1, were written to depict physiological and behavioral patterns of nicotine dependence. Particularly during its earlier years, the FTQ acquitted itself quite well as a predictor of smoking cessation and as a predictor of enhanced response to nicotine gum (Fagerström, 1978; Fagerström & Schneider, 1989). Because of reports regarding the psychometric limitations of the FTQ (Lichtenstein & Mermelstein, 1986; Pomerleau, Majchrzak, & Pomerleau, 1989) a revised version, the six-item Fagerström Test for Nicotine Dependence (FTND), also shown in Table 2.1, was introduced (Heatherton, Kozlowski, Frecker, & Fagerström, 1991) Improved test–retest and internal reliability have been reported for the FTND (Pomerleau, Carton, Lutzke, Flesslan, & Pomerleau, 1994).

The *DSM–III* approach was operationalized in the Diagnostic Interview Schedule (DIS, Robins, Helzer, & Croughan, 1981) and has been used in a number of epidemiologic studies. These reports have provided information about the prevalence and the demographic distribution of nicotine dependence in the general population (Anthony et al., 1995) and its association with psychiatric illnesses such as major depression, anxiety, alcoholism, and other substance dependencies (Breslau et al., 1991). Much less is known, however, about the relationship of nicotine dependence level as defined by the *DSM* with the ability to stop smoking or with biological indicators of smoking intake such as the level of breath carbon monoxide or the level

TABLE 2.1
Fagerström Tolerance Questionnaire and Fagerström Test for Nicotine Dependence: Items and Scoring

	FTQ	*FTND*
1. How soon after you wake up do you smoke your first cigarette?	0. After 30 minutes 1. Within 30 minutes	0. After 30 minutes 1. 31–60 minutes 2. 6–30 minutes 3. Within 5 minutes
2. Do you find it difficult to refrain from smoking in places where it is forbidden?	0. No 1. Yes	0. No 1. Yes
3. Which cigarette would you hate to give up?	0. Any other 1. The first one in the morning	0. Any other 1. The first one in the morning
4. How many cigarettes per day do you smoke?	0. 1–15 1. 16–25 2. 26 or more	0. 10 or less 1. 11–20 2. 21–30 3. 31 or more
5. Do you smoke more frequently during the first hours after waking than during the rest of the day?	0. No 1. Yes	0. No 1. Yes
6. Do you smoke if you are so ill that you are in bed most of the day?	0. No 1. Yes	0. No 1. Yes
7. What is the nicotine content of your cigarettes?	0. <1 mg 1. 1.0–1.2 mg 2. >1.2 mg	
8. Do you inhale the smoke?	0. Never 1. Sometimes 2. Always	

Note. Adapted from Fagerström et al. (1996).

of nicotine or cotinine (a metabolite of nicotine) which are detectable in blood, saliva, or urine.

In 1993, my colleagues and I began an effort to develop a questionnaire that would depict the *DSM–III–R* (APA, 1987) and the *DSM–IV* (APA, 1995) substance abuse criteria in language that pointedly reflects addicted cigarette smoking behavior, as opposed to a generic drug abuse/dependence syndrome. After conducting focused interviews that helped us construct questionnaire items, testing successive versions of a multiple-item instrument, and performing psychometric analysis, we developed a set of items that together represented the themes specified in the *DSM–IV* criteria for substance dependence. Analysis of responses from 160 smokers who had come to a smoking cessation program indicated that the *DSM* criteria for nicotine dependence would evoke reliable responses in a test–retest administered 1 week apart; and, taken together in linear combination, correlate with subjects' blood level of cotinine ($R = .47$, $F = 3.99$, $p = .000$), breath carbon monoxide level ($R = .43$, $F = 3.17$, $p = .0003$), number of cigarettes smoked daily ($R = 0.51$, $F = 4.90$, $p < .001$), the Fagerström Tolerance Questionnaire (FTQ) ($R = 0.61$, $F = 8.47$, $p < .001$), and the quit rate at the end of the treatment program ($R = .38$, $F = 2.40$, $p = .005$). (Covey, L. S., Struening, E. L., unpublished data).

Researchers at the Mayo Clinic in Minnesota have also developed a nicotine dependence measure that they named the Self-Administered Nicotine Dependence Scale (SANDS) (Davis et al., 1994). Drawing on their clinical experience with nicotine dependent patients, the authors operationalized six composite domains including self-efficacy, social skills deficit, loss of control, consequences of use, social support for smoking, and concern for healthy life-style, which together were represented by 79 items. Further psychometric analysis yielded two nonoverlapping subscales, which the authors labeled as social skills deficit (SSD) and self-efficacy (SE). The item sets displayed modest internal consistency, and the SSD subscore was significantly associated with smoking status at the end of a smoking cessation program.

The SANDS and the *DSM–IV* substance dependence criteria offer a broader conceptualization of nicotine dependence than the FTQ. What neither the *DSM* nor the FTQ model has measured however, is an emotional dimension.

In another research study recently conducted by our group, we explored the idea that an emotional domain is a core feature of nicotine dependence. The rationale for an emotional dependence domain grew out of clinical work with smokers who, despite an ability to stop smoking in the short term, repeatedly return to smoking when faced with emotionally provoking life experiences. To test this speculation, we developed and administered a 65-item measure that depicted subjects' attributions of mood-regulating functions to smoking while also capturing the established physiological and behavioral patterns described in previous nicotine dependence models such as the FTQ and the *DSM–IV* criteria. The results of our first study, based on 330 participants in smoking cessation programs held in New York City and Loma Linda, CA, confirmed the presence of such a mood-regulation factor and its association with physiological and behavioral factors (Covey et al., 1997). Examples of mood regulation items are: *I depend on cigarettes to raise my spirits when I feel down; Smoking cigarettes improves my mood; I find smoking cigarettes very relaxing; Smoking cigarettes is a source of comfort; I fear losing control of my emotions if I do not smoke; If I stopped smoking, I would feel I've lost a best friend.* We are continuing our research to elucidate the nature of nicotine dependence and to understand the relevance of emotional factors and their juxtaposition with physiological and behavioral dependence factors. If the evidence from this research convincingly demonstrates the importance or centrality of a mood-regulation factor or "emotional dependence" in persistent tobacco use, this would imply the need for treatments that specifically address the presence of such emotional factors.

Nicotine Withdrawal Syndrome

The nicotine withdrawal syndrome is a pattern of uncomfortable signs and symptoms that regularly follows cessation of smoking. The most common of these is craving, a condition marked by an intense desire for tobacco and persistent thoughts about smoking. A high level of craving has been consistently shown to influence the likelihood of relapse. The other common withdrawal symptoms are depressed mood, irritability, restlessness, anxiety, difficulty concentrating, increased appetite, and sleep disturbance (APA, 1995; Hughes & Hatsukami, 1986). Of these symptoms, depressed mood appears to be among the least common for most smokers, but tends to occur frequently when smoking cessation is attempted by the smoker who is prone to depression (Breslau, Kilbey, & Andreski, 1992; Covey, Glassman, & Stetner, 1990). Recognizing the presence of depressed mood during the acute nicotine withdrawal period is important because this phenomenon has been shown to exert an adverse influence on smoking cessation outcome (Covey et al., 1990; Hughes, 1992; West, Hajek, & Belcher, 1989).

Withdrawal symptoms begin within 12 hours of quitting or reducing cigarette intake. The period of highest difficulty is around the first 3 days of abstinence. From here on, if abstinence continues, withdrawal symptoms begin to decline, although craving may continue to peak from time to time (Shiffman, 1979). In general, the first 2 weeks will be marked by high levels of psychological discomfort. About 4 weeks after quitting, and almost certainly by 6 weeks, the smoker's psychological state is often back to the precessation level. In fact, many of those who manage to sustain nicotine abstinence up to this time experience enhanced feelings of self-esteem and self-pride in having achieved what once appeared to be an impossible goal. It is not surprising, however, for the ex-smoker to continue to experience intermittent waves of craving to smoke even weeks later when all other signs of withdrawal have abated.

Relapse

A characteristic shared by persons who are nicotine dependent with persons dependent on alcohol or heroin is a marked tendency to relapse (Hunt, Barnett, & Branch, 1971). The most relapse-prone period is the first few days after quitting. During the first few days or weeks after quitting, among the strongest precipitants of relapse is the availability of cigarettes. A related factor, therefore, is smoking by others, especially those with whom the would-be smoker is in close contact, such as a spouse or other household member. Smoking even a few cigarettes during the first week jeopardizes a smoking cessation attempt. Conversely, the ability to stop smoking completely during the targeted quit day and to sustain abstinence during the first week (Hurt et al., 1994; Kenford et al., 1994; Schneider et al., 1995; Westman, Behm, Simel, & Rose, 1997) is a positive predictor of the quitter's continued long-term abstinence. The odds for long-term abstinence generally improve as the number of days since quit day increases.

With regard to long-term abstinence, weight gain plays a paradoxical role. The average weight gain for those who stop smoking is 5 to 10 pounds for men and is slightly higher for women (Flegal, Troiano, Pamuk, Kuczmarski, & Campbell, 1995; Gross, Stitzer, Maldonado, 1989). Weight gain results because stopping smoking is followed by a decrease in the metabolic rate, which leads to increased absorption of ingested food. Not helping matters is the fact that cessation is usually followed by increased appetite, which begins within a few days of stopping smoking and often continues beyond the normal 2- to 4-week duration of the withdrawal syndrome. For some quitters, the added weight is so unacceptable that they give up their efforts to stay off cigarettes. For others, a simultaneous attention to preventing weight gain may sabotage their struggle to avoid a return to smoking. Indeed, it has been repeatedly found that quitters who gain weight are the ones most likely to maintain nicotine abstinence over time (Perkins, 1995).

Origins of Nicotine Dependence

The precise causes of nicotine dependence are unknown. Nevertheless, evidence exists indicating that environmental and genetic factors are involved in the likelihood of a person's becoming a smoker, the amount smoked, and the level of difficulty involved when attempts to quit are made. Among the strongest environmental determinants of smoking behavior are smoking by friends and siblings, the availability of cigarettes in the community, and the acceptability of smoking by the person's peers. Parental smoking has also been identified as a predictor of smoking behavior, although the environmental or genetic nature of that exposure is not clear.

Recent investigations into the genetics of smoking suggest a substantial contribution of heritable factors to the likelihood of initiating regular smoking, the amount of cigarettes smoked, and the persistence of smoking behavior. This conclusion was drawn by Heath and Madden (1994) in their review of large-scale twin studies conducted in Scandinavia, Australia, and the United States. These researchers further suggested that the influence of genetic factors may be particularly strong on the smoker's ability to stop smoking.

MAJOR DEPRESSION

Most of the evidence on the co-occurrence or comorbidity of nicotine dependence and psychiatric states has concerned major depression, a condition characterized by persistent negative feelings such as sadness, loss of pleasure, hopelessness, low self-esteem, and inappropriate guilt, which are accompanied by various physical signs that may include decreased or increased appetite, sleep disturbance, fatigue, restlessness, concentration difficulty, and possibly suicidal thoughts or actions (APA, 1994).

In 1988, in the course of conducting a trial of the antihypertensive drug clonidine for smoking cessation, Alexander Glassman and his colleagues at Columbia University and the New York State Institute observed that, in spite of an exclusionary criterion that required the absence of current symptoms of serious depression, 60% of the participants said that they had experienced the full syndrome of major depression at least 6 months before they came to the study (Glassman et al., 1988). This was a remarkably impressive figure because at that time, community-based prevalence estimates of lifetime major depression were about 10–20% (Baldesarrini, 1984). Having observed such a high prevalence of major depression history in the study sample, Glassman and colleagues then examined whether this history would influence the smoking cessation rate. This post hoc hypothesis was supported by the data. Although the cessation rate among smokers with no past history of major depression who did not receive the experimental drug was 40%, the success rate in those with the history was 10%. A high proportion of persons with a history of major depression has also been reported in three other smoking trials. A large-scale trial of clonidine by our group (Glassman et al., 1993), a test of behavior therapies in California (Hall, Munoz, & Reuz, 1992), and a clinical trial of fluoxetine (Niaura et al., 1995), all of which involved heavy smokers with previous experiences of cessation failure, found rates of past major depression that were 35–41%. Although these figures are less than the 60% observed in the initial clonidine trial by Glassman et al. (1988), they are still markedly higher than the rates of major depression that are commonly seen in the general population. Moreover, all three studies also found that major depression history was associated with a higher rate of smoking cessation failure.

Studies based on treatment samples such as those just described are subject to the errors of what has been called the "clinician's illusion" (Cohen & Cohen, 1984). This is an inappropriate generalization of findings based on the special populations that make their way to treatment clinics to the population of persons who, for various reasons, do not seek treatment. The latter generally make up the larger group and may not share the same characteristics as the clinical samples. Because of the possibility that Glassman's 1988 study of clonidine was biased because it was conducted in the specialized setting of a university-based treatment clinic, the research group examined the question with a community-based and randomly selected sample of 3,200 individuals from the St. Louis, MO, site of the multicenter psychiatric epidemiological study conducted by the National Institute of Mental Health (Glassman et al., 1990). Subjects for this study were selected in a manner that avoided the selectivity that could bias findings from studies conducted in the specialized settings of treatment centers. Indeed, the data from this representative sample replicated the original clinical finding. The study found that a history of regular smoking was significantly more frequent among persons with a history of depression compared with nondepressed individuals. Among persons with a history of major depression, 80% of the men and 72% of the women had been regular smokers; in contrast, among persons with no history of major depression, significantly fewer men and women, 68% and 49%, respectively, had been regular smokers at some time in their life. Also in support of the 1988 clinical study, these community-based data showed that 28% of smokers with no history of major depression were able to stop smoking for at least 1 year, whereas only 14% of those with past major depression managed to do so.

Other data based on representative samples have shown similar results. A study of 1,200 members of a health maintenance organization, aged 21–30 years, in Detroit, MI (Breslau, Kilbey, & Andreski, 1991), and a study of 1,566 female twins conducted at the Virginia Medical College (Kendler et al., 1993) both demonstrated an association between major depression and cigarette smoking even when the additional co-occurrence of anxiety and/or alcoholism was taken into consideration in multivariate analyses. Both these studies also showed a dose-response relationship; that is, higher rates of depression were observed with increasing amounts of cigarettes smoked, and vice versa.

The studies of major depression that have been cited thus far extended several previous reports that linked depressed mood with cigarette smoking in adults. In a study based on a nationally representative sample of 2,000 persons, elevated ratings on a measure of depressed mood (the Center for Epidemiologic Studies Depression Scale, CES-D), occurred more frequently among smokers compared with nonsmokers (Anda et al., 1990). Elevated depression scores also predicted who would still be smoking 16 years later in that study. In a similar finding, higher rates of depressed mood, anxiety, and tension were observed among smokers compared with nonsmokers in a community-based study conducted in New Zealand, (Waal-Manning & de Hamel, 1978).

Age and the Association Between Depression and Smoking

Several studies have observed this relationship as early as the adolescent years. A study of male and female 11th graders by Covey and Tam (1990) found that high scores on a depression inventory were associated with a higher prevalence of smoking at least one cigarette daily and with increased number of cigarettes smoked. This association remained after controlling for other psychological factors such as anxiety and life satisfaction, as well as smoking by peers and being raised in a single-parent home. Similarly, a study based on a randomized sample of high-school students in Melbourne, Australia, found that those with high levels of depression and anxiety were twice as likely as those with low levels to be smokers (Patton et al., 1996). Other investigators have found a higher prevalence of depressed mood among male smokers attending a rural high school (Malkin & Allen, 1980). More recently, David Fergusson and colleagues (Ferguson, Lynskey, & Horwood, 1996) reported on a study that used instruments that more specifically measure nicotine dependence and depressive disorders (major depression and dysthymia) according to the *DSM–III–R* criteria. Examining data obtained from birth until the age of 16 years from 1,265 children born in New Zealand during 1977, these investigators found that the association between depression and cigarettes smoking had become well established by the time of adolescence.

A little-known yet intriguing study, reported in the 1991 annual convention of the American Psychiatric Association by Zimmerman and colleagues, found that the association between major and depression was age related. It was greatest among the youngest age group (20–29 years), then declined until the association was no longer apparent among those 45 and older (Zimmerman, Coryell, & Black, 1991). In a study that extended this finding, Salive and Blazer (1996) found no association between major depression and smoking in their sample of men aged 65 years or older but, surprisingly, found that same-aged women with past major depression were less likely to be smokers than those without the history! The possibility that depression and smoking interact differently according to age level has implications for treatment and requires clarification.

Gender and the Association Between Depression and Smoking

The evidence on this issue has been inconsistent. Some studies have observed an effect of depressed mood or major depression on the prevalence of regular smoking among both genders (Anda et al., 1990; Breslau et al., 1991; Covey & Tam, 1990; Glassman et al., 1990), others have found it only among women (Frederick, Frerichs, & Clark, 1988; Perez-Stable, Marin, Marin, & Katz, 1990), whereas other studies have found the association to be stronger among women than men (Covey, Hughes, Glassman, Blazer, & George, 1994; Glassman et al., 1993). Nevertheless, it is noteworthy that studies based on adolescents (Covey & Tam, 1990; Fergusson et al., 1996; Patton et al., 1996) and young adults (Breslau et al., 1991) have consistently found the association to be present regardless of gender. It could be that the mechanisms linking depression and smoking are similar among men and women, but that the higher lifetime frequency of depressive conditions among women (Weissman, Bruce, Leaf, Florio, & Holzer, 1991) makes the relationship among women more readily apparent.

Can Cessation Provoke Depression?

The medical benefits of smoking cessation results are clear: Stopping smoking reduces the risk of multiple smoking-related illnesses including cardiovascular disease, cancer, chronic bronchitis, and emphysema (U.S. Department of Health and Human Services, 1990). For smokers with past major depression, however, some evidence suggests that smoking cessation carries particular psychological and psychiatric risks. These risks apply to various levels of negative or dysphoric feelings, from depressed mood to more severe depressive states requiring treatment, that could emerge during the postcessation period. It also appears that the period of risk that begins within days of nicotine withdrawal may extend to several months after cessation.

As we noted earlier, smoking cessation entails a 2- to 4-week period of nicotine withdrawal symptoms for most smokers. Our research that focused on the first week after quitting has suggested that (except for increased appetite and craving, which were experienced by all smokers) each of these withdrawal symptoms, but most significantly depressed mood, is experienced more severely by quitters with a history of depression (Covey et al., 1990). As shown in Fig. 2.1, we found that among 36 smokers who had been assigned to the placebo condition in a drug trial, 75% of smokers with past major depression experienced depressed mood within the first week of nicotine

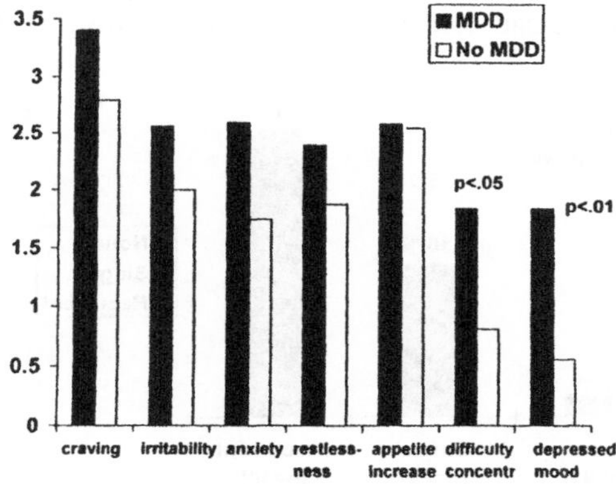

FIG. 2.1. Mean ratings of withdrawal symptom intensity (range = 0 to 5) 1 week after quit day by history of major depression.

abstinence. In contrast, depressed mood occurred among only 15% of the nondepressed smokers. Breslau reported a similar observation among participants in a health maintenance organization (Breslau et al., 1992).

Additionally, it has become apparent that depression following smoking cessation entails more than minor and transient states of dysphoria. As reported in another paper by Glassman and colleagues, the development of severe depressions within a few weeks of cessation was observed in eight patients within a few weeks of stopping smoking, while the subjects were still in treatment (Glassman et al., 1993). Six of these cases occurred among 113 subjects with a history of major depression, and 1 occurred among 34 subjects without that history but who had reported a history of alcoholism. The eighth case did not have previous major depression but did report a suicidal attempt at age 13 years and frequent although sporadic bouts of depressed mood. All eight cases resumed smoking within days of experiencing the depression and quickly felt relief.

The duration of risk for experiencing severe depression after smoking cessation is not yet clear. My colleagues and I have been able to report, nonetheless, that the period of risk for a new major depressive episode for smokers with prior histories of major depression may extend to several months following cessation. In an examination of events during the first 3 months after 126 smokers had successfully ended a 10-week treatment, we observed the statistically significant finding that although a serious depressive episode occurred in 2 of 99 smokers (or 2%) without past major depression within that period, such an event occurred in 2 of 25 persons (16%) who had experienced major depression once previously, and in 3 of 10 persons (30%) who had experienced multiple depressive episodes in the past (Covey, Glassman, Stetner, 1997) (Fig. 2.2). Although it can be argued that persons with prior depression are at great risk of a recurrent depression regardless of smoking or smoking cessation status, the 20% rate of new postcessation

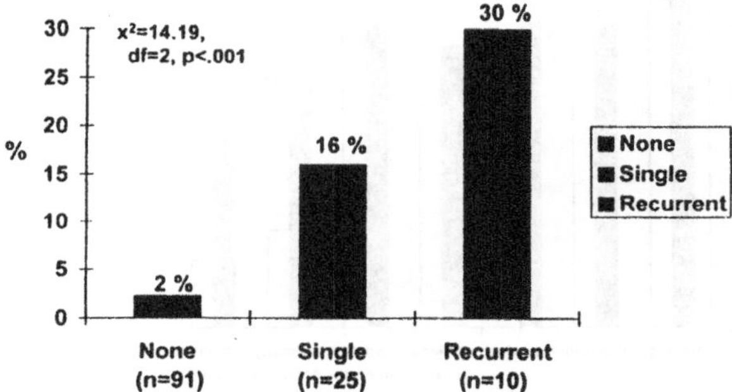

FIG. 2.2. Incidence of major depression 3 months after completing smoking cessation treatment by history of major depression.

depressions among our sample of 35 nicotine abstainers who had been free of the diagnosis for at least 6 months and an average of 2 years is unusually high. Rather, it resembles the rate of new depressive episodes among persons treated for depression. In sum, it does appear that, despite the huge physical benefits of stopping smoking, individuals with a prior history of major depression carry a risk for a recurrence of the illness when they stop smoking.

Mechanisms Underlying the Association Between Depression and Smoking

Attempts to understand the mechanisms underlying the association between nicotine dependence and major depression have suggested the effect of common predisposing factors. This explanation argues against a situation where one condition is the cause of the other. In their data set cited earlier, Breslau and colleagues followed up their subjects after 13 months and found two related observations: (a) a higher incidence of major depressive episodes during that time among nicotine-dependent smokers than among nonsmokers, and (b) an increased severity of nicotine dependence among persons with major depression (Breslau, Kilbey, & Andreski, 1993). This evidence points to a shared vulnerability. Although that study did not point to the nature of that shared factor, the data from 1,566 female twins by Kendler et al. (1993) suggested that, compared with environmental factors, common genes exerted a stronger influence on the frequent co-occurrence of depression and smoking. Thus, although evidence exists for the heritability of nicotine dependence and for the genetic origins of depressive disorders, the physiological mechanisms underlying the genetic causation of either condition remain to be identified. The commonality of their genetic origin is a hypothesis that has yet to be confirmed.

ALCOHOLISM

About 80–90% of individuals with alcoholism have smoked cigarettes regularly at some time in their lives, and alcoholic individuals smoke more heavily than do nonalcoholics (DiFranza & Guerrera, 1983). A number of explanations for this relationship have been proposed:

1. The ingestion of one substance precipitates craving for the other.
2. Dependence to one addictive substance enhances the individual's reactivity to the rewarding effects of other psychoactive agents.
3. As with depression, nicotine dependence and alcohol dependence share common etiological factors that may be genetic or environmental in nature.

It is of course plausible that both genetic and environmental factors interact to maximize a person's vulnerability to both alcohol abuse and cigarette use. The frequent clustering of smoking and alcohol during adolescence (along with drug use and truancy), has been noted by Jessor and Jessor (1977).

Are Alcoholics More or Less Able to Stop Smoking Compared With Nonalcoholic Smokers?

The answer, it seems, depends on whether or not the alcoholism is active and whether there is further psychiatric comorbidity. In our clinical work, we have seen that alcoholics with substantial levels of sobriety, particularly those with intense or long-term involvement with Alcoholics Anonymous, have a high ability to stop smoking that, in the short-term, may exceed that of nonalcoholic smokers. Of course, whether this observation generalizes to other populations of alcoholic smokers remains to be known. On the other hand, our clinical data also suggest that the nicotine relapse rate may be worse among smokers with an alcohol history compared with nonalcoholics (Covey, Glassman, Stetner, & Becker, 1993).

That the likelihood of smoking cessation is greatly improved when the alcoholism is no longer active was demonstrated in a study by Breslau and her group (Breslau, Peterson, Schultz, Andreski, & Chilcoat, 1996). Additionally, our research group has collected data indicating that increasing psychopathology among alcoholics is associated with a decreased ability to stop smoking. In a smoking cessation study we found that a history of major depression is an especially severe barrier to smoking cessation among recovered alcoholics. Of 39 alcoholic males who had been free of alcohol for at least 6 months before they came to the study, those who had not experienced depression in the past stopped smoking at a rate of 25%, similar to the 27% rate found among nonalcoholic males. However, the success rate among the 14 alcoholic males with a history of major depression was zero (Covey, Glassman, & Stetner, 1993). Further light on this issue was shed by a recent study that my colleagues and I conducted with a sample of 78 recovering alcoholics, all of whom had been alcohol free for at least 1 year but were still participating in an outpatient rehabilitation program. We found that the more severe form of depression, characterized by earlier onset (prepubertal depression) and recurrence (multiple episodes), was associated with higher levels of nicotine dependence (Covey, Larino, Asencio, & Allen, 1997b).

Will Smoking Cessation Provoke an Alcoholic Relapse?

The conventional lore in alcohol treatment settings has been that smoking cessation threatens alcohol sobriety. That presumption, however, has not been documented in empirical data. In fact, existing evidence, albeit derived mainly from alcoholics in remission, does not support that assumption (Bobo, 1989). In our own clinic work, for example, we have successfully treated over a hundred alcoholics who had been free of the diagnosis for at least 6 months without observing a relapse to alcohol use in all but three cases. Thus, at least among sober alcoholics, relapse to alcohol following smoking cessation may be a rare occurrence rather than the rule. More studies are needed in order to clarify this important issue.

Benefits of Smoking Cessation for Alcoholics

Although it has been known for some time that combined exposure to alcohol and tobacco increases the risk in a multiplicative fashion for several medical disorders such as cancers of the oral cavity, larynx, esophagus, and liver, and cardiovascular disease, compared with the risk from either alcohol or tobacco alone (U.S. Department of Health and Human Services, 1990), a hidden statistic, until recently, has been that the largest cause of mortality among alcoholics has not been cirrhosis of the liver as might be expected, but the smoking-related diseases including emphysema, lung cancer, and cardiovascular disorders (Hurt et al., 1996). This medical fact underscores the importance of smoking cessation for individuals with alcoholism. Additionally, as expressed by some recovering alcoholic smokers whom I have seen in our clinic, an important impetus for smoking cessation has been their awareness that by smoking cigarettes in an effort to self-medicate emotionally, they continue to avoid making the changes necessary for emotional progress.

ANXIETY

Symptoms of anxiety, like depressed mood, are among the expressions of "negative affect" that have been associated with an increased likelihood of being a smoker. Many smokers report that they smoke in order to relieve tension or stress. That smoking relieves anxiety is highly plausible because studies have shown that anxiety reduction is among the pharmacological effects of nicotine (Balfour, 1991; Pomerleau, 1986).

It is not surprising therefore that an association between anxiety disorders and cigarette smoking has been observed in epidemiological studies (Breslau et al., 1991; Covey et al., 1993). The term *anxiety disorders* as used in the *DSM–IV* (APA, 1994) includes several disorders, of which phobias (e.g., simple phobia, social phobia, and agoraphobia) are the most common. Obsessive-compulsive disorders, panic disorder, generalized anxiety disorder, and posttraumatic stress disorder are also classified in the *DSM–IV* as anxiety disorders. Taken as a group, anxiety disorders are among the most prevalent of the psychiatric illnesses. Overall, the frequency of anxiety disorders is higher in women and tends to decline with age (Robins & Regier, 1991). Only a few studies have examined the association between cigarette smoking and anxiety, either as diagnosis or symptom.

In their study of 1,200 young adults, Breslau and colleagues found that the diagnosis of nicotine dependence was more frequently observed among those with a history of obsessive compulsive disorder, agoraphobia, and phobia, than among individuals without a psychiatric diagnosis (Breslau et al., 1991). In a survey involving 3,000 individuals in the NIMH-ECA study in Durham, NC, men and women with generalized anxiety disorder (GAD) were more likely to have become regular smokers in their lifetime, compared with individuals without that disorder (Covey et al., 1993). A significant relationship was evident even when the co-occurrence of alcoholism and major depression was controlled for in multivariate analyses. Individuals with generalized anxiety disorder in this sample were also found less likely to be ex-smokers. In contrast with the data on major depression, where the association with the inability to stop smoking was strong among women but not men, the reduced ability to stop smoking in the presence of GAD was stronger among men (Covey et al., 1993).

The outcome of cessation according to subjects' level of anxiety symptoms, however, was examined in a trial of the anxiolytic medication buspirone as a cessation aid (Cinciripini et al., 1995). Subjects with evidence of serious psychopathology were excluded at screening (including, presumably, smokers with severe anxiety disorders); nevertheless, the data analysis stratified subjects according to level of anxiety symptoms as measured by the Profile of Moods Inventory (POMS). Results obtained from the smokers treated with placebo provide some indication of the relationship between anxiety symptoms and smoking cessation outcome without the confounding effect of the anxiolytic drug. During the first week of treatment, quit rates were similar in subjects with low or high levels of anxiety symptoms. Nine weeks later, however, fewer subjects who scored high on the anxiety measure were still abstinent and the difference, when compared with low anxiety scorers, increased over time. Although this study does not add to our knowledge regarding the association between anxiety disorders and smoking because subjects with evidence of serious psychopathology were excluded, the study results do suggest that high levels of anxiety symptoms may be an impediment to smoking cessation. Regarding the effect of the experimental drug, buspirone was found to be helpful for the high-anxiety subjects, but somewhat detrimental to cessation efforts of the low anxiety subjects. The authors concluded that the effect of buspirone occurred not through the general alleviation of nicotine withdrawal symptoms but by specific influences on characteristically anxious smokers. For the low-anxiety subjects, on the other hand, the authors suggest that drug effects may have interfered with efforts to stop as abstinence rates were seen to improve when the drug was withdrawn (see also chap. 8).

It is noteworthy that although individuals with major depression or alcoholism have been overrepresented in clinical samples of smokers compared with their frequency in the general population, the frequency of individuals with anxiety disorders in smoking cessation clinic samples has been lower than one would expect. Of more than 1,000 smokers treated during the past 10 years in our clinic, for example, fewer than 20 smokers have met a diagnosis of GAD. This frequency rate of 2% is considerably lower than the 6–10% rate of generalized anxiety disorder usually seen among the adult population in the United States (Blazer, Hughes, George, Swartz, & Boyer, 1991). This lower representation in smoking cessation clinics may reflect severely low feelings of self-efficacy about quitting among chronically anxiety-riven individuals. To counter this negative expectation, stronger and more reliable evidence for the efficacy of cessation treatments would seem necessary.

If a persistent anxiety disorder hinders smoking cessation, the converse, unfortunately, may also be true. That is, if tension relief is a frequent motivator of smoking, it is possible that by using cigarettes to alleviate their symptoms, persons who need treatment for their anxiety disorder prevent themselves from getting that treatment. In other words, the attribution of emotionally medicative qualities to nicotine may, in the long run, impede recovery from a psychiatric disability. This would be an example of a reciprocally deleterious relationship between smoking and a psychiatric illness.

SCHIZOPHRENIA

Schizophrenia affects about 1% of the general population. It is clear from clinical and community-based data that cigarette smoking is highly prevalent among individuals with schizophrenia, occurring at rates of 85–90% (Covey et al., 1993; Glynn & Sussman, 1993; Hughes et al., 1986). These estimates of smoking among persons with schizophrenia are more than three times today's smoking prevalence rate of roughly 28% in the general U.S. population. Furthermore, former smokers among this group are rare. In community-based data from Durham, NC, the quit rate among all ever smokers was 30%, but it was 0% among the group with a diagnosis of schizophrenia, male or female (Covey et al., 1993). In a study of smokers with schizophrenia who wanted to quit, Dalack and Meador-Woodruff (1996) reported little success with even short-term abstinence. Indeed, family, friends, and clinical staff frequently described individuals with schizophrenia as "chain smokers" who typically smoke up to 40 or more cigarettes daily.

Why do individuals with schizophrenia smoke so much? It has been suggested that the biological effects of nicotine—in particular, the stimulation of dopamine release—may be especially reinforcing for schizophrenics (Glassman, 1993; Ziedonis, Kosten, Glazer, & Francis, 1994). Additionally, Adler and colleagues noted that cigarette smoking appears to ameliorate perceptual deficits suffered by many individuals with schizophrenia (Adler, Hoffer, Griffith, Waldo, & Freedman, 1992). It has also been suggested that schizophrenic individuals smoke for a variety of reasons, some of which are shared by smokers from the general population and some of which are unique to their clinical condition. A survey by Glynn and Sussman (1990), for instance, found that, like other smokers, individuals with schizophrenia smoke for relaxation, out of "habit," or to settle their nerves, but that they also smoke for specific psychiatric reasons such as to mitigate auditory hallucinations or to reduce the adverse effects of their neuroleptic medication. Another group of researchers, Lavin, Siris, and Mason (1996), suggested that the "psychological tool" model whereby cigarettes are used to regulate a variety of uncomfortable emotional states may be particularly applicable to patients with schizophrenia. Just as many smokers will use cigarettes interchangeably to increase arousal, to improve attention and vigilance, or to reduce anxiety and anger, persons with schizophrenia may use cigarettes to self-medicate their positive symptoms, such as delusions or hallucinations, as well as their negative symptoms, such as blunted affect and depression. Gilbert and Gilbert (1996) suggested that the "finger-tip" control over nicotine administration available to the smoker provides a fine-grain modulatory control over the release of neurotransmitters, such as dopamine, which play a central role in the development of schizophrenia. These authors note that this ability is not as readily possible with drugs that are not administered as frequently, making cigarettes a favored psychoactive agent.

Smoking may also help diminish the adverse effects of neuroleptic drugs, including movement disorders consequent to medications, such as tardive dyskinesia, neuroleptic-induced parkinsonism, and akithisia. A study comparing 58 schizophrenic smokers with 20 nonsmokers found the former to have significantly less parkinsonism and more akithisia than did the nonsmokers (Goff, Henderson, & Amico, 1992). On the other hand, one study found an increased incidence of tardive dyskinesia among schizophrenic smokers (Yassa, Lal, Lopassy, & Ally, 1987) and another found that smoking exacerbated those symptoms (Menza, Grossman, Van Horn, Cody, & Forman, 1991).

Cigarette smoking is known to increase the metabolism of neuroleptic drugs. This has important implications on the management of psychotropic treatment. Patients with schizophrenia who smoke appear to need higher neuroleptic doses than do nonsmokers to achieve comparable treatment effects (Goff et al., 1992). Thus it is important to monitor cigarette use because both increases and reductions in smoking intake have potential effects on experienced symptoms as well as on the appropriate level of neuroleptic treatments. In particular, cessation of smoking can result in increased blood levels of neuroleptic medications and produce greater side effects. Abrupt abstinence could also precipitate severe withdrawal or exacerbate symptoms that might have been partially alleviated by nicotine. Unfortunately, there is limited knowledge to date about the effects of smoking cessation among patients with schizophrenia. The mostly anecdotal papers that have been published report varying degrees of disruptions, from none or little to very serious events, in hospital settings where smoking was banned.

Although more information is needed, there have been reports regarding the usefulness of the nicotine patch for smoking cessation by patients with schizophrenia. The use of nicotine gum seems to have been less productive, but this may be related to problems of compliance because many patients may find it difficult to follow the precise instructions in order to chew nicotine gum correctly.

ATTENTION DEFICIT/HYPERACTIVITY DISORDER

Attention deficit/hyperactivity disorder (ADHD) is a disorder whose onset begins in childhood and is characterized by inattention, distractibility, impaired concentration, organizational difficulty, impulsivity, and hyperactivity (APA, 1994). Its prevalence has been estimated to be about 5% among adolescent populations, and about half of that rate among adults (Shelley-Tremblay & Rosen, 1996). Compared with members of the general population, individuals with ADHD smoke in larger numbers (Downey, Pomerleau, & Pomerleau, 1996; Milberger, Biderman, Faraone, Chen, & Jones, 1997), have an earlier onset of cigarette smoking (Downey et al., 1996; Milberger et al., 1997), and have a lower quit rate (Pomerleau, Downey, Stelson, & Pomerleau, 1995). It has been suggested that individuals with ADHD resort to smoking in an attempt to modulate the severe attentional and memory deficits that are symptoms of the disorder (Pomerleau et al., 1995). This notion was supported by findings from an experiment involving adults with ADHD who were given a nicotine patch. ADHD symptoms improved both in smokers who had not smoked overnight and in nonsmokers (Levin et al., 1996). That the improvements occurred regardless of past smoking intake indicated that the favorable nicotine effects were not merely a function of relief from withdrawal symptoms.

Whether or not the observed association between cigarette smoking and ADHD actually results from the effect of another condition that is often found among ADHD patients, for example, conduct disorder, remains to be clarified. In a 15-year longitudinal study of 900 children in New Zealand (Lynskey & Fergusson, 1995), 8-year-old children who scored high on a scale of conduct problems were found to be 3.8 times more likely to smoke cigarettes by the age of 15 years than were children without significant conduct problems. In fact, when conduct problems were controlled for, the association between smoking and attention deficit behaviors was no longer statistically significant, although a statistical trend remained ($p < .10$). This contrasted with the finding that children with attention deficit behaviors were three times more likely to use illicit drugs than those without those symptoms ($p < .005$). The authors concluded that there is a lack of evidence linking childhood attention deficit behaviors with later substance abuse unless it occurs in the presence of conduct problems.

On the other hand, a recent 4-year prospective study of 6- to 17-year-old boys with or without ADHD found that the higher prevalence of smoking and the earlier age of smoking initiation among ADHD individuals was observed even after controlling for socioeconomic status, IQ, and the co-occurrence of psychiatric disorders. Nevertheless, this study did find that among the boys with ADHD, the risks associated with cigarette smoking were greater in the presence of conduct, major depressive, and anxiety disorders (Milberger et al., 1997).

These juxtaposed conditions—the relative high prevalence of ADHD, its early childhood onset, findings regarding the increased risk for smoking and early age of smoking initation associated with ADHD, and the tendency of early age of smoking initiation to influence the likelihood of becoming a regular smoker and becoming a highly dependent smoker (Breslau, Fenn, & Peterson, 1993; Taioli & Wynder, 1991)—highlight the importance of smoking prevention programs for children and adolescents with ADHD.[1]

TREATMENT IMPLICATIONS

Available knowledge about smoking cessation treatment for patients with a psychiatric history has been mainly on smokers with a disposition to depression. My colleagues and I at the Columbia University–New York Psychiatric Institute Smoking Cessation Clinic have treated several hundred smokers with past major depression. The treatment recommendations given here are based largely on that experience.

The clinician seeking to help smokers with a known history of psychiatric comorbidity needs to be aware of their patients' twofold liability: They are likely to have a difficult time when they stop smoking, and if they do manage to quit, they are at risk of severe withdrawal symptoms as well as a prolonged period of psychological discomfort. In some cases, the postcessation psy-

[1]Research for this section was conducted by Fay Stetner.

chiatric episode may be so severe as to require its own treatment. In a study of smokers with past major depression completed by our group at the Smoking Cessation Research Clinic of the New York State Psychiatric Institute, 20% of subjects who successfully completed smoking cessation treatment experienced a variety of psychiatric events (including major depression, panic disorder, uncontrolled eating, and compulsive behaviors) during the next 6 months. Given these risks, some guidelines for the treatment of the hard-core smoker with concomittant psychiatric illness are the following:

1. Obtain a detailed smoking history, including an assessment of the patient's level of nicotine dependence. In clinical and research data, I have seen that smokers with psychiatric histories will score highly on physiological dependence measures such as the Fagerström Tolerance Questionnaire (FTQ) or the *DSM–IV* substance dependence criteria. When physiological dependence is high, as indicated by an FTQ score greater than 6 or the physiological criteria in *DSM–IV* (i.e., Criterion 1, tolerance, and Criterion 2, characteristic withdrawal symptoms) are endorsed, nicotine replacement therapy is recommended.

2. Assess psychiatric history and inquire about previous use of psychotropic medications. A past history of major depression or previous use of antidepressant medication, in particular, indicates a potential benefit of adjunctive treatment with an antidepressant medication. In my work with the psychiatrist Alexander Glassman, we have had regular success with the serotonin reuptake inhibitors sertraline (Zoloft) and fluoxetine (Prozac) for smokers with a history of depression. We have also successfully used bupropion (Wellbutrin), a dopaminergic antidepressant whose indication for smoking cessation was approved by the Federal Drug Administration in 1997 and which is marketed for smoking cessation as Zyban. Bupropion was found to be highly effective both by itself and in combination with the nicotine patch as a cessation drug in clinical trials involving smokers regardless of depression history (Johnston & Ascher, 1996). Generally high success rates with bupropion would suggest its usefulness for smokers with depression.

If the pretreatment assessment indicates that the smoker is also seriously in the midst of a psychiatric condition such as a major depressive episode, severe anxiety, active alcoholism, or drug dependence, the patient should be referred for appropriate treatment, and a decision should be made regarding a course of treatment in which both the nicotine dependence and the comorbid disorder are addressed in a timely manner.

3. Once nicotine abstinence has begun, monitor the patient's psychological status during and beyond the first 2 to 4 weeks of nicotine withdrawal. This requires extended contact through office visits and periodic telephone

calls throughout the first 6 months after stopping smoking. If the patient reports continued high levels of withdrawal discomfort beyond the 4 to 6 weeks following stopping smoking cessation, consider prophylactic treatment to alleviate the dysphoric condition. As seen in our clinical data, the persistence of such postcessation discomfort is a potential harbinger of postcessation psychiatric event (Covey, Glassman, & Stetner, 1997). Of course, if a psychiatric episode does occur (or recur), treat, or refer the patient, immediately for appropriate treatment.

4. Psychological counseling. Although pharmacological treatments comprise the first line of intervention for the smoker with a psychiatric history, the influence of psychological factors on sustaining the patient's felt need to smoke requires the concomittant application of intensive and supportive psychological treatment. In a process analogous to the relief provided by nicotine replacement therapy for physiological withdrawal, this type of clinical support can provide the temporary emotional replacement to help the ex-smoker avert or reduce psychological disequilibrium when the ex-smoker is still learning to function without relying on cigarettes.

For the smoker with or without an underlying psychiatric condition, achieving the goal of long-term nicotine abstinence requires more than not smoking again. In order to sustain abstinence, certain patterns of behaviors, cognitions, and affect management need to be transformed. Some ways of behaving, thinking and feeling need to be changed or eliminated because they serve as irresistible cues to smoking again; new behaviors need to be established as part of a "recovered" lifestyle that promotes nonsmoking. Psychological treatment is important because it can facilitate such changes.

In some cases, psychological counseling that takes place over 8 to 10 weeks with concomitant pharmacological treatment (nicotine replacement therapy or an antidepressant), followed by booster sessions every few months, may be adequate for assisting the patient to stop smoking and maintain long-term abstinence. However, I have also seen many instances when smoking cessation patients seek more frequent and longer clinical support after the cessation-related counseling has terminated. Although some of those patients used resources such as Nicotine Anonymous and, when applicable, Alcoholics or Narcotics Anonymous, others have asked to be referred for individual psychotherapy. I have been impressed by the fact that when cigarette smoking had served to alleviate or to mask underlying psychological difficulties and motivation to continue not smoking is high, smoking cessation often provides a spur to beginning a course of psychotherapy. The good news is, as I have seen during the past 10 years of working with addicted smokers, that such postcessation referral for psychotherapy often results in an improved quality of life over and above simply quitting smoking.

New Psychiatric Events After Cessation Among Smokers With No Previous Psychiatric History

An important clinical group are those smokers with no known history of a psychiatric condition for whom a psychiatric condition emerges after stopping smoking. Case reports of severe depressive episodes occurring after cessation have been published (Bock, Goldstein, & Marcus, 1996; Flanagan & Maany, 1982; Stage, Glassman, & Covey, 1996). We have also seen a number of cases where a debilitating depressive condition became apparent only when the nicotine abstinence period had lasted for several months, although not during previous abstinence periods of shorter duration. A reliable fund of knowledge on how to identify this type of smoker at the beginning of treatment is not yet available. Based on clinical experience, I believe that a pronounced tendency to attribute mood-regulating functions to cigarette smoking and a history of relapse associated with painful emotions or stressful events are indicators of this emotional vulnerability. As mentioned earlier in this article and in chapter 9, my colleagues and I have begun to develop an instrument for detecting a core emotional component of nicotine dependence.

CONCLUSION

Scientific knowledge on the association between nicotine dependence and psychiatric disorders is still at an early stage and new information is continuing to emerge. For example, early results from an analysis of data from the National Anxiety Screening Survey, currently being conducted by Elmer Struening and colleagues at Columbia University, show an increasing prevalence of cigarette smoking with the number of comorbid anxiety disorders (i.e., phobia, panic disorder, generalized anxiety disorder, posttraumatic disorder, and obsessive-compulsive disorders). Several investigations in this country and abroad are underway that will hopefully shed more information on why it is that smoking is so prevalent among individuals with schizophrenia and on how the new generation of neuroleptics (such as clozapine and olanzapine) may be helpful for reducing patients' use of tobacco. Within the last few years, the National Institute on Alcoholism and Alcohol Abuse has launched studies to develop treatments for patients who are dually addicted to alcohol and nicotine. Findings from ongoing genetic studies of nicotine dependence may also provide another resource that will illuminate pathways by which prevention and treatment of both nicotine dependence and the psychiatric conditions may be improved.

For now, abundant evidence strongly suggests that when delving beneath the exterior of the smoker who wishes to stop smoking but seems unable to do so, the clinician may unmask a psychiatric vulnerability. This is not a moral or social indictment; rather, it is a challenge and a call for vigilance for the clinician who seeks to help the hard-core smoker.

REFERENCES

Adler, L. E., Hoffer, L. J., Wiser, A., & Freedman, R. (1993). Cigarette smoking normalizes auditory physiology in schizophrenics. *American Journal of Psychiatry, 150,* 1856–1861.

Adler, L. E., Hoffer, L. J., Griffith, J., Waldo, M. C., & Freedman, R. (1992). Normalization by nicotine of deficient auditory sensory gating in the relatives of schizophrenics. *Biological Psychiatry, 32,* 607–616.

American Psychiatric Association. (1987). *Diagnostic and statistical manual of mental disorders* (3rd ed., rev.). Washington, DC: American Psychiatric Association.

American Psychiatric Association. (1980). *Diagnostic and statistical manual of mental disorders* (3rd ed.). Washington, DC: American Psychiatric Association.

American Psychiatric Association. (1994). *Diagnostic and statistical manual of mental disorders* (4th ed.). Washington, DC: American Psychiatric Association.

Anda, R. F., Williamson, D. F., Escobedo, L. G., Mast, E. E., Giovino, G. A., & Remington, P. L. (1990). Depression and the dynamics of smoking: A national perspective. *JAMA, 264,* 1541–1545.

Anthony, J. C., Warner, L. A., & Kessler, R. C. (1994). Comparative epidemiology of dependence on tobacco, alcohol, controlled substances, and inhalants. *Experimental Clinical Psychopharmacology, 2,* 244–268.

Baldesarrini, R. J. (1984). Risk rates for depression. *Archives of General Psychiatry, 41,* 103–104.

Balfour, D. J. K. (1991). The influence of stress on psychopharmacological responses to nicotine. *British Journal of Addictions, 86,* 489–493.

Blazer, D. G., Hughes, D. C., George, L. K., Swartz, M., & Boyer, R. (1991). Generalized anxiety disorder. In L. N. Robinson & D. A. Regier (Eds.), *Psychiatric disorders in America* (pp. 180–203). New York: The Free Press.

Bobo, J. K. (1989). Nicotine dependence and alcoholism epidemiology and treatment. *Journal of Psychoactive Drugs, 21,* 323–329.

Bock, B. C., Goldstein, M. G., & Marcus B. H. (1996). Depression following smoking cessation in women. *Journal of Substance Abuse, 8,* 137.

Breslau, N., Fenn, N., & Peterson, E. (1993). Early smoking initiation and nicotine dependence in a cohort of young adults. *Drug and Alcohol Dependence, 33,* 129–137.

Breslau, N., Kilbey, M. M., & Andreski, P. (1991). Nicotine dependence, major depression, and anxiety in young adults. *Archives of General Psychiatry, 48,* 1069–1074.

Breslau, N., Kilbey, M. M., & Andreski, P. (1992). Nicotine withdrawal symptoms and psychiatric disorders: Findings from an epidemiologic study of young adults. *American Journal of Psychiatry, 149,* 464–469.

Breslau, N., Kilbey, M. M., & Andreski, P. (1993). Nicotine dependence and major depression: New evidence from a prospective investigation. *Archives of General Psychiatry, 50,* 31–35.

Breslau, N., Peterson, E., Schultz, L., Andreski, P., & Chilcoat, H. (1996). Are smokers with alcohol disorders less likely to quit? *American Journal of Public Health, 86*(7), 985–990.

Cinciripini, P. M., Lapitzky, L., Seay, S., Wallfisch, A., Meyer, W. J., & Van Vunakis, H. (1995). A placebo-controlled evaluation of the effects of buspirone on smoking cessation: Differences between high-and low-anxiety smokers. *Journal of Clinical Psychopharmacology, 15*, 182–191.

Cohen, P., & Cohen, J. (1984). The clinician's illusion. *Archives of General Psychiatry, 41*, 1178–1182.

Covey, L. S., Glassman, A. H., & Stetner, F. (1990). Depression and depressive symptoms in smoking cessation. *Comprehensive Psychiatry, 31*, 350–354.

Covey, L. S., Glassman, A. H., & Stetner, F. (1993, November). *A nicotine dependence scale based on psychiatric criteria.* Paper presented at the 6th Annual Conference on Nicotine Dependence, American Society Addiction Medicine, Atlanta GA.

Covey, L. S., Glassman, A. H., & Stetner, F. (1997). Major depression following smoking cessation. *American Journal of Psychiatry, 154*, 263–265.

Covey, L. S., Glassman, A. H., Stetner, F., & Becker, J. (1993). Effect of history of alcoholism or major depression on smoking cessation. *American Journal of Psychiatry, 150*, 1546–1547.

Covey, L. S., Hughes, D. C., Glassman, A.H., Blazer, D.G., & George, L. K. (1994). Ever-smoking, quitting, and psychiatric disorders: Evidence from the Durham, North Carolina, Epidemiologic Catchment Area. *Tobacco Control, 3*, 222–227.

Covey, L. S., Larino, M., Asencio, R., & Allen, G. B. (1997b, June). *Major depression and nicotine dependence among recovering alcoholics.* Paper presented at the 3rd Annual Scientific Conference of the Society for Research on Nicotine and Tobacco, Nashville, TN.

Covey, L. S., Struening, E. L., Larino, M., DePena, M., Glassman, A. H., Ferry, L. H., & Saunders, B. (1997a, June). *Is there more to nicotine dependence than the DSM–IV criteria?* Presented at the 3rd Annual Meeting of the Society Research on Nicotine and Tobacco, Nashville, TN.

Covey, L. S., & Tam, D. (1990). Depressive mood, the single-parent home, and adolescent cigarette smoking. *American Journal of Public Health, 80*, 1330–1333.

Dalack, G. W., & Meador-Woodruff, J. H. (1996). Smoking, smoking withdrawal, and schizophrenia: Case reports and a review of the literature. *Schizophrenia Research, 22*, 133–141.

Davis, L. J., Hurt, R. D., Offord, K. P., Lauger, G. G., Morse, R. M., & Bruce, B. K. (1994). Self-administered nicotine-dependence scale (SANDS): Item selection, reliability estimation, and initial validation. *Journal of Clinical Psychology, 50*, 918–930.

DiFranza, J. R., & Guerrera, M. P. (1983). Alcoholism and smoking. *Journal of Studies on Alcohol, 51*, 130–135.

Downey, K. K., Pomerleau, C. S., & Pomerleau, O. F. (1996). Personality differences related to smoking and adult attention deficit hyperactivity disorder. *Journal of Substance Abuse, 8*, 129–135.

Fagerström, K. O. (1978). Measuring degree of physical dependence to tobacco with reference to individualization of treatment. *Addictive Behaviors, 3*, 235–241.

Fagerström, K. O. (1996). Nicotine dependence versus smoking prevalence comparisons among countries and categories of smokers. *Tobacco Control, 5*, 52–56.

Fagerström, K. O., & Schneider, N. G. (1989). Measuring nicotine dependence: A review of the Fagerström Tolerance Questionnaire. *Journal of Behavioral Medicine, 12*, 159–182.

Fergusson, D. M., Lynskey, M. T., & Horwood, L. F. (1996). Comorbidity between depressive disorders and nicotine dependence in a cohort of 16-year olds. *Archives of General Psychiatry, 53*, 1043–1047.

Flanagan, J., & Maany, I. (1982). Smoking and depression (letter). *American Journal of Psychiatry, 139*, 541.

Flegal, K. M., Troiano, R. P., Pamuk, E. R., Kuczmarski, R. J., & Campbell, S. M. (1995). The influence of smoking cessation on the prevalence of overweight in the United States. *New England Journal of Medicine, 333*, 1165–1170.

Frederick, T., Frerichs, R. R., & Clark, V. A. (1988). Personal health habits and symptoms of depression at the community level. *Preventive Medicine, 17*, 173–182.

Gilbert, D. G., & Gilbert, B. O. (1996). Personality, psychopathology, and nicotine response as mediators of the genetics of smoking. *Behavior Genetics, 25*, 133–147.

Glassman, A. H. (1993). Cigarette smoking: Implications for psychiatric illness. *American Journal of Psychiatry, 150*, 546–553.

Glassman, A. H., Covey, L. S., Dalack, G. W., et al. (1993). Smoking cessation, clonidine, and vulnerability to nicotine. *Clinical Trials and Therapy, 54*, 670–679.

Glassman, A. H., Helzer, J., Covey, L. S., Cottler, L. B., Stetner, F., Tipp, J. E., & Johnson, J. (1990). Smoking, smoking cessation, and major depression. *JAMA, 264*, 1546–1549.

Glassman, A. H., Stetner, F., Walsh, B. T., Raizman, P. S., Fleiss, J. L., Cooper, T. B., & Covey, L. S. (1988). Heavy smokers, smoking cessation, and clonidine. *JAMA, 259*, 2863–2866.

Glynn, S. M., & Sussman, S. (1990). Why patients smoke (letter). *Hospital and Community Psychiatry, 41*, 1027–1028.

Goff, D. C., Henderson, D. C., & Amico, E. (1992). Cigarette smoking in schizophrenia: Relationship to psychopathology and medication side effects. *American Journal of Psychiatry, 149*, 1189–1194.

Gross, J., Stitzer, M. L., & Maldonado, J. (1989). Nicotine replacement: Effects on postcessation weight gain. *Journal Consulting Clinical Psychology, 57*, 87–92.

Hall, S. M., Munoz, R. F., & Reus, V. I. (1992). Depression and smoking treatement: A clinical trial of an affect regulation treatment. *NIDA Research Monographs, 119*, 326.

Heath, A. C., & Madden, P. A. (1995). Genetic influences on smoking behavior. In R. Turner, Jr., L. R. Cardon, & J. K. Hewitt (Eds.), *Behavior genetic approaches in behavioral medicine.* New York: Plenum Press.

Heatherton, T. F., Kozlowski, L. T., Frecker, R. C., & Fagerström, K. O. (1991). The Fagerström Test for Nicotine Dependence: A revision of the Fagerström Tolerance Questionnaire. *British Journal of Addiction, 86*, 1119–1127.

Hughes, J. R. (1992). Tobacco withdrawal in self-quitters. *Journal of Consulting Clinical Psychology, 60*, 689–697.

Hughes, J. R., & Hatsukami, D. K. (1986). Signs and symptoms of nicotine withdrawal. *Archives of General Psychiatry, 43*, 280–294.

Hughes, J. R., Hatsukami, D. K., Mitchell, J. E., et al. (1986). Prevalence of smoking among psychiatric outpatients. *American Journal of Psychiatry, 143*, 993–997.

Hunt, W. A., Barnett, L. W., & Branch, L. G. (1971). Relapse rates in addiction programs. *Journal of Clinical Psychology, 27*, 455–456.

Hurt, R. D., Dale, L. C., Frederickson, P. A., Caldwell, C. C., Lee, G. A., Offord, K. P., Lauger, G. G., Marusic, Z., Neese, L. W., & Lundberg, T. G. (1994). Nicotine patch therapy for smoking cessation combined with physician advice and nurse follow-up. *JAMA, 271*, 595–600.

Hurt, R. D., Offord, K. P., Croghan, I. T., Gomez-Dahl, L. C., Kottke, T. E., Morse, R. M., Melton III, L. J. (1996). Mortality following inpatient addiction treatment: Role of tobacco use in a communibased cohort. *JAMA, 275*, 1097–1103.

Jessor, R., & Jessor, S. L. (1977). *Problem behavior and psychological development: A longitudinal study of youth.* New York: Academic Press.

Johnston, J. A., & Ascher, J. A. (1996, December). *Bupropion SR for smoking cessation.* Presented at the FDA Drug Abuse Advisory Committee Meeting, Washington, DC.

Kendler, K. S., Neale, M. C., MacLean C. J., Heath, A. C., Eaves, L. J., & Kessler, R. C. (1993). Smoking and major depression: A casual analysis. *Archives of General Psychiatry, 50*, 36–43.

Kenford, S. L., Fiore, M. C., Jorenby, D. E., Smith, S. S., Wetter, D., & Baker, T. B. (1994). Predicting smoking cessation. Who will quit with and without the nicotine patch. *JAMA, 271*, 589–594.

Kozlowski, L. T., Skinner, W., & Kent, C. (1989). Prospects for smoking treatment in individuals seeking treatement for alcohol and other drug problems. *Addictive Behaviors, 14*, 273–278.

Lavin, M. R., Siris, S. G., & Mason, S. E. (1996). What is the clinical importance of cigarette smoking in schizophrenia. *American Journal of Addictions, 5*, 189–208.

Levin, E. D., Conners, C. K., Sparrow, E., & Hinton, S. C. (1996). Nicotine effects on adults with attention-deficit/hyperactivity disorder. *Psychopharmacology, 123,* 55–66.

Lichtenstein, E., & Mermelstein, R. J. (1986). Some methodological cautions in the use of the Tolerance Questionnaire. *Addictive Behaviors, 11,* 439–442.

Lynskey, M. T., & Fergusson, D. M. (1995). Childhood conduct problems, attention deficit behaviors, and adolescent alcohol, tobacco, and illicit drug use. *Journal of Abnormal Child Psychology, 23,* 281–302.

Malkin, S. A., & Allen, D. L. (1980). Differential characteristics of adolescent smokers and non-smokers. *Journal of Family Practice, 10,* 437–440.

Menza, M. A., Grossman, N., Van Horn, M., Cody, R., & Forman, N. (1991). Smoking and movement disorders in psychiatric patients. *Biological Psychiatry, 30,* 109–115.

Milberger, S., Biderman, J., Faraone, S. V., Chen, L., & Jones, J. (1997). ADHD is associated with early initiation of cigarette smoking in children and adolescents. *Journal of the American Academy of Child and Adolescent Psychiatry, 36,* 37–44.

Niaura, R. S., Goldstein, M. G., Depue, J., Keuthen, N., Kristeller, J., & Abrams, D. B. (1995). Fluoxetine, symptoms of depression, and smoking cessation (abstract). *Annals of Behavioral Medicine, 17,* Suppl. S061.

Patton, G. C., Hibbert, M., Rosier, M. J., Carlin, J. B., Caust, J., & Bowes, G. (1996). Is smoking associated with depression and anxiety in teenagers? *American Journal of Public Health, 86,* 225–230.

Perez-Stable, E. J., Marin, G., Marin, B. V., & Katz, M. D. (1990). Depressive symptoms and cigarette smoking among Latinos in San Franciso. *American Journal of Public Health, 80,* 1500–1502.

Perkins, K. A. (1995). Weight gain following smoking cessation. *Journal of Consulting Clinical Psychology, 61,* 768–777.

Pomerleau, C. S., Carton, S. M., Lutzke, M. L., Flesslan, K. A., & Pomerleau, O. V. (1994). Reliability of the Fagerström Tolerance Questionnaire and the Fagerström Test for Nicotine Dependence. *Addictive Behaviors, 19,* 33–39.

Pomerleau, C. S., Majchrzak, M. J., & Pomerleau, O. F. (1989). Nicotine dependence and the Fagerström Tolerance Questionnaire: A brief review. *Journal of Substance Abuse, 1,* 471–477.

Pomerleau, O. F. (1986). Nicotine as a psychoactive drug: Anxiety and pain reduction. *Psychopharmacology Bulletin, 22,* 865–869.

Pomerleau, O. F., Downey, K. K., Stelson, F. W., & Pomerleau, C. S. (1995). Cigarette smoking in adult patients diagnosed with attention deficit hyperactivity disorder. *Journal of Substance Abuse, 7,* 373–378.

Robins, L. N., Helzer, J. E., & Croughan, J. (1981). NIMH–DIS: Its history, characteristics and validity. *Archives of General Psychiatry, 38,* 381–390.

Robins, L. N., & Regier, D. A. (Eds.). (1991). *Psychiatric Disorders in America: The epidemiologic catchment area study.* New York: The Free Press.

Salive, M. E., & Blazer, D. G. (1996). Depression and smoking cessation in older adults—A longitudinal study. *Journal of the American Geriatric Society, 41*(12), 13–16.

Schneider, N. G., Olmstead, R. E., Mody, F. V., Doan, K., Franzon, M., Jarvik, M. E., & Steinberg, C. (1995). Efficacy of a nasal nicotine spray in smoking cessation: A placebo-controlled double-blind trial. *Addiction, 90,* 1671–1682.

Shelley-Tremblay, J. F., & Rosen, L. A. (1996). Attention deficit hyperactivity disorder: An evolutionary perspective. *Journal of Genetic Psychology, 157,* 443–453.

Shiffman, S. M. (1979). The tobacco withdrawal syndrome. In N. A. Krasenegor (Ed.), *Cigarette smoking as a dependence process* (NIDA Research Monograph 23, pp. 153–184). Rockville, MD: Public Health Service.

Stage, K. B., Glassman, A. H., & Covey, L. S. (1996). Depression after smoking cessation: Case reports. *Journal of Clinical Psychiatry, 57,* 467–469.

Taioli, E., & Wynder, E. L. (1991). Effect of the age at which smoking begins on frequency of smoking in adulthood (letter). *New England Journal of Medicine, 325,* 968–969.

U.S. Department of Health and Human Services. (1988). *The health consequences of smoking: Nicotine addiction. A report of the Surgeon General* (Publication No. [CDC] 88-8046). Rockville, MD: Center for Disease Control.

U.S. Department of Health and Human Services. (1990). *The health benefits of smoking cessation* (Publication No. [CDC] 90-8416). Rockville, MD: Center for Disease Control.

Waal-Manning, H. J., & de Hamel, F. A. (1978). Smoking habit and psychometric scores: A community study. *New Zealand Medical Journal, 88,* 188–191.

Weissman, M. M., Bruce, M. L., Leaf, P. J., Florio, L. P., & Holzer, C. (1991). Affective disorders. In L. N. Robins & D. A. Regier (Eds.), *Psychiatric disorders in America* (pp. 53–80). New York: The Free Press.

West, R. J., Hajek, R., & Belcher, M. (1989). Severity of withdrawal symptoms as a predictor of outcome of an attempt to quit smoking. *Psychological Medicine, 19,* 981–985.

Westman, E. C., Behm, F. M., Simel, D. L., & Rose, J. E. (1997). Smoking behavior on the first day of a quit attempt predicts long-term abstinence. *Archives of Internal Medicine, 157,* 335–340.

Yassa, R., Lal, S., Lopassy, A., & Ally, J. (1987). Nicotine exposure and tardive dyskinesia. *Biological Psychiatry, 22,* 67–72.

Ziedonis, D. M., Kosten, T. R., Glazer, W. M., & Frances, R. J. (1994). Nicotine dependence and schizophrenia. *Hospital and Community Psychiatry, 45,* 204–206.

Zimmerman, M., Coryell, W. H., & Black, D. W. (1991, May). *Cigarette smoking and psychiatric illness.* Meeting Program of the 144th Annual Meeting of the American Psychiatric Association, New Orleans, LA, p. 167.

Part III

Assessment and Treatment: Special Populations

CHAPTER THREE

Preventing Cigarette Smoking Among Children and Adolescents

Gilbert J. Botvin
Jennifer A. Epstein
Institute for Prevention Research, Cornell University Medical College

Each day 3,000 adolescents start smoking in the United States. According to recent projections, an estimated 5 million people aged 17 years or under in 1995 will die prematurely from a smoking-related illness (Centers for Disease Control, 1996). Despite the concerted efforts of educators and health professionals, cigarette smoking continues to be one of the most serious health problems facing this nation. Although cigarette smoking has been on the decline among adults, adolescent smoking has been steadily on the rise since 1992. Recent national survey data indicate that more than one third of high-school seniors smoked in the past 30 days (Johnston, O'Malley, & Bachman, in press; Kann et al., 1996). Perhaps of greatest concern is the fact that steady increases in cigarette smoking over the past few years were evident for 8th, 10th, and 12th graders in the Monitoring the Future survey (Johnston et al., in press). Initiation and development of cigarette smoking begins in the early teens, increases in the middle teens, and levels off by the late teens (Botvin & Botvin, 1992). Regular use of cigarettes usually begins in mid-adolescence and continues to progress. By late adolescence, some youth are smoking at levels comparable to adult smokers. Furthermore, adolescent smoking trends have important implications because 77% of adult smokers became daily smokers before age 20 (U.S. Department of Health and Human Services, 1994).

Consequently, the task of developing effective approaches to adolescent smoking prevention takes on great importance. This task has lasted more than two decades. Empirical evidence from early evaluation studies showed either limited success and or complete ineffectiveness. More recent efforts from a growing number of carefully designed and methodologically sophisticated research studies clearly indicates that certain types of approaches to smoking prevention work. Moreover, some of these approaches have demonstrated long-term effectiveness. This chapter concentrates on what is currently known about the effectiveness of adolescent smoking prevention efforts. Its primary focus is on careful evaluation research published in peer-reviewed journals using acceptable scientific methods. Finally, possible applications of prevention approaches to smoking cessation in older adolescents are covered.

CONSTRUCTING A SOLID FOUNDATION FOR PREVENTION

Smoking prevention research has progressed during the past 20 years. Early research consisted of small-scale pilot studies designed to test the acceptability, feasibility, and preliminary efficacy of promising approaches. Recent state-of-the-art prevention research involves large-scale randomized field trials designed to provide the strongest possible evidence of effectiveness. This range of evaluation studies provides substantial evidence for the effectiveness of certain approaches to smoking prevention. The best contemporary prevention research has three distinguishing features. First, the most promising approaches are based on an understanding of what is known about the etiology of smoking. Second, these approaches are conceptualized within a theoretical framework. Finally, evaluations of these approaches consist of empirical testing using appropriate research methods. Although all three are critically important aspects of prevention research, an understanding of the etiology of smoking is fundamental.

Antecedents and Correlates of Smoking

Elucidation of the causes of smoking and its developmental progression is critical to the nature and timing of potentially effective prevention approaches. Extensive research related to smoking etiology has been conducted over the past 20 years. Surprisingly, many prevention efforts appear to have been developed without any acknowledgment or appreciation of this work. Despite research indicating that smoking is multiply determined, the most ubiquitous prevention approaches, until recently, focused on factual information about cigarettes and the adverse consequences of smoking.

Reviews of the smoking etiology literature clearly indicate that smoking results from a complex interaction of a number of different etiologic factors including knowledge, attitudes, social, personality, and developmental factors (Botvin & Botvin, 1992; Conrad, Flay, & Hill, 1992; Hawkins, Catalano, & Miller, 1992; U.S. Department of Health and Human Services, 1994). Promising prevention approaches go beyond incorporating the complex etiology of smoking through an appreciation of the importance of social factors in promoting the initiation of smoking.

Parents (Bauman, Foshee, Linzer, & Koch, 1990; Chassin, Presson, Sherman, Montello, & McGrew, 1986), siblings (Botvin et al., 1992; Chassin, Presson, Sherman, Corty, & Olshavsky, 1984; Mittlemark et al., 1987; Swan, Creeser, & Murray, 1990), and peers and friends (Bauman et al., 1990; Botvin, Epstein, Schinke, & Diaz, 1994; Elder, Molgaard, & Greshan, 1988; Hunter, Vizelberg, & Berenson, 1991; O'Connell et al., 1981; Ogawa, Tominaga, Gellert, & Aoki, 1988; Shean, 1991), as well as the media (Tye, Warner, & Glantz, 1987; Whelan, 1984), serve as powerful social influences to promote and sustain smoking during childhood and early adolescence. Adolescents who perceive smoking as something "everyone is doing" are at increased risk of becoming smokers (Chassin, Presson, Sherman, Corty, & Olshavsky, 1984; Chassin et al., 1990; Collins et al., 1987; Gerber & Newman, 1989). Psychological characteristics such as low self-esteem, self-image, social confidence, assertiveness, personal control, and self-efficacy have been found to be associated with smoking (Ahlgren, Norem, Hochhauser, & Garvin, 1982; Botvin, Baker, Botvin, Dusenbury, Cardwell, & Diaz, 1993; Botvin et al., 1994; Chassin et al., 1990; Ellickson & Hays, 1990-91; Lawrance & Rubinson, 1986; Stacy, Sussman, Dent, Burton, & Flay, 1992; Young & Werch, 1990).

Developmental factors associated with the adolescent period appear to increase risk for smoking. Adolescence is characterized by dramatic change and readjustment (Mussen, Conger, & Kagan, 1974), often resulting in new stresses and anxieties that may increase vulnerability to peer pressure. During puberty, striking and rapid physical changes occur that may disturb self-image and self-esteem. Psychosocial changes occurring immediately prior to or during the beginning of the adolescent period also increase the likelihood that an adolescent will try cigarettes. These developmental changes often increase adolescents' susceptibility to direct and indirect social influences to smoke. When cigarette use is consistent with the norms of their friends or other important reference groups and is combined with a tendency to conform to group norms, then adolescents are more likely to smoke.

Furthermore, cognitive developmental changes can undermine previously acquired knowledge of the potential risks of smoking. Adolescents may notice inconsistencies between adult warnings and behavior or discover logical flaws in the arguments adults advance against smoking. Finally, issues relating to identity and public image may substantially increase general susceptibility to advertising appeals and other social influences promoting smoking.

Transition From Etiology to Intervention

Clearly, smoking is not the result of a single etiologic factor. Many different factors apparently interact with one another to produce a complex probabilistic risk to smoke. Prevention cannot simply target a single cause of smoking. The task is much more difficult because interventions must target multiple risk and protective factors. According to smoking etiology research, effective prevention programs targeting children and adolescents must impact on social factors as well as knowledge, attitudes, norms, skills, and personality. Understanding the etiology of smoking also helps explain why some prevention approaches were not effective in reducing smoking.

SMOKING PREVENTION APPROACHES

Most smoking prevention research evaluated interventions in school settings. Generally, the interventions were conducted within the classroom (usually in the form of a curriculum). School-based smoking prevention programs fall into three major approaches: (a) information dissemination approaches, (b) social influences approaches, and (c) competence enhancement approaches. Although the first approach is discussed briefly, the main emphasis of this chapter is on the last two approaches because they meet the distinguishing features for prevention research discussed earlier. Specifically, etiologic findings and psychological theory are the basis of these latter two approaches. In addition, evaluations using appropriate research methods attest to their effectiveness.

Health Information Approaches

The most conventional smoking education approaches attempt to prevent adolescent smoking through increased awareness and knowledge of the negative consequences of cigarettes. In many cases, these approaches rely on fear-arousal methods. Reviews of these approaches highlighted their ineffectiveness (Thompson, 1978; Goodstadt, 1978). Although results indicate that these approaches can increase knowledge and sometimes change attitudes toward smoking, they did not change smoking behavior. Although developmentally appropriate and personally relevant health information has a place in smoking prevention programs, clearly information alone is not effective.

Social Influence Approaches

Psychological Inoculation. In a major departure from previous approaches, Evans and his colleagues developed and tested a different type of smoking prevention intervention. Their approach focused on the social and psychological factors believed to be involved in the initiation of cigarette smoking (Evans, 1976; Evans et al., 1978). Specifically, their prevention program was the first to concentrate on teaching adolescents skills to resist social influences to smoke based on theory. Understanding the causes of smoking is helpful but insufficient in devising effective smoking prevention approaches. It is necessary to develop some sense of how the various risk factors fit together and which factors are potentially amenable to intervention, and then to design an intervention based on a comprehensive understanding of these different elements. Evans and his colleagues realized this and attempted to devise an appropriate smoking prevention program.

The program was derived from persuasive communications theory and a concept called *psychological inoculation* (McGuire, 1964, 1968). This concept is analogous to inoculation in infectious disease prevention. Thus, persuasive prosmoking communications designed to alter attitudes, beliefs, and behavior related to smoking are a psychosocial analogue of germs. To prevent "infection" it is necessary to expose the individual to a weak dose of those germs in a way that facilitates the development of "antibodies" and thereby increases resistance to any future exposure to persuasive messages in their more virulent form. From the perspective of psychological inoculation, cigarette smoking is the result of social influences (persuasive messages) to smoke from peers and the media, which are either direct (i.e., offers to smoke from other adolescents or cigarette advertising) or indirect (i.e., exposure to high-status role models who smoke). An underlying assumption of Evans' approach was that adolescents could be effectively inoculated against social influences to smoke by gradually exposing them to progressively more intense prosmoking social influences. By equipping adolescents with the appropriate skills to resist social influences, they should be less likely to become smokers.

Consistent with this, the intervention was designed to increase adolescents' awareness of the various social pressures to smoke likely to be encountered as they progressed through junior high school. The program included demonstrations of specific techniques to effectively resist various pressures to smoke. The prevention strategy also incorporated two other important components: (a) feedback designed to correct the misperception that everybody is smoking and (b) information about the immediate physiological effects of smoking. Results showed that the prevention group had 50% fewer smokers than the control group (Evans et al., 1978).

Resistance Skills Training. A number of research teams have developed and tested variations on the social influence model over the years (Arkin, Roemhild, Johnson, Luepker, & Murray, 1981; Hurd et al., 1980; Luepker, Johnson, Murray, & Pechacek, 1983; Perry, Killen, Slinkard, & McAlister, 1983; Telch, Killen, McAlister, Perry, & Maccoby, 1982). Although these interventions also included material to increase awareness of the various social influences to smoke, they placed much greater emphasis on teaching specific skills for effectively resisting both peer and media pressures than the original Evans social influence model. Several names have been used for these approaches, including the broad term *social influence approach* (because they target the social influences promoting smoking), *refusal skills training* (because a central feature of these programs is that they teach adolescents how to say "No" to cigarette offers), and *resistance skills training*.

Resistance skills training approaches stress the fundamental importance of social factors in promoting the initiation of smoking among adolescents. Family (parents and older siblings), peers, and the mass media are the major social influences. All social influences are a product of the interaction between individual learning histories and forces in both the community and the larger society (Bandura, 1977). On the individual level, influences related to specific behaviors arise from learned expectations and skills regarding those behaviors. For example, adolescents may smoke because they expect relatively immediate positive outcomes such as increased alertness, relief from anxiety, or enhanced social status. Logically, if adolescents did not expect to receive rewarding consequences from smoking or if they had the ability to resist specific social pressures to smoke, then they would not smoke. People learn expectations and skills from observation and direct experience. Adolescents receiving resistance skills training learn how to recognize, handle, or avoid situations in which they have a high likelihood of experiencing peer pressure to smoke. They learn both what to say in response to a peer pressure situation (i.e., the specific content of a refusal message) and how to say it in the most effective way possible.

Peer Leader Program Providers. Social influence approaches generally incorporate *peer leaders* as program providers. Peer leaders are usually older students (e.g., 10th graders might serve as peer leaders for 7th graders). Sometimes peer leaders are the same age as participants and may even be from the same class. The reason to include peer leaders is that peers often appear to have higher credibility with adolescents than adults do. Peer leaders are useful as discussion leaders, nonsmoking role models, and trainers in demonstrations of the cigarette refusal skills in these prevention programs.

Correcting Normative Expectations. Adolescents typically overestimate the prevalence of smoking (Fishbein, 1977). Therefore, correcting normative expectations is another important component of social influence approaches. To correct these misperceptions about smoking norms, participating students receive information about actual smoking prevalence rates. For example, social influence approaches allow students to compare their inaccurate estimates with actual smoking prevalence rates from national, school-wide, or classroom surveys. In addition, social influence prevention programs have also typically included a component designed to increase students' awareness of the techniques advertisers use to promote the sale of cigarettes and to teach techniques for formulating counterarguments to advertising.

Competence Enhancement Approaches

Smoking prevention research has extensively evaluated a prevention model that teaches general personal and social skills in combination with components of the social resistance skills model (Botvin, Baker, Filazzola, & Botvin, 1990; Botvin, Baker, Renick, Filazzola, & Botvin, 1984; Botvin & Eng, 1980; Botvin, Eng, & Williams, 1980; Botvin, Renick, & Baker, 1983; Gilchrist & Schinke, 1983; Pentz, 1983; Schinke & Gilchrist, 1983, 1984). These *competence enhancement approaches* are more comprehensive than either health information or social influence approaches. Unlike affective education approaches that rely on experiential classroom activities, these approaches emphasize the use of proven cognitive/behavioral skills training methods. They are based on social learning theory (Bandura, 1977) and problem behavior theory (Jessor & Jessor, 1977). According to these theories, smoking, like other behaviors, is socially learned and functional, resulting from the interplay of social and personal factors. Modeling and reinforcement of smoking and prosmoking cognition, attitudes, and beliefs influence adolescents to smoke.

Competence enhancement approaches typically teach two or more of the following:

1. General problem-solving and decision-making skills.
2. General cognitive skills for resisting interpersonal or media influences.
3. Skills for increasing self-control and self-esteem.
4. Adaptive coping strategies for relieving stress and anxiety through the use of cognitive coping skills or behavioral relaxation techniques.
5. General social skills.
6. General assertive skills.

Adolescents learn these skills using a combination of instruction, demonstration, feedback, reinforcement, behavioral rehearsal (practice during class), and extended practice through behavioral homework assignments.

A primary aim of personal and social skills training programs is to enhance general competence by teaching skills for coping with life that have a relatively broad application. In contrast, the social influence approaches are designed to teach information, norms, and refusal skills with a problem-specific focus. Personal and social skills training programs stress the application of general skills to situations directly related to smoking (e.g., applying general assertive skills to situations involving peer pressure to smoke). These same skills can be applied to the many challenges adolescents face in their everyday lives, including but not limited to smoking.

Broad-based competence enhancement approaches may not be effective unless they also contain some resistance skills training material according to one study (Caplan et al., 1992). Inclusion of resistance skills training may be necessary because such material both includes a focus on providing accurate peer and adult norms and helps students apply generic personal and social skills to smoking-related situations. Thus the most effective prevention approaches appear to be those that combine the features of the problem-specific social influence model and the broader competence enhancement model.

An example of this type of competence enhancement approach is the Life Skills Training (LST) program that has been tested at Cornell University Medical College (e.g., Botvin et al., 1983; Botvin, Baker, Dusenbury, Botvin, & Diaz, 1995). The LST program is a school-based approach to tobacco, alcohol, and drug abuse prevention. It is designed for middle/junior high school students and has three major components. The first component teaches health information, promotes nonsmoking and non-drug-use norms, and trains students how to handle social influences to smoke, drink, or use illicit drugs. The second component teaches a set of self-management skills for assessing strengths/weaknesses, setting and achieving goals, making decisions, and coping with anxiety. The final component teaches general social skills such as how to communicate more effectively, develop friendships, and handle situations warranting an assertive response.

EMPIRICAL EVIDENCE OF EFFECTIVENESS

Short-Term Effectiveness

Both the social influence and the competence enhancement approaches reduced cigarette smoking relative to controls. A number of studies document the effectiveness of social influence approaches. These studies show that social influence approaches reduced the rate of smoking by between 35 and 45% after the initial intervention. Most of these prevention studies have focused primarily on preventing the onset of cigarette smoking—that is, preventing the transition from nonsmoking to smoking. The results reported range from reductions of 30–40% in the proportion of individuals beginning to smoke (comparing the proportion of new smokers in the prevention group with that of the control group). Several studies have demonstrated reductions in the overall prevalence of cigarette smoking among the participating students both for experimental smoking (less than one cigarette per week) and for regular smoking (one or more cigarettes per week). In these studies, the impact on the prevalence of regular smoking has typically been in the 40–50% range.

Competence enhancement approaches to smoking prevention reduced new experimental smoking from 40 to 75%. Data from two early studies with a promising program called Life Skills Training (Botvin & Eng, 1982; Botvin et al., 1983) demonstrated reductions ranging from 56% to 66% in the proportion of pretest nonsmokers becoming regular smokers at the 1-year follow-up without additional booster sessions. With booster sessions these reductions have been as high as 87% (Botvin et al., 1983). Moreover, initial reductions of an equal magnitude have also been reported for regular smoking (Botvin et al., 1983; Botvin & Eng, 1982).

Long-Term Effectiveness

The durability of effectiveness of smoking prevention approaches over time has become an extremely important issue. Follow-up studies using school-based approaches indicate that the positive behavioral effects for cigarette smoking are evident for up to 3 years after the conclusion of these programs (Luepker et al., 1983; McAlister, Perry, & Maccoby, 1979; Sussman, Dent, Stacy, & Sun, 1993; Telch et al., 1982), and multicomponent studies have found prevention effects for up to 7 years (Perry & Kelder, 1992). Despite these impressive effects, the results of most long-term follow-up studies of school-based approaches indicate that prevention effects are typically not maintained (Flay et al., 1989; Murray, Davis-Hearn, Goldman, Pirie, & Luepker, 1988). Consequently, some critics conclude that school-based prevention approaches may simply not be powerful enough to produce lasting effects (Dryfoos, 1993). Defenders argue that the prevention approaches tested in these studies had deficiencies subverting their long-term effectiveness (Resnicow & Botvin, 1993).

An absence of long-term prevention effects in some studies should not be taken as an indictment of all school-based prevention programs. Lack of long-term prevention effects may reflect factors related to either the type of intervention tested or the implementation of these interventions. Some reasons for the lack of durable prevention effects in several long-term follow-up studies are that:

1. The length of the intervention was too short (i.e., the prevention approach was effective, but the initial prevention "dosage" was too low to produce a long-term effect).

2. Booster sessions were either inadequate or not included (i.e., the prevention approach was effective, but it eroded over time because of the absence or inadequacy of ongoing intervention).
3. The intervention was not implemented with enough fidelity to the intervention model (i.e., the correct prevention approach was used, but it was implemented incompletely, improperly, or both).
4. The intervention was based on faulty assumptions, was incomplete, or was otherwise deficient (i.e., the prevention approach was ineffective).

Long-term follow-up data from one of the largest school-based prevention studies ever conducted found reductions in smoking 6 years after the initial baseline assessment (Botvin et al., 1995). This randomized, controlled, field trial involved nearly 6,000 seventh graders from 56 public schools in New York State. After random assignment of schools to prevention and control conditions, students in the prevention condition received the Life Skills Training (LST) program during the seventh grade (15 prevention sessions) with booster sessions in the eighth grade (10 sessions) and ninth grade (5 sessions). No intervention was provided during Grades 10 to 12. Participants completed follow-up surveys in class, by mail, and/or by telephone at the end of the 12th grade and beyond for those students not available for the school survey. Results indicated that there were significantly fewer smokers for students who received the LST prevention program during seventh, eighth, and ninth grades. In addition, results showed that the prevention program had an impact on more serious levels of smoking beyond monthly or weekly cigarette use. According to the results of this study, the LST program delivered during junior high school reduced pack-a-day smoking at the end of high school by 25% when compared with untreated controls. With annual smoking-related mortality exceeding 400,000 deaths per year, this prevention approach offers the potential for saving over 100,000 lives per year.

Prevention effects were also found for hypothesized mediating variables in the direction of decreased risk. Students who received the most complete implementation of the prevention program showed the strongest prevention effects. In addition, prevention effects were found using both the individual and school as the unit of analysis. Attrition rates were equivalent for prevention and control conditions, as were pretest levels of smoking for the final analysis sample. This supports the conclusion that prevention effects were the result of the intervention and not due to differential attrition, or pretest nonequivalence. The results of this study suggest that, to be effective, school-based interventions need to be more comprehensive and have a stronger initial dosage than most studies using the social influence approach have had. Prevention programs also need to include at least 2 additional years of intervention (booster sessions) and be implemented in a manner that is faithful to the underlying intervention model.

Generalizability to Ethnic Minority Youth

Most smoking prevention research has been conducted with predominantly White, middle-class, suburban populations. Racial/ethnic minority youth have been underserved with respect to prevention services and underrepresented in prevention evaluation studies. Relatively little is known concerning the etiology of smoking among minority youth. Existing evidence indicates that there is substantial overlap in the factors promoting and maintaining smoking among predominantly Hispanic and African-American populations relative to White populations, including social influences to smoke and psychological characteristics (Bettes, Dusenbury, Kerner, James-Ortiz, & Botvin, 1990; Botvin, Baker, Botvin, Dusenbury, Cardwell, & Diaz, 1993; Botvin et al., 1994; Botvin, Goldberg, Botvin, & Dusenbury, 1993; Dusenbury et al., 1992; Dusenbury, Epstein, Botvin, & Diaz, 1994). This suggests that prevention approaches found to be effective with one population should also be effective with others.

An example is research with a competence enhancement approach called Life Skills Training (described in the Competence Enhancement Approaches section), which has been shown to be effective in decreasing smoking and risk factors associated with smoking among ethnic-minority youth. Qualitative research with parents, teachers, and students found high acceptance and perceived utility for this prevention approach among African-American and Hispanic populations. Where appropriate, the language, examples, and behavioral rehearsal scenarios were modified to increase cultural sensitivity and relevance to each of the target populations. But no modifications were made to the underlying prevention approach, which focused on teaching generic personal and social skills, antismoking norms, cigarette refusal skills, and prevention-related knowledge and information.

Studies conducted with inner-city Hispanic youth (Botvin, Dusenbury, Baker, James-Ortiz, & Kerner, 1989; Botvin et al., 1992) and African-American youth (Botvin, Batson, Witts-Vitale, Bess, Baker, & Dusenbury, 1989; Botvin & Cardwell, 1992) have consistently shown that the Life Skills Training approach can decrease cigarette smoking relative to a control group in the 7th grade. Long-term studies conducted with Hispanic youth who received the initial intervention in 7th grade and booster sessions in 8th and 9th grade have demonstrated the continued presence of less frequent cigarette smoking through the end of the 10th grade (Botvin, 1994).

IMPLEMENTATION ISSUES

Timing of Intervening

A critical time for experimentation with cigarettes occurs at the beginning of adolescence, according to etiology of smoking and adolescent development research (Botvin & Botvin, 1992). That is why most prevention research studies focus on middle school (sixth, seventh, and to eighth grade) or junior high school (seventh, eighth, and ninth grade) students. Even though many researchers agree that at least some of the risk factors for smoking may have their roots in early childhood (arguing for beginning interventions at a younger age), the low base rates of smoking prior to adolescence preclude testing the effectiveness of prevention approaches at younger ages. To adequately test the impact of prevention programs it is necessary to select an age range that not only makes sense from an intervention perspective, but also is old enough to include individuals who are likely to begin smoking in sufficient numbers for researchers to detect statistically significant differences between prevention and control groups. Generally speaking, this mens that meaningful evaluation of prevention effects based on smoking behavior cannot be conducted prior to the seventh grade.

Universal or High-Risk Interventions

Additional research should address whether prevention programs should be "universal" interventions targeted at all available individuals (e.g., all the students in the seventh grade) or should only be targeted at "high-risk" populations (e.g., a subgroup of seventh graders identified using some established criteria of high risk). One obvious difficulty concerns the definition of risk. Another is that less is known about the potential of even the most effective contemporary prevention approaches with high-risk individuals. Because researchers have generally not attempted to identify those individuals who are the most likely to become smokers and or to examine the relative effectiveness of existing prevention approaches with different risk groups, it is difficult to determine the extent to which these interventions would be effective with those individuals at the highest risk. Thus, although it might be a more efficient utilization of available resources to target prevention interventions at high-risk adolescents, the most prudent strategy at this point is to include everyone available.

Program Providers

Considerable variation exists among the individuals responsible for implementing school-based prevention programs. College students, research project staff, and classroom teachers have all implemented prevention programs. Same-age or older peer leaders have been included in nearly all of the studies testing social influence approaches and in some of the studies testing the personal and social skills training approaches. In general, evidence supports the addition of peer leaders for this type of prevention strategy (Arkin et al., 1981; Perry et al., 1983).

Although peer leaders have been used successfully to varying degrees in these programs, they usually assist adult program providers and have specific and well-defined roles. The primary providers in most of these studies have been either research project staff members or teachers. There is also evidence to suggest that peer-led programs may not be uniformly effective for all students. For example, the results of one study suggest that social influence programs conducted by teachers affect boys and girls similarly, whereas peer-led programs may influence girls more than boys (Fisher, Armstrong, & deKler, 1983).

Project staff, peer leaders, and classroom teachers are all capable of successfully implementing competence enhancement prevention approaches, according to past research (Botvin & Botvin, 1992). However, not all adult program providers are equally effective (Botvin, Baker, Filazzola, & Botvin, 1990). Additional research is needed to identify the characteristics of the most effective providers, as well as the optimal match between the characteristics of providers and prevention program participants.

Intervention Components and Their Efficacy

Contemporary smoking prevention programs contain a variety of components. Progress has clearly been made toward identifying effective prevention approaches. Yet little is known concerning the extent to which different intervention components contribute to smoking prevention. It is necessary to identify the relative efficacy of specific program components to increase our understanding of why the most effective interventions work and to facilitate the development of more effective interventions. This may not only prove helpful in guiding practitioners concerning the "active ingredients" or essential elements in prevention programs, but may also enable program developers to identify nonessential components and decrease the length of interventions, thereby increasing the likelihood of utilization by schools. Effective smoking prevention programs may work because of a few key components, or they may be the result of the synergistic interactions of all program components.

Although there is a paucity of knowledge about the relative effectiveness of various intervention components, some studies have addressed this issue. For example, many prevention approaches based on the social influence model have included a public commitment component; however, at least one study suggests that this component may not contribute to the effectiveness of these programs (Hurd et al., 1980). Similarly, many of these programs have used films or videotapes similar to those initially developed by Evans and his colleagues (Evans et al., 1978). It is not yet clear what type of media material is the most effective or the extent to which it is necessary as a component. In addition to studies testing the effectiveness of approaches in school settings, studies have also tested this intervention approach along with media (Flynn et al., 1992), parent (Rohrbach, Hodgson, Broder, & Montgomery, 1994), or media and parent (Pentz et al., 1989; Perry, Kelder, Murray, & Klepp, 1992) components. These studies indicate that the inclusion of additional intervention components produces stronger prevention effects than the school-based intervention alone.

Program Length

A basic practical consideration in developing preventive interventions for adolescents concerns the amount of time necessary for implementation. At this point, it is difficult to specify how long prevention programs should be. The evaluation literature contains programs ranging from as few as 3 or 4 sessions to as many as 20. A consensus meeting of smoking prevention experts convened by the National Cancer Institute concluded that the minimum program length for adolescent smoking prevention programs should be at least 5 sessions (Glynn, Anderson, & Schwarz, 1991).

Several factors may affect program length. One factor affecting program length is the type of prevention program. Prevention programs teaching domain-specific skills (i.e., skills specific to resisting social influences to smoke) require less time to implement than competence enhancement approaches. Programs that combine both specific and generic skills training approaches are longer still. Although there is some evidence to suggest that longer programs are more effective, it is not yet clear what the optimal program length is for producing a meaningful and lasting reduction in smoking.

Booster Sessions

As discussed earlier, prevention effects tend to erode over time without additional intervention. At the same time, when booster sessions or ongoing preventive interventions have been provided, preventive gains have generally been maintained and, in some instances, have even been enhanced (Botvin et al., 1983; Botvin, Baker, Dusenbury, Tortu, & Botvin, 1990). For prevention programs targeted at adolescents, booster sessions should be implemented throughout the middle/junior high school period. It may also be necessary to provide preventive interventions throughout high school. Booster sessions generally build on the material covered previously in the prevention program, providing both a review of program content and an opportunity to practice the skills taught in the program. The developmental appropriateness of the material taught in the various years of the prevention program may warrant the introduction of new material in one or more of the booster years. Typically, booster sessions require fewer prevention sessions than those involved in the primary intervention.

ADOLESCENT SMOKING CESSATION

Smoking prevention programs tend to be conducted with adolescents in the seventh grade when smoking prevalence rates are too low and infrequent to adequately test the effects for smoking cessation. In high school, adolescent smokers are regular smokers and some youth smoke at levels comparable to adults. Adolescents of this age continue to smoke for a variety of reasons, including stress and anxiety, social influences to smoke (peers, parents, and relatives), boredom, pleasure/affect, addiction, and desire (Sarason, Mankowski, Peterson, & Dinh, 1992; Tuakli, Smith, & Heaton, 1990). Most daily young smokers (74%) reported that they continued to smoke due to the difficulty of quitting (Barker, 1994). Numerous surveys indicate that many adolescent smokers have tried to quit smoking and failed (Ershler, Leventhal, Fleming & Glynn, 1989; Moss, Allen, Giovino, & Mills, 1992; Tuakli et al., 1990). National data attest to the difficulty of quitting smoking among adolescents. For example, 44% of high school seniors who were daily smokers during 1976–1986 believed that they would not be smoking in 5 years, yet 73% of them remained daily smokers 5 to 6 years later (U.S. Department of Health and Human Services, 1994).

Although progress has been made in developing effective smoking prevention approaches for younger adolescents, there is a pressing need for smoking cessation approaches for older adolescents. Concentrating on high-school-age smokers is a way of targeting smokers early on and may maximize success in cessation. Yet virtually no research has focused on development and evaluation of adolescent smoking cessation approaches.

Reviews (Thompson, 1978; Seffrin & Bailey, 1985) of early attempts to develop antismoking campaigns to encourage smoking cessation among youth indicate that these attempts had many problems (e.g., education was didactic, evaluations tended to be anecdotal or descriptive). A report of the Surgeon General (U.S. Department of Health and Human Services, 1989) called for further research and continued program development in adolescent smoking cessation, yet little progress has been made as studies that evaluated smoking cessation programs suffered from a variety of methodological problems. Some research has examined self-initiated smoking cessation during late adolescence. A longitudinal study found that high school students who quit smoking had responded to peer influences (Chassin, Presson, & Sherman, 1984). Specifically, future quitters had fewer friends who smoked. Furthermore, quitting led to changes in their social environment that reinforced cessation (fewer friends who smoked, less positive peer attitudes toward smoking). Another study also found that having fewer friends that smoked predicted self-initiated smoking cessation (Hansen, Collins, Johnson, & Graham, 1985). These findings suggest that adolescent smoking cessation programs need to include methods for changing peer influences to smoke similar to those included in effective smoking prevention programs.

Psychosocial Skills Approach to Smoking Cessation for Adolescents

Theoretical models, such as social learning theory (Bandura, 1977), that serve as the basis for effective prevention approaches may also be relevant for development of smoking cessation interventions. Such interventions need to (a) be adapted for older adolescents who have become regular smokers and (b) integrate effective techniques from smoking cessation research with adults. Using a psychosocial skills model for smoking cessation based on social learning theory (Bandura, 1977), such an intervention for adolescents would include material to increase awareness of social influences to continue smoking, teach cigarette refusal skills, help break associations with smoking, teach how to elicit appropriate social support to quit smoking, and demonstrate a variety of cognitive-behavioral techniques to quit smoking and prevent relapse.

SUMMARY AND CONCLUSION

This chapter has focused on smoking prevention efforts among children and adolescents. Specifically, we described how smoking develops in children and summarized the main factors associated with becoming a smoker. We also detailed the most common prevention approaches and reviewed evaluation results of these approaches. Finally, we discussed the implications for designing smoking cessation programs for older adolescents. Much progress has been made in the smoking prevention field. More is now known about the etiology of smoking, which helps to better guide the development of effective prevention approaches. In addition, evidence exists for what kinds of prevention approaches work and under what conditions.

Smoking prevention approaches that rely on providing students with information about the adverse consequences of cigarettes have consistently been found to be ineffective—when the standard of effectiveness is deterring smoking. The only prevention approaches demonstrated to effectively impact on smoking behavior are those that teach adolescents social resistance skills and antismoking norms, either alone (social influence approaches) or in combination with teaching generic personal and social skills (competence enhancement approaches). Both approaches stress skills training and deemphasize health information related to the adverse health consequences of smoking. These approaches have been shown to work with different program providers and different target populations, including racial/ethnic minority youth. Despite generally impressive initial prevention effects, it is evident that without booster sessions these effects decay over time. Thus to produce lasting prevention effects, it is necessary to have ongoing prevention activities throughout the early adolescent years.

Smoking prevention work progressed greatly as a result of an appreciation of smoking etiology research and more dependence on a theoretical framework. Empirical evidence from a number of methodologically sophisticated evaluation studies demonstrates for the first time that specific school-based prevention models are effective. Yet despite these promising findings, additional research is needed to further refine current prevention models to optimize their effectiveness and elucidate how they work. Health care professionals, educators, community leaders, and policymakers should move expeditiously toward wide dissemination and utilization of these approaches. It is equally important for research to continue to refine existing prevention models and to increase our understanding of the causes of smoking.

REFERENCES

Ahlgren, A., Norem, A. A., Hochhauser, M., & Garvin, J. (1982). Antecedents of smoking among pre-adolescents. *Journal of Drug Education, 12,* 325–340.

Arkin, R. M., Roemhild, H. J., Johnson, C. A., Luepker, R. V., & Murray, D. M. (1981). The Minnesota smoking prevention program: A seventh grade health curriculum supplement. *Journal of School Health, 51,* 616–661.

Bandura, A. (1977). *Social learning theory.* Englewood Cliffs, NJ: Prentice-Hall.

Barker, B. (1994). Reasons for tobacco use and symptoms of nicotine withdrawal among adolescent and young adult tobacco users—United States, 1993. *Morbidity and Mortality Weekly Report, 43,* 745–750.

Bauman, K. E., Foshee, V. A., Linzer, M. A., & Koch, G. G. (1990). Effect of parental smoking classification on the association between parental and adolescent smoking. *Addictive Behaviors, 15*(5), 413–422.

Bettes, B. A., Dusenbury, L., Kerner, J. F., James-Ortiz, S., & Botvin, G. J. (1990). Ethnicity and psychosocial factors in alcohol and tobacco use in adolescence. *Child Development, 61,* 557–565.

Botvin, G. J. (1994). *Final report to the National Cancer Institute: Smoking Prevention among New York Hispanic youth.* New York: Cornell University Medical College.

Botvin, G. J., Baker, E., Botvin, E. M., Dusenbury, L., Cardwell, J., & Diaz, T. (1993). Factors promoting cigarette smoking among black youth: A causal modeling approach. *Addictive Behaviors, 18,* 397–405.

Botvin, G. J., Baker, E., Dusenbury, L., Botvin, E. M., & Diaz, T. (1995). Long-term follow-up results of a randomized drug abuse prevention trial in a White middle-class population. *Journal of the American Medical Association, 273,* 1106–1112.

Botvin, G. J., Baker, E., Dusenbury, L., Tortu, S., & Botvin, E. M. (1990). Preventing adolescent drug abuse through a multimodal cognitive-behavioral approach: Results of a 3-year study. *Journal of Consulting and Clinical Psychology, 58,* 437–446.

Botvin, G. J., Baker, E., Filazzola, A. D., & Botvin, E. M. (1990). A cognitive-behavioral approach to substance abuse prevention: A one-year follow-up. *Addictive Behaviors, 15,* 47–63.

Botvin, G. J., Baker, E., Renick, N. L., Filazzola, A. D., & Botvin, E. M. (1984). A cognitive-behavioral approach to substance abuse prevention. *Addictive Behaviors, 9,* 137–147.

Botvin, G. J., Batson, H. W., Witts-Vitale, S., Bess, V., Baker, E., & Dusenbury, L. (1989). A psychosocial approach to smoking prevention for urban black youth. *Public Health Reports, 104*, 573–582.

Botvin, G. J., & Botvin, E. M. (1992). Adolescent tobacco, alcohol, and drug abuse: Prevention strategies, empirical findings, and assessment issues. *Journal of Developmental and Behavioral Pediatrics, 13*, 290–301.

Botvin, G. J., & Cardwell, J. (1992). Primary prevention (smoking) of cancer in Black populations. Grant contract number N01-CN-6508. Final Report to National Cancer Institute. Cornell University Medical College.

Botvin, G. J., Dusenbury, L., Baker, E., James-Ortiz, S., Botvin, E. M., & Kerner, J. F. (1992). Smoking prevention among urban minority youth: Assessing effects on outcome and mediating variables. *Health Psychology, 11*, 290–299.

Botvin, G. J., Dusenbury, L., Baker, E., James-Ortiz, S., & Kerner, J. F. (1989). A skills training approach to smoking prevention among Hispanic youth. *Journal of Behavioral Medicine, 12*, 279–296.

Botvin, G. J., & Eng, A. (1980). A comprehensive school-based smoking prevention program. *Journal of School Health, 50*, 209–213.

Botvin, G. J., & Eng, A. (1982). The efficacy of a multicomponent approach to the prevention of cigarette smoking. *Preventive Medicine, 11*, 199–211.

Botvin, G. J., Eng, A., & Williams, C. L. (1980). Preventing the onset of cigarette smoking through life skills training. *Preventive Medicine, 9*, 135–143.

Botvin, G. J., Epstein, J. A., Schinke, S. P., & Diaz, T. (1994). Predictors of cigarette smoking among inner-city minority youth. *Journal of Developmental and Behavioral Pediatrics, 15*, 67–73.

Botvin, G. J., Goldberg, C. J., Botvin, E. M., & Dusenbury, L. (1993). Smoking behavior of adolescents exposed to cigarette advertising. *Public Health Reports, 108*, 217–224.

Botvin, G. J., Renick, N. L., & Baker, E. (1983). The effects of scheduling format and booster sessions on a broad-spectrum psychosocial approach to smoking prevention. *Journal of Behavioral Medicine, 6*, 359–379.

Caplan, M., Weissberg, R. P., Grober, J. S., Sivo, P., Grady, K., & Jacoby, C. (1992). Social competence promotion with inner-city and suburban young adolescents: Effects on social adjustment and alcohol use. *Journal of Consulting and Clinical Psychology, 60*, 56–63.

Centers for Disease Control. (1996). Projected smoking-related deaths among youth—United States. *Morbidity and Mortality Weekly Reports, 45*, 971–974.

Chassin, L. A., Presson, C. C., & Sherman, S. J. (1984). Cigarette smoking and adolescent psychosocial development. *Basic and Applied Social Psychology, 99*, 722–742.

Chassin, L. A., Presson, C. C., Sherman, S. J., Corty, E., & Olshavsky, R. W. (1984). Predicting the onset of cigarette smoking in adolescents: A longitudinal study. *Journal of Applied Social Psychology, 14*, 224–243.

Chassin, L. A., Presson, C. C., Sherman, S. J., & Edwards, D. (1990). The natural history of cigarette smoking: Predicting young-adult outcomes from adolescent smoking patterns. *Health Psychology, 9*, 701–716.

Chassin, L. A., Presson, C. C., Sherman, S. J., Montello, D., & McGrew, J. (1986). Changes in peer and parent influence during adolescence: Longitudinal versus cross-sectional perspectives on smoking initiation. *Developmental Psychology, 22*, 327–334.

Collins, L. M., Sussman, S., Rauch, J. M., Dent, C. W., Johnson, C. A., Hansen, W. B., & Flay, B. R. (1987). Psychosocial predictors of young adolescent cigarettte smoking: A sixteen-month three-wave longitudinal study. *Journal of Applied Social Psychology, 17*, 554–573.

Conrad, K. M., Flay, B. R., & Hill, D. (1992). Why children start smoking cigarettes: Predictors of onset. *British Journal of Addiction, 87*(12), 1711–1724.

Dryfoos, J. G. (1993). Common components of successful interventions with high-risk youth. In N. J. Bell & R. W. Bell (Eds.), *Adolescent risk taking* (pp. 131–147). Newbury Park, CA: Sage.

Dusenbury, L., Epstein, J. A., Botvin, G. J., & Diaz, T. (1994). The relationship between language spoken and smoking among Hispanic-Latino youth in New York City. *Public Health Reports, 109,* 421–427.

Dusenbury, L., Kerner, J. F., Baker, E., Botvin, G. J., James-Ortiz, S., & Zauber, A. (1992). Predictors of smoking prevalence among New York Latino youth. *American Journal of Public Health, 82,* 55–58.

Elder, J. P., Molgaard, C. A., & Gresham, L. (1988). Predictors of chewing tobacco and cigarette use in a multiethnic public school population. *Adolescence, 23,* 689–702.

Ellickson, P. L., & Hays, R. D. (1990). Beliefs about resistance self-efficacy and drug prevalence: Do they really affect drug use? *International Journal of the Addictions, 25,* 1353–1378.

Ershler, J., Leventhal, H., Fleming, R., & Glynn, K. (1989). The quitting experience for smokers in sixth through twelfth grades. *Addictive Behaviors, 14,* 365–378.

Evans, R. I. (1976). Smoking in children: Developing a social psychological strategy of deterrence. *Preventive Medicine, 5,* 122–127.

Evans, R. I., Rozelle, R. M., Mittlemark, M. B., Hansen, W. B., Bane, A. L., & Havis, J. (1978). Deterring the onset of smoking in children: Knowledge of immediate physiological effects and coping with peer pressure, media pressure, and parent modeling. *Journal of Applied Social Psychology, 8,* 126–135.

Fishbein, M. (1977). Consumer beliefs and behavior with respect to cigarette smoking: A critical analysis of the public literature. In *Federal Trade Commission Report to Congress pursuant to the Public Health Cigarette Smoking Act of 1976* (pp. 1–113). Washington, DC: U.S. Government Printing Office.

Fisher, D. A., Armstrong, B. K., & deKler, N. H. (1983, August). *A randomized-controlled trial of education for prevention of smoking in 12-year-old children.* Paper presented at the Fifth World Conference on Smoking and Health, Winnipeg, Canada.

Flay, B. R., Keopke, D., Thomson, S. J., Santi, S., Best, J. A., & Brown, K. S. (1989). Long-term follow-up of the first Waterloo smoking prevention trial. *American Journal of Public Health, 79,* 1371–1376.

Flynn, B. S., Worden, J. K., Secker-Walker, S., Badger, G. J., Geller, B. M., & Costanza, M. C. (1992). Prevention of cigarette smoking through mass media intervention and school programs. *American Journal of Public Health, 82,* 827–834.

Gerber, R. W., & Newman, I. M. (1989). Predicting future smoking of adolescent experimental smokers. *Journal of Youth and Adolescence, 18,* 191–201.

Gilchrist, L. D., & Schinke, S. P. (1983). Self-control skills for smoking prevention. In P. F. Engstrom & P. Anderson (Eds.), *Advances in cancer control* (pp. 125–130). New York: Alan R. Liss.

Glynn, T. J., Anderson, D. M., & Schwarz, L. (1991). Tobacco-use reduction among high-risk youth: Recommendations of a National Cancer Institute Expert Advisory panel. *Preventive Medicine, 20,* 279–291.

Goodstadt, M. S. (1978). Alcohol and drug education: Models and outcomes. *Health Education Monographs, 6,* 263–279.

Hansen, W. B., Collins, L. M., Johnson, C. A., & Graham, J. W. (1985). Self-inititated smoking cessation among high school students. *Addictive Behaviors, 10,* 265–271.

Hawkins, J. D., Catalano, R. F., & Miller, J. Y. (1992). Risk and protective factors for alcohol and other drug problems in adolescence and early adulthood: Implications for substance abuse prevention. *Psychological Bulletin, 112,* 64–105.

Hunter, S. M., Vizelberg, I. A., & Berenson, G. S. (1991). Identifying mechanisms of adoption of tobacco and alcohol use among youth: the Bogalusa heart study. *Social Networks, 13,* 91–104.

Hurd, P., Johnson, C. A., Pechacek, T. F., Bast, C. P., Jacobs, D., & Luepker, R. V. (1980). Prevention of cigarette smoking in 7th grade students. *Journal of Behavioral Medicine, 3,* 15–28.

Jessor, R., & Jessor, S. L. (1977). *Problem behavior and psychosocial development: A longitiudinal study of youth*. New York: Academic Press.

Johnston, L. D., O'Malley, P. M., & Bachman, J. G. (in press). *National survey results on drug use from the Monitoring the Future Study, 1975–1996, Vol. I. Secondary school students*. Washington, DC: U.S. Department of Health and Human Services.

Kann, L., Warren, C. W., Harris, W. A., Collins, J. L., Williams, B. I., Ross, J. G., Kilbe, L. J., State & Local YRBSS coordinators (1996). Youth risk behavior surveillance—United States, 1995. In CDC Surveillance Summaries, September 27, 1996. *Morbidity and Mortality Weekly Reports, 45*(SS-4), 1–26.

Lawrance, L., & Rubinson, L. (1986). Self-efficacy as a predictor of smoking behavior in young adolescents. *Addictive Behaviors, 11*, 367–382.

Luepker, R. V., Johnson, C. A., Murray, D. M., & Pechacek, T. F. (1983). Prevention of cigarette smoking: Three year follow-up of educational programs for youth. *Journal of Behavioral Medicine, 6*, 53–61.

McAlister, A. L., Perry, C., & Maccoby, N. (1979). Adolescent smoking: Onset and prevention. *Pediatrics, 63*, 650–658.

McGuire, W. J. (1964). Inducing resistance to persuasion: Some contemporary approaches. In L. Berkowitz (Ed.), *Advances in experimental social psychology* (pp. 192–227). New York: Academic Press.

McGuire, W. J. (1968). The nature of attitudes and attitude change. In G. Lindzey & E. Aronson (Eds.), *Handbook of social psychology* (pp. 136–314). Reading, MA: Addison-Wesley.

Mittlemark, M. B., Murray, D. M., Luepker, R. V., Pechacek, T. F., Pirie, P. L., & Pallonen, U. E. (1987). Predicting experimentation with cigarettes: The Childhood Antecedents of Smoking Study (CASS). *American Journal of Public Health, 77*, 206–208.

Moss, A. J., Allen, K. F., Giovino, G. A. & Mills, S. L. (1992). *Recent trends in adolescent smoking, smoking-uptake correlates, and expectations about the future. Advance Data.* No. 221. Atlanta, GA: U.S. Department of Health and Human Services, Public Health Service, Centers for Disease Control and Prevention, National Center for Health Statistics.

Murray, D. M., Davis-Hearn, M., Goldman, A. I., Pirie, P. L., & Luepker, R. V. (1988). Four and five year follow-up results from four seventh-grade smoking prevention strategies. *Journal of Behavioral Medicine, 11*, 395–405.

Mussen, P., Conger, J., & Kagan, J. (1974). *Child development and personality* (4th ed.). New York: Harper & Row.

O'Connell, D. L., Alexander, H. M., Dobson, A. J., Lloyd, D. M., Hardes, G. R., Springthorpe, H. J., & Leeder, S. R. (1981). Cigarette smoking and drug use in schoolchildren: II. Factors associated with smoking. *International Journal of Epidemiology, 10*, 223–231.

Ogawa, H., Tominaga, S., Gellert, G., & Aoki, K. (1988). Smoking among junior high school students in Nagoya, Japan. *International Journal of Epidemiology, 17*, 814–820.

Pentz, M. A. (1983). Prevention of adolescent substance abuse through social skill development. In T. J. Glynn, C. G. Leukefeld, & J. B. Ludford (Eds.), *Preventing adolescent drug abuse: Intervention strategies* (NIDA Research Monograph No. 47, pp. 195–232). Washington, DC: U.S. Government Printing Office.

Pentz, M. A., Dwyer, J. H., MacKinnon, D. P., Flay, B. R., Hansen, W. B., Wang, E. Y., & Johnson, C. A. (1989). A multicommunity trial for primary prevention of adolescent drug abuse. Effects on drug prevalence. *Journal of American Medical Association, 261*, 3259–3266.

Perry, C. L., Killen, J., Slinkard, L. A., & McAlister, A. L. (1983). Peer teaching and smoking prevention among junior high students. *Adolescence, 9*, 277–281.

Perry, C. L., & Kelder, S. H. (1992). Models for effective prevention. *Journal of Adolescent Health, 13*, 355–363.

Perry, C. L., Kelder, S. H., Murray, D. M., & Klepp, K. I. (1992). Community-wide smoking prevention: Long-term outcomes of the Minnesota heart health program and the class of 1989 study. *American Journal of Public Health, 82*(9), 1210–1216.

Resnicow, K., & Botvin, G. J. (1993). School-based substance use prevention programs: Why do effects decay? *Preventive Medicine, 22*(4), 484–490.

Rohrbach, L. A., Hodgson, C. S., Broder, B. I., & Montgomery, S. B. (1994). Parental participation in drug abuse prevention: Results from the Midwestern Prevention Project [Special issue: Preventing alcohol abuse among adolescents: Preintervention and intervention research]. *Journal of Research on Adolescence, 4,* 295–317.

Sarason, I. G., Mankowski, E. S., Peterson, A. V., Jr., & Dinh, K. T. (1992). Adolescents' reasons for smoking. *Journal of School Health, 62,* 185–190.

Schinke, S. P., & Gilchrist, L. D. (1983). Primary prevention of tobacco smoking. *Journal of School Health, 53,* 416–419.

Seffrin, J. R., & Bailey, W. J. (1985). Approaches to adolescent smoking cessation and education. *Special Services in the Schools, 1,* 25–38.

Shean, R. E. (1991). *Peers, parents and the next cigarette: smoking acquisition in adolescence.* Unpublished dissertation, University of Western Australia, Nedlands.

Stacy, A. W., Sussman, S., Dent, C. W., Burton, D., & Flay, B. R. (1992). Moderators of peer social influence in adolescent smoking. *Personality and Social Psychology Bulletin, 18,* 163–172.

Sussman, S., Dent, C. W., Stacy, A. W., & Sun, P. (1993). Project Towards No Tobacco Use: 1-Year behavior outcomes. *American Journal of Public Health, 83,* 1245–1250.

Swan, A. V., Creeser, R., & Murray, M. (1990). When and why children first start to smoke. *International Journal of Epidemiology, 19,* 323–330.

Telch, M. J., Killen, J. D., McAlister, A. L., Perry, C. L., & Maccoby, N. (1982). Long-term follow-up of a pilot project on smoking prevention with adolescents. *Journal of Behavioral Medicine, 5,* 1–8.

Thompson, E. L. (1978). Smoking education programs 1960–1976. *American Journal of Public Health, 68,* 250–257.

Tuakli, N., Smith, M. A., & Heaton, C. (1990). Smoking in adolescence: Methods for health education and smoking cessation. *Journal of Family Practice, 31,* 369–374.

Tye, J., Warner, K., & Glantz, S. (1987). Tobacco advertising and consumption: Evidence of a causal relationship. *Journal of Public Health Policy,* 492–507.

U.S. Department of Health and Human Services. (1989). *Reducing the health consequences of smoking: 25 Years of progress: A report of the Surgeon General* (DHHS Publication No. (CDC) 89-8411). Atlanta, GA: Public Health Service, Centers for Disease Control.

U.S. Department of Health and Human Services. (1994). *Youth and tobacco: Preventing tobacco use among young people.* Atlanta, GA: Public Health Service, Centers for Disease Control, U.S. Department of Education.

Whelan, E. M. (1984). *A smoking gun: How the tobacco industry gets away with murder.* Philadelphia, PA: George F. Stickley.

Young, M., & Werch, C. E. (1990). Relationship between self-esteem and substance use among students in fourth through twelfth grade. *Wellness Perspectives: Research, Theory and Practice, 7,* 31–44.

CHAPTER FOUR

Issues for Women Who Wish to Stop Smoking

Cynthia S. Pomerleau
University of Michigan Department of Psychiatry

American women were slower than men to adopt cigarette smoking and never reached the smoking rates achieved by men in the 1940s and 1950s, when up to 70% of the male population smoked. By 1965, smoking prevalence among women had reached 34%; probably at least in part as a result of the publication of the 1964 Surgeon General's Report documenting the health hazards of smoking (U.S. Public Health Service, 1964), followed by increasingly stringent societal measures designed to discourage smoking, the percentage of women smokers leveled off rather than continuing to rise. Starting in 1978, smoking prevalence in women began declining to its current rate of 23%—still slightly lower than the prevalence in men, although the two have nearly converged.

Although women have been, to some extent, the beneficiaries of changes in public policy that came too late to protect men, there is meager cause for celebration. Early hopes that women might be spared the ravages of tobacco-related illness that men have suffered have long since been dispelled. In 1986, lung cancer surpassed breast cancer as the leading cause of cancer death in women, a change that is almost completely attributable to increases in smoking among women. Smoking is also a major contributor to other cancers, chronic obstructive pulmonary disease (COPD), cardiovascular disease, and—especially in oral contraceptive users over 35—stroke (Pomerleau, Berman, Gritz, Marks, & Goeters, 1994).

Moreover, despite the apparent steady decline in smoking among women over the past two decades, some ominous signs have recently appeared on the horizon—most notably the alarming rates of initiation among younger women. Clearly there is no cause for complacency, or for assuming that the downward trend is irreversible.

A controversial notion that persists in the literature is that women have a harder time than men quitting and staying quit. Much ink has been spilled on both sides of this issue (Husten, Chrismon, & Reddy, 1996), and perhaps the most important observation is that the dismal quit rates in both sexes swamp minor differences between men and women. Nonetheless, although a number of studies have shown no differences, in those studies that do show differences, it is generally the women who fare worse, experiencing more difficulty in quitting, especially in the initial quit period, and being slightly more prone to relapse.

Whether poor outcomes for women result from a lack of sensitivity to the special needs and problems women face when they attempt to quit is not known. Although the idea that targeted interventions will enhance quit rates is seductive, there is little empirical evidence to support this proposition. On the other hand, the lack of evidence may be more indicative of a failure to develop *successful* targeted interventions than of a lack of validity of the concept of targeting per se. Even in the absence of definitive answers to all these questions, however, it seems likely that attention to issues of special relevance to women—that is, attempting to address as well as identify the problems—will be helpful to therapists in maximizing successful quitting in their women patients. The remainder of this chapter is devoted to an examination of gender differences in smoking that might suggest ways in which the needs of women smokers wishing to stop smoking may be met more effectively.

SMOKING CESSATION ACROSS THE LIFE CYCLE

Because women's lives are more punctuated, sociobiologically speaking, than are men's—by menarche and menopause, by the monthly cycle of ovulation and bleeding, by pregnancy and childbirth, and by the accompanying assaults of these life changes on body image—looking at women as a block may blur differences in women's smoking cessation needs across the life cycle. The special needs of women at different life stages will require much more attention if we are to be maximally helpful to women smokers. Nevertheless, sufficient research has been done in a few aspects of the female life cycle to offer at least some guidance to the clinician.

Helping Adolescent Girls Stop Smoking

Discussions of adolescents and smoking tend to focus on ways of preventing smoking initiation, a topic covered in chapter 5 of this volume. The average age of smoking initiation for girls has declined to around 12 or 13 years

(Pomerleau, Berman, Gritz, Marks, & Goeters, 1994), however, so prevention efforts may already be too late for many girls even by junior high school. By the time they are high school seniors, 28% report having smoked within the past month (Elders, Perry, Eriksen, & Giovino, 1994), a prevalence that has remained stable for several years (Johnston, O'Malley, & Bachman, 1994).

Teenagers are even less susceptible than their elders to scare messages about the long-delayed and dicey consequences of smoking (O. F. Pomerleau, 1981). In a 1991 survey, 3 out of 10 high school seniors did not believe that heavy smoking poses a serious health risk (U.S. Department of Health and Human Services, 1994). For girls in this age group, therefore, emphasis on current symptoms and immediate consequences may be particularly relevant. In addition to adverse effects that do not discriminate between the sexes (e.g., more colds, coughing spells, and sore throats; shortness of breath; Epps, Manley, Grande, & Lynch, 1996), a consequence specific to women—dysmenorrhea, which has been reported in both adolescents and adult women (Brown, Vessey, & Stratton, 1988; Jensen & Coambs, 1994; Procopé & Timonen, 1971; Sloss & Frerichs, 1983)—may help to discourage smoking.

Adolescent girls are particularly concerned with body image and also highly susceptible to advertising efforts intended to link smoking with thinness. A substantial minority engage in abnormal eating and dieting practices (Abraham, Mira, Beumont, Sowerbutts, & Llewellyn-Jones, 1983). There is also considerable evidence of smoking initiation as a weight-control strategy in adolescent women (Charlton, 1984). Therefore, much of the material on weight concerns (see Weight Gain and Strategies for Weight Control) has particular relevance to young women. Reminders that smoking causes bad breath, discolored teeth, smelly clothes, and so on may help to deflect concerns with body image from the weight issue.

In view of recent evidence of nicotine dependence in a substantial percentage of adolescent smokers (U.S. Department of Health and Human Services, 1994), the possibility that nicotine replacement strategies effective in adult women (see Women With High Levels of Nicotine Dependence) might also be helpful in girls should probably be explored. Young women who smoke in excess of a pack per day, who smoke shortly after waking up, or who have been unable to quit because of withdrawal symptomatology should be considered as potentially eligible for this approach.

Menstrual Cycle Phase and Smoking Cessation

Although the idea that smoking may vary across the menstrual cycle in response to hormonal fluctuations has a certain intuitive appeal, there is little evidence to support this presumption, except in women with premenstrual dysphoric disorder (PDD; Marks, Hair, Klock, Ginsburg, & Pomerleau, 1994) and perhaps other forms of depression. Smoking abstinence, however, appears to unmask the effects of menstrual cycle on nicotine addiction, and the mild increase in discomfort occurring during the premenstruum even in women without PDD is magnified by nicotine withdrawal—an effect that has been demonstrated in both laboratory and clinical settings (O'Hara, Portser, & Anderson, 1989; Pomerleau, Garcia, Pomerleau, & Cameron, 1992). Although these findings are complicated by a considerable overlap between menstrual and nicotine abstinence symptomatology, there is also evidence that craving for a cigarette increases during abstinence in the premenstrual phase (Pomerleau et al., 1992), suggesting that this phenomenon is not simply the result of the generalized dysphoria (anxiety, depression, etc.) common to both menstrual and smoking withdrawal symptomatology.

This discomfort may translate into increased difficulty in quitting. In one study, women smokers tested in the premenstrual phase were significantly less successful than either women smokers at tested at mid cycle or men smokers in abstaining from smoking for 2 days (Craig, Parrott, & Coomber, 1992). In another study, however, women were found to be at higher risk of lapsing during the menses, regardless of phase of quit date (Frye, Ward, Bliss, & Garvey, 1992). All these studies tend to the recommendation that if possible, women should time quit attempts so that the first few difficult days do not coincide with the perimenstrual phase; it may increase likelihood of success, and it will almost certainly reduce discomfort during the period of peak withdrawal symptomatology. If it is not convenient or possible to control the quit date—for example, in a group treatment setting—particular attention to coping with withdrawal symptomatology is probably warranted. Women who plan to use nicotine polacrilex should probably be encouraged to use the 4 mg strength, since 2 mg gum has been shown to be relatively ineffective in relieving withdrawal symptomatology in women (Hatsukami, Skoog, Allen, & Bliss, 1995; see Women With High Levels of Nicotine Dependence).

A footnote: Little is known about the applicability of data on menstrual cycle to oral contraceptive users. Smoking potentiates the risk of cardiovascular disease, cerebrovascular disease, and other conditions in oral contraceptive users (Pomerleau, Berman, Gritz, Marks, & Goeters, 1994), yet nearly one quarter of oral contraceptive users are smokers (Barrett et al., 1994). There is therefore a serious need to address smoking in this population.

Smoking Cessation Approaches for Pregnant Women

About 20–25% of pregnant American women continue to smoke throughout pregnancy (Benowitz, 1991). Although scare tactics are not generally effective, pregnant women need to know that smoking is the largest modifiable risk factor for poor pregnancy outcomes in the United States (Novello, 1990), including spontaneous abortion (Kline, Stein, Susser, & Warburton, 1977), low birth weight (Kramer, 1987), neurobehavioral deficits in the offspring

(Butler & Goldstein, 1973), Sudden Infant Death Syndrome (SIDS; Haglund & Cnattingius, 1990), and numerous other prenatal and perinatal complications. For women who have not wished to quit or who have previously been unable to quit, pregnancy may constitute a "teachable moment," when concern about the harmful effects of smoking on the fetus becomes immediate and real (Ockene, 1993), and weight and body image issues are reframed if not submerged.

Nicotine binding sites increase rapidly in human fetal brain between 12 and 19 weeks (Cairns & Wonnacott, 1988). Moreover, fetal growth restriction can be largely prevented by cessation of nicotine use by 16–18 weeks of gestation (Butler & Goldstein, 1973). These and other data argue strongly for vigorous intervention efforts early in pregnancy (Oncken, 1996). If nausea and vomiting during the first trimester provoke spontaneous quitting, as sometimes occurs (Gritz, Nielsen, & Brooks, 1996), the opportunity to capitalize on this situation by providing reinforcement for sustained abstinence should not be missed.

The question of nicotine replacement during pregnancy is a thorny one. Unfortunately, not only can it *not* be said that nicotine replacement is safe during pregnancy, it cannot even be said definitively that nicotine replacement is safer than smoking. Although the fetus is spared the effects of CO and other toxic constituents of tobacco, a woman smoker may get more nicotine via medication than she does via smoking (especially if she smokes while using nicotine replacement), and the fetus may be exposed more chronically to nicotine when administered by gum or especially patch than by smoking. The Food and Drug Administration has approved the use of gum only if "risks cannot be ruled out" (Category C) and warned that the patch is associated with "positive evidence of risk" (Category D). Although these products are deemed acceptable if "the benefits outweigh the risks," there is little evidence from human studies on which to base a decision as to either the benefits or the risks relative to smoking. Certainly, at the present moment it must be considered only as an aid in quitting in properly motivated pregnant women, not as a safer substitute for smoking in pregnant women who will not or cannot stop smoking. Conservative practice dictates starting with a nonpharmacologic approach—although the desirability of cessation early in pregnancy must also be weighed. If behavioral methods fail, the benefits of nicotine replacement probably outweigh the risks of continued smoking, at least in women who smoke 20 or more cigarettes per day (Benowitz, 1991). Nicotine gum is probably preferable to the patch, since dosing is less sustained, ceases at night, and generally results in lower nicotine levels than achieved with the patch (Benowitz, 1991).

Although, as noted earlier, the deferral of weight and body image concerns necessitated by pregnancy may facilitate quitting at this time, a caveat must be added: Weight and nutritional status are affected by both smoking cessation and pregnancy and therefore need to be addressed concurrently. Current guidelines for acceptable weight gain during pregnancy favor a 25- to 30-pound gain in normal-weight women (a few pounds less in overweight women and a few pounds more in underweight women). Because many women are accustomed to using smoking as a weight management strategy, care must be taken to avoid placing the need to control weight in competition with the need to quit smoking, which in virtually all instances must be regarded as the higher priority. Even in women who are not inclined to use smoking as a weight management tool, however, the potential enhancement of weight gain caused by quitting and the possibility of increased intake of sweet foods cannot be neglected altogether, because they may render delivery more difficult, increase risk of postpartum relapse, and in some instances predispose to gestational diabetes. For these and other reasons, it is important to coordinate delivery of prenatal care with smoking cessation counseling.

Although the spontaneous quit rate during pregnancy exceeds that in the general population of women (U.S. Department of Health and Human Services, 1988), a tragic sequel (for both mother and infant) is that postpartum relapse rates are extremely high, exceeding 50% at 3 months and 70% after a year (Ockene, 1993). Therefore, strong attention to relapse prevention is critical in women who succeed in quitting during pregnancy (Mullen, Quinn, & Ershoff, 1990). The stress of caring for an infant, the desire to recover prepregnancy slimness, the reinstatement of prepregnancy cues for smoking (e.g., resumption of alcohol and/or caffeine use if discontinued during pregnancy)—all these should be regarded as potential relapse triggers and their possible impact rehearsed with the woman who wishes to remain a lifelong nonsmoker. Reminders about the dangers of passive smoke exposure in children and increased likelihood of smoking in the children of smoking adults (Epps et al., 1996) may be especially poignant to the woman who has recently given birth.

Quitting in Menopausal and Postmenopausal Women

The probable impact of smoking on menopause has been well documented, with most studies showing an earlier age of menopause in women who smoke, an effect that is dose related (see Midgette & Baron, 1990). It is also possible that smoking aggravates the "symptoms" of menopause (Greenberg, Thompson, & Meade, 1987). The impact of menopause on smoking, by contrast, has received little attention, and the potential special needs of menopausal and postmenopausal women have been largely untouched. It has been suggested that women may find it especially difficult to quit during the perimenopausal years because of the endocrine changes they are experiencing, which may be associated with mood swings, weight gain, and changes in affect, and which are often accompanied by changes or dislocations in social role (Gritz et al., 1996). Statistics showing a drop in the odds ratio for quitting in women in this age group relative to men (Jarvis, 1994) tend to support this speculation. Although there is currently little in the literature to guide treatment of women in this life stage, we may hope that the increasing salience of their needs (as baby-boom women reach the age of menopause) will spur research in this area.

WEIGHT GAIN AND STRATEGIES FOR WEIGHT CONTROL

The Importance of Weight Concerns

Unfortunately, the increasingly negative image of smoking has not competed successfully with an apparent secular trend toward increasing societal pressures for a degree of thinness attainable only by a small percentage of women, a percentage that will dwindle further as the population ages over the coming years. Reluctance to contemplate weight gain following cessation, although well documented as a barrier to quitting or even considering quitting (Klesges & Klesges, 1988; Klesges et al., 1988), is a problem whose importance and intransigence have, if anything, been underestimated. This opinion was recently echoed in an editorial in the *New England Journal of Medicine* by Joseph Califano, Secretary of Health, Education, and Welfare in the late 1970s: "I am often asked whether I would have done anything differently. Yes—I would have focused far more attention on the relation between smoking and weight and the importance American women attach to being thin. . . . Even though I gained 30 pounds in 1975 after [quitting], I did not appreciate the great importance to women of the link between quitting smoking and gaining weight" (Califano, 1995, p. 1215).

The therapeutic community remains at a serious disadvantage on this issue because it is trying to discourage the use of a product that actually does suppress weight when used as directed by the manufacturer. There is evidence to indicate that many women are deterred from quitting by fear of weight gain, and that some adolescents start smoking to avoid weight gain (Charlton, 1984; Klesges & Klesges, 1988; Klesges et al., 1988). Depending on the measure used, 25–40% of all women smokers strongly endorse "weight control" as a reason for smoking (Pomerleau et al., 1993), compared with only a handful of men. Although sociocultural factors undoubtedly contribute to this phenomenon, there is also considerable evidence that women gain more than men following cessation, that they tend to be the "supergainers" (13 kg or more; Williamson et al., 1991), and that gender differences in eating persist for several months following cessation (Hall, McGee, Tunstall, Duffy, & Benowitz, 1989). When women smokers were asked how much weight they would be willing to gain if they stopped smoking, a full three-quarters expressed unwillingness to gain more than 5 pounds; the modal value—40%—was zero (Pomerleau & Kurth, 1996).

Dealing with this "reality gap" is perhaps the most formidable challenge facing the intervention community today. Although advertising for smokers who want to quit without gaining weight brings a large response (Pirie et al., 1992), even sophisticated programs combining smoking cessation therapy with behavioral weight control techniques have not been successful (Hall, Tunstall, Vila, & Duffy, 1992; Pirie et al., 1992). Although exercise is helpful in controlling weight (Marcus, Albrecht, Niaura, Abrams, & Thompson, 1991; Rodin, 1987; Talcott et al., 1995), motivating anyone to exercise, let alone people who engage in a habit that compromises respiratory function, is a difficult task. Pharmacological interventions may be helpful for women who have serious postcessation eating problems (Pomerleau, Berman, Gritz, Marks, & Goeters, 1994) but do answer the needs of nonobese women who simply are not willing to gain 10 pounds. Advocates of cognitive restructuring to promote acceptance of modest increases in weight (Grunberg, Winders, & Wewers, 1991; Perkins, 1994) seriously underestimate the intensity of the aversion to weight gain harbored by many if not most women. A recent suggestion that women diet off a few pounds *before* they attempt to stop smoking cessation (French & Jeffery, 1995) also seems ill advised, because smoking and the reinforcing value of nicotine may actually increase when eating is restricted (see Perkins, 1994).

What, then, can be done? Despite the lack of proven techniques, the following measures can be recommended:

1. History of weight gain during previous quit attempts should be queried; it may provide guidance in developing a strategy for controlling postcessation weight gain.

2. The probabilistic nature of postcessation weight gain should be explained. The average amount of postcessation weight gain is just that—an average. A better approach is to describe it as being distributed along a continuum: (a) Approximately 20–30% of women will gain less than 5 pounds, with few maintaining or losing weight (Nides et al., 1994; Pirie et al., 1992). They are the lucky ones. For these women, nothing further need be done, unless there is reason to believe that depression or severe dieting are involved. (b) Around half will gain 5–15 pounds, an amount that can be addressed by dietary changes (e.g., reducing fat intake and snacking) and exercise (which may become more enjoyable once lung function is no longer compromised by smoking). Some women may also find themselves more able to accept the fact than the prospect of weight gain, as suggested by the paradox that weight gain during cessation predicts continued subsequent abstinence (Gritz, Berman, Read, Marcus, & Siau, 1990; Hall,

Ginsberg, & Jones, 1986; Norregaard, Tonnesen, & Petersen, 1993). (c) Approximately 25% of women will gain more than 15 pounds (Nides et al., 1994), with approximately half of these women gaining more than 30 pounds (Williamson et al., 1991). For these women, metabolic changes alone are unlikely to account for the weight gain; these women were probably using smoking to control a tendency to overeat (Pomerleau et al., 1993) and may need an intensive intervention.

After around 6 months, weight gain will have stabilized for most women (Nides et al., 1994; Pirie et al., 1992), assuming nicotine replacement has terminated. Thus, if possible, women should be encouraged to put their weight concerns on hold temporarily, and in the interim to concentrate on quitting smoking. After a few months, a much better assessment of their weight-gain problems and therapeutic needs can be made. On the other hand, it is important to avoid misrepresenting the likelihood of weight gain, as the smoking cessation community did for years when it promulgated the notion that only about a third of ex-smokers gain weight. As indicated earlier, almost all smokers gain at least some weight upon quitting, and 70% to 80% will reach the 5-pound cutoff that defines the upper limit of what the majority of women state they would be willing to tolerate. One hopeful note: Although obese women are even less willing to gain weight than normal-weight women, they are also at lower risk of postcessation weight gain (Williamson et al., 1991)—a fact that may be helpful in persuading them to adopt the wait-and-see approach.

3. Because most relapse occurs early (Hunt, Barnett, & Branch, 1971), and because weight gain has been shown to be associated with early relapse (Borrelli, Mermelstein, & Shadel, 1995; Swan, Ward, Carmelli, & Jack, 1993), deferring the moment at which women reach the 5-pound limit for acceptable weight gain until cessation is well established may also be helpful. Strategies for minimizing early weight gain include beginning quit attempts immediately following the offset of menses, so that the critical first few days of abstinence aren't compounded by perimenstrual bloating and weight gain—a fact that may account for increased relapse at this time. Use of pharmacological aids known to attentuate postcessation weight gain, such as nicotine replacement products (e.g., Gross, Stitzer, & Maldonado, 1989) and sustained release buproprion (Hurt, Sachs, Glover, Offord, Johnston, Dale, et al., 1998), may also be effective. (Unfortunately, sustained release buproprion is contraindicated in individuals with current or past eating disorders.)

4. Exercise should be encouraged if the prospective quitter is receptive.

5. Trivializing the weight-gain issue will not be well received. It is important for health professionals to treat the desire for thinness respectfully and to avoid using such phrases as "unwanted cosmetic effects" (Williamson et al., 1991) to describe a deep-seated cultural and psychological aversion on the part of women (Batten, 1993). And messages like "You'd have to

gain 100 pounds to equal the dangers of smoking" probably contain the seeds of their own defeat because the overt content seems at odds with the graphically objectionable image they evoke. A more promising strategy would be to contextualize rather than deprecate the desire for thinness. Body image consists of a whole constellation of factors; body shape is an important component, but it is not the only one. Looking youthful, looking healthy, looking womanly and feminine, being athletic and capable may also be involved; having a nice voice, nice skin, nice teeth/nice smile, nice breath, and flattering clothes are important to many women. They may also perceive these things as being important to their partners or prospective partners. Cigarette smoking is detrimental to all but one of these. The tobacco industry and its advertisers hold only one ace, but they have played it so effectively that they have essentially reduced the body image question to one of weight and thinness. Not only have they tapped into the prevailing cultural preference for thinness, they may have contributed to it as well. They have understood what Califano articulated in the editorial quoted earlier—that the weight control issue speaks differently to men and women: For men, 6 or 8 pounds is a shrug of the shoulders; for women, it's a dress size. Attempts to divert attention to other categories of reasons for not smoking, such as concerns about health or the effects of passive smoking, may successfully appeal to some women but are not likely to make the problem go away. Smoking cessation professionals are more likely to make headway if they can reframe the body image question so that it encompasses the negative as well as the "positive" effects of smoking on body image.

Racial Differences in Weight Concerns

Black women appear to be more willing than White women to tolerate postcessation weight gain (Pomerleau & Kurth, 1996). Because White women tend to be slimmer than Black women (and indeed, than women in most other racial or ethnic groups; Kumanyika, Wilson, & Guilford-Davenport, 1993), it is likely that cultural factors (e.g., a weaker cultural preference for thinness) may be protective. On the other hand, Black women are more likely to gain weight in dangerous amounts upon smoking cessation (Williamson et al., 1991), so it may be necessary to monitor weight gain and intervene if weight gain becomes uncontrolled.

Weight Concerns in Eating-Disordered Individuals

Smoking, interestingly, is not strongly associated with anorexia nervosa (Bulik et al., 1992)—which is, however, a relatively rare disorder. By contrast, bulimia and binge-eating, and subclinical manifestations of these conditions, are widely distributed in the general population and have been shown to be overrepresented in smokers (Pomerleau & Krahn, 1993).

Although these disorders are sometimes regarded as phenomena of youth, research in adult women smokers suggests that they frequently persist into adulthood. For example, when the Dieting and Bingeing Severity Scale (DBSS; Krahn, Kurth, Demitrack, & Drewnowski, 1992), a questionnaire designed to assess eating behavior in college students and validated using the SCID (Kurth, Krahn, Nairn, & Drewnowski, 1995), was administered to a sample of 184 moderately dependent adult female smokers, only 10.2% of the adult women smokers were found to be not dieting at all; 31.2% were classified as casual dieters, and 28.0% as intense dieters. Another 17.2% fell into the severe dieting category, 11.3% were at-risk dieters, and 2.2% gave responses consistent with a clinical diagnosis of bulimia nervosa—almost as many as seen in a comparable sample of college women (unpublished data). Women in the higher DBSS categories were significantly more likely to qualify as weight-control smokers and to give retrospective reports of weight gain, increased eating, and binge eating during previous periods of abstinence from smoking than were women in the lower DBSS categories. They were willing to tolerate significantly less weight gain on quitting. Further confirmation is provided by Hall and colleagues (1986), who found that high scores on measures of disinhibited eating are predictive of postcessation eating and weight gain among abstinent smokers, making it likely that such women will include an excess of "supergainers."

These findings suggest that the DBSS or some comparable instrument may be a potentially useful tool for identifying women smokers likely to experience problems with postcessation eating and weight gain and in triaging patients to appropriately tailored interventions. Unfortunately, data to provide guidance on treatment strategies are scanty, because many early trials of pharmacological agents as potential adjuncts to smoking cessation were conducted in unselected samples, with cofactors inadequately assessed or present in inadequate numbers—possibly even leading to their premature dismissal as possible aids in smoking cessation in targeted populations. Nonetheless, it may be worthwhile to consider cognitive behavioral therapy or administration of appropriate medications in patients judged to be at high risk for postcessation bulimia or binge eating and concomitant high weight gain or harmful compensatory behaviors such as purging (Pomerleau, Berman, Gritz, Marks, & Goeters, 1994).

COFACTORS FOR SMOKING IN WOMEN

The relationship between smoking and a variety of comorbid conditions is discussed in chapter 2 and is not reviewed in detail here. It is worth observing, however, that two of these conditions, depression and anxiety, are major women's public health problems in their own right. A third important category of cofactors overrepresented in women, eating disorders, was discussed earlier in the context of weight concerns. If women with these cofactors use nicotine to manage affective states (Lerman et al., 1996), the underlying problem may reemerge or be exacerbated when they try to stop smoking, and instead of being transient may persist and become increasingly troublesome (Covey, Glassman, & Stetner, 1990, 1997; Dalack, Glassman, Rivelli, Covey, & Stetner, 1995; Glassman, 1993). Alternatively, the would-be quitter may become so uncomfortable or discouraged that she returns to smoking. The emergence of postcessation depression constitutes a particularly poor prognosis for quitting (Hughes, 1992; Anda et al., 1990). Thus, any treatment plan for such individuals should take the comorbid condition into account; in more severely affected individuals, it may be helpful to treat the cofactor concomitantly or sequentially.

WOMEN SMOKERS WITH HIGH LEVELS OF NICOTINE DEPENDENCE

A smoker who smokes more than 20 cigarettes a day, who smokes within 30 minutes of awakening, and who experiences severe withdrawal symptomatology on abstinence from smoking is likely to be highly dependent upon nicotine. The prevalence of nicotine dependence among female tobacco smokers, using criteria published in the *Diagnostic and Statistical Manual of Mental Disorders*, 3rd edition, revised (*DSM–III–R*; APA, 1987), has been estimated at 30.9%, compared with 32.7% among their male counterparts (Anthony, Warner, & Kessler, 1994), suggesting that the likelihood of becoming highly dependent, once one has become a smoker, does not differ materially between men and women. Another recent epidemiological study, however, indicates that a higher percentage of women than men endorse a number of signs of dependence, including feeling dependent, inability to cut down, and smoking within 30 min of awakening (Husten et al., 1996). Although figures are likely to vary considerably depending on what measure of dependence is used, it seems reasonable to conclude that women smokers are at least as likely as men to become highly dependent, and moreover that the treatment needs of the highly dependent female smoker may differ from those of the highly dependent male smoker.

1. Pharmacological interventions may be differentially effective in women and men. The most widely used pharmacological intervention, and until recently the only approved pharmacological intervention, is some form of nicotine replacement. At least two studies have indicated that the 2 mg dose of nicotine gum is less effective in suppressing withdrawal symptomatology in women than in men (Hatsukami et al., 1995; Killen, Fortmann, Newman,

& Varady, 1990). In one of these studies, women showed more severe withdrawal symptomatology from nicotine gum regardless of dose (Hatsukami et al., 1995). In a large study of predictors of quitting and relapse, 69% of the women who smoked at all in the first 4 months after their quit day had relapsed to smoking by 12 months, compared with 59% of the men (Bjornson et al., 1995), suggesting that even apparently minor lapses in women should be taken very seriously. Prolonged gum use was a predictor of late relapse (probably indicating that gum use simply postponed relapse). Taken together, these data suggest that women may benefit from higher doses of gum than men, may need to be tapered more slowly, and in some instances may even require long-term maintenance. By contrast, there have been no reports to date of gender differences in withdrawal with transdermal nicotine.

Nonnicotine pharmacological aids in cessation, including various antidepressants and antianxiety medications, have also been tested with varying degrees of success. A promising recent development is the FDA approval of sustained release buproprion as an aid in smoking cessation (Hurt et al., 1998). Originally marketed as an antidepressant, it has been demonstrated to be effective for smoking cessation and also, as noted above, to attenuate postcessation weight gain.

2. Withdrawal symptomatology may be more likely to interfere with cessation in women than in men. Although a number of retrospective studies have reported that women experience more or more severe withdrawal symptomatology than men (see Shiffman, 1979), prospective studies have consistently shown little evidence of gender differences (Hughes, 1992; Hughes, Gust, Skoog, Keenan, & Fenwick, 1991; Hughes & Hatsukami, 1986; Svikis, Hatsukami, Hughes, Carroll, & Pickens, 1986; Tate, Pomerleau, & Pomerleau, 1993). A possible explanation for this discrepancy is offered by a study comparing prospective and retrospective reports in the same subjects, in which women recalled withdrawal symptomatology during past quit attempts not only more vividly but also apparently more accurately than did men (Pomerleau, Tate, Lumley, & Pomerleau, 1994). Thus, recollections of past discomfort may undermine their confidence in their ability to remain abstinent (the "abstinence phobia"; Hall, 1979). Moreover, at least one study has shown withdrawal distress to be predictive of treatment outcome in women but not in men (Gunn, 1986). These studies suggest that withdrawal symptomatology is more salient for women than for men, and that behavioral or pharmacological methods to relieve withdrawal are especially relevant for women trying to quit. The clinician should be especially alert for the possible emergence of postcessation depression—a symptom, as noted earlier, that constitutes a particularly poor prognosis for quitting—in light of evidence, albeit retrospective, that depression is more likely to emerge in women than in men (Husten et al., 1996; Pomerleau & Pomerleau, 1994).

CONCLUSIONS

Helping women quit will continue to be challenging to clinicians. The weight issue is one of the major unresolved problems facing the intervention community today. Depression, another serious barrier to quitting and staying quit, is much more prevalent in women than in men. Because women in general have a greater tendency toward "negative-affect" smoking (Sorenson & Pechacek, 1987) and to be more responsive than men to the mood-altering effects of smoking (Bjornson et al., 1995; Gritz et al., 1996), treatment of dependence per se is likely to be complicated by the greater likelihood that women are "self-medicating" and will consequently find withdrawal symptomatology more difficult to cope with.

But helping women quit will also be rewarding. Women are more willing than men to participate in assisted quitting programs (Fiore et al., 1990; Owen & Davies, 1990) and can therefore be expected to respond positively to efforts on their behalf. Success will not only confer substantial health benefits on women themselves, but will also be magnified in succeeding generations. Although women and men smokers are probably more alike than different in the kinds of help they need to quit smoking, there are many areas in which attention to the special needs of women may reduce the likelihood of treatment failure. For this reason, it important to persist in our search for better ways of helping women to quit smoking.*

ACKNOWLEDGMENTS

Preparation of the manuscript was supported by National Heart, Lung, and Blood Institute grant HL52981 to Cynthia S. Pomerleau and NCI grant CA42730 to Ovide F. Pomerleau.

REFERENCES

Abraham, S. F., Mira, M., Beumont, P. J. V., Sowerbutts, T. D., & Llewellyn-Jones, D. (1983). Eating behaviours among young women. *Medical Journal of Australia, 2,* 225–228.

American Psychiatric Association. (1987). *Diagnostic and statistical manual of mental disorders* (3rd ed., rev.). Washington, DC: Author.

Anda, R. F., Williamson, D. F., Escobedo, L. G., Mast, E. E., Giovino, G. A., & Remington, P. L. (1990). Depression and the dynamics of smoking: A national perspective. *JAMA, 264,* 1541–1545.

**Editor's Note:* For recent developments in the use of buproprion related to weight gain and pregnancy issues, see chapter 8, p. 167.

Anthony, J. C., Warner, L. A., & Kessler, R. C. (1994). Comparative epidemiology of dependence on tobacco, alcohol, controlled substances, and inhalants: Basic findings from the National Comorbidity Survey. *Experimental and Clinical Psychopharmacology, 2*, 244–268.

Barrett, D. H., Anda, R. F., Escobedo, L. G., Croft, J. B., Williamson, D. F., & Marks, J. S. (1994). Trends in oral contraceptive use and cigarette smoking. *Archives of Family Medicine, 3*, 438–443.

Batten, L. (1993). Respecting sameness and difference: Taking account of gender in research on smoking. *Tobacco Control, 2*, 185–186.

Benowitz, N. L. (1991). Nicotine replacement therapy during pregnancy. *JAMA, 22*, 3174–3177.

Bjornson, W., Rand, C., Connett, J. E., Lindgren, P., Nides, M., Pope, F., Buist, A. S., Hoppe-Ryan, C., & O'Hara, P. (1995). Gender differences in smoking cessation after 3 years in the Lung Health Study. *American Journal of Public Health, 82*, 223–230.

Borrelli, B., Mermelstein, R. J., & Shadel, W. G. (1995). The role of weight concern and self-efficacy in smoking cessation and weight gain. *Annals of Behavioral Medicine, 17*, S096.

Brown, S., Vessey, M., & Stratton I. (1988). The influence of method of contraception and cigarette smoking on menstrual patterns. *British Journal of Obstetrics and Gynaecology, 95*, 905–910.

Bulik, C. M., Sullivan, P. F., Epstein, L. H., McKee, M., Kaye, W. H., Dahl, R. E., & Weltzin, T. E. (1992). Drug use in women with anorexia and bulimia nervosa. *International Journal of Eating Disorders, 3*, 213–225.

Butler, N. R., & Goldstein, H. (1973). Smoking in pregnancy and subsequent child development. *British Medical Journal, 4*, 573–575.

Cairns, N. J., & Wonnacott, S. (1988). [^{3}H] (-)nicotine binding sites in fetal human brain. *Brain Research, 475*, 1–7.

Califano, J. A. (1995). The wrong way to stay slim. *New England Journal of Medicine, 333*, 1214–1216.

Charlton, A. (1984). Smoking and weight control in teenagers. *Public Health, 98*, 277–281.

Covey, L. S., Glassman, A. H., & Stetner, F. (1990). Depression and depressive symptoms in smoking cessation. *Comprehensive Psychiatry, 31*, 350–354.

Covey, L. S., Glassman, A. H., & Stetner, M. A. (1997). Major depression following smoking cessation. *American Journal of Psychiatry, 154*, 263–265.

Craig, D., Parrott, A., & Coomber, J. (1992). Smoking cessation in women: Effects of the menstrual cycle. *International Journal of Addiction, 27*, 697–706.

Dalack, G. W., Glassman, A. H., Rivelli, S. K., Covey, L. S., & Stetner, F. (1995). Mood, major depression and fluoxetine response in cigarette smokers. *American Journal of Psychiatry, 152*, 398–403.

Elders, M. J., Perry, C. L., Eriksen, M. P., & Giovino, G. A. (1994). The report of the Surgeon General: Preventing tobacco use among young people. *American Journal of Public Health, 84*, 543–547.

Epps, R. P., Manley, M. W., Grande, D., & Lynch, B. S. (1996). How clinicians can affect patient smoking behavior through community involvement and clinical practice. *JAMWA, 51*, 43–47.

Fiore, M. C., Novotny, T. E., Pierce, J. P., Giovino, G. A., Hatziandreu, E. J., Newcomb, P. A., Surawicz, T. S., & Davis, R. M. (1990). Methods used to quit smoking in the United States. *JAMA, 263*, 2760–2765.

French, S. A., & Jeffery, R. W. (1995). Weight concerns and smoking: A literature review. *Annals of Behavioral Medicine, 17*, 234–244.

Frye, C. A., Ward, K. D., Bliss, R. E., & Garvey, A. J. (1992). Influence of the menstrual cycle on smoking relapse and withdrawal symptoms [abstract]. *Proceedings of the 13th Annual Scientific Sessions of the Society of Behavioral Medicine*, 107.

Glassman, A. H. (1993). Cigarette smoking: Implications for psychiatric illness. *American Journal of Psychiatry, 150*, 546–553.

Greenberg, G., Thompson, S. G., & Meade, T. W. (1987). Relation between cigarette smoking and use of hormonal replacement therapy for menopausal symptoms. *Journal of Epidemiology and Community Health, 41,* 26–29.

Gritz, E. R., Berman, B. A., Read, L. L., Marcus, A. C., & Siau, J. (1990). Weight change among registered nurses in a self-help smoking cessation program. *American Journal of Health Promotion, 5,* 115–121.

Gritz, E. R., Nielsen, I. R., & Brooks, L. A. (1996). Smoking cessation and gender: The influence of physiological, psychological, and behavioral factors. *JAMWA, 51,* 35–42.

Gross, J., Stitzer, M. L., & Maldonado, J. (1989). Nicotine replacement: Effects on postcessation weight gain. *Journal of Consulting Clinical Psychology, 57,* 87–92.

Grunberg, N. E., Winders, S. E., & Wewers, M. E. (1991). Gender differences in tobacco use. *Health Psychology, 10,* 43–53.

Gunn, R. C. (1986). Reactions to withdrawal symptoms and success in smoking cessation clinics. *Addictive Behaviors, 11,* 49–53.

Haglund, B., & Cnattingius, S. (1990). Cigarette smoking as a risk factor for sudden infant death syndrome: A population-based study. *American Journal of Public Health, 80,* 29–32.

Hall, S. M. (1979). The abstinence phobia. In N. Krasnegor (Ed.), *Behavioral treatment and analyses of substance abuse* (NIDA Research Monograph Series No. 25, pp. 55–67). Washington, DC: Department of Health, Education, and Welfare.

Hall, S. M., Ginsberg, D., & Jones, R. T. (1986). Smoking cessation and weight gain. *Journal of Consulting Clinical Psychology, 54,* 342–346.

Hall, S. M., McGee, R., Tunstall, C. D., Duffy, J., & Benowitz, N. (1989). Changes in food intake and activity after quitting smoking. *Journal of Consulting Clinical Psychology, 57,* 81–86.

Hall, S. M., Tunstall, C. D., Vila, K. L., & Duffy, J. (1992). Weight gain prevention and smoking cessation: Cautionary findings. *American Journal of Public Health, 82,* 799–803.

Hatsukami, D., Skoog, K., Allen, S., & Bliss, R. (1995). Gender and the effects of different doses of nicotine gum on tobacco withdrawal symptoms. *Experiments in Clinical Psychopharmacology, 3,* 163–173.

Hughes, J. R. (1992). Tobacco withdrawal in self-quitters. *Journal of Consulting Clinical Psychology, 60,* 689–697.

Hughes, J. R., Gust, S. W., Skoog, K., Keenan, R. M., & Fenwick, J. W. (1991). Symptoms of tobacco withdrawal. *Archives of General Psychiatry, 48,* 52–59.

Hughes, J. R., & Hatsukami, D. (1986). Signs and symptoms of tobacco withdrawal. *Archives of General Psychiatry, 43,* 289–294.

Hunt, W. A., Barnett, L. W., & Branch, L. G. (1971). Relapse rates in addiction programs. *Journal of Clinical Psychology, 27,* 455–456.

Hurt, R. D., Sachs, D. P. L., Glover, E. D., Offord, K. P., Johnston, J. A., Dale, L. C., Khayrallah, M. A., Schroeder, D. R., Glover, P. N., Sullivan, C. R., Croghan, I. T., & Sullivan, P. M. (1998). Sustained-release buproprion and placebo for smoking cessation. *N Engl J Med, 337,* 1195–1202.

Husten, C. G., Chrismon, J. H., & Reddy, M. N. (1996). Trends and effects of cigarette smoking among girls and women in the United States, 1965–1993. *JAMWA, 51,* 11–18.

Jarvis, M. J. (1994). Gender differences in smoking cessation: Real or myth? *Tobacco Control, 3,* 324–328.

Jensen, P. M., & Coambs, R. B. (1994). Cigarette smoking and adolescent menstrual disorders. *Canadian Woman Studies, 14*(3), 57–60.

Johnston, L. D., O'Malley, P. M., & Bachman, J. G. (1994). *National survey results on drug use from Monitoring the Future Study, 1992–1995: Vol. 1, Secondary school students.* Bethesda, MD: U.S. Department of Health and Human Services, Public Health Service, National Institutes of Health, National Institute on Drug Abuse.

Killen, J. D., Fortmann, S. P., Newman, B., & Varady, A. (1990). Evaluation of a treatment approach combining nicotine gum with self-guided behavioral treatments for smoking relapse prevention. *Journal of Consulting Clinical Psychology, 58*(1), 85–92.

Klesges, R. C., & Klesges, L. M. (1988). Cigarette smoking as a dieting strategy in a university population. *International Journal of Eating Disorders, 7*, 413–419.

Klesges, R. C., Somes, G., Pascale, R. W., Klesges, J. M., Murphy, M., Brown, K. S., & Williams, E. (1988). Knowledge and beliefs regarding the consequences of cigarette smoking and their relationships to smoking status in a biracial sample. *Health Psychology, 7*, 387–401.

Kline, J., Stein, Z. A., Susser, M., & Warburton, D. M. (1977). Smoking as a risk factor for spontaneous abortion. *New England Journal of Medicine, 297*, 793–796.

Krahn, D. D., Kurth, C. L., Demitrack, M., & Drewnowski, A. (1992). The relationship of dieting severity and bulimic behaviors to alcohol and other drug use in young women. *Journal of Substance Abuse, 4*, 341–353.

Kramer, M. S. (1987). Determinants of low birth weight: Methodological assessment and metaanalysis. *Bulletin of the World Health Organization, 6*, 663–737.

Kumanyika, S., Wilson, J. F., & Guilford-Davenport, M. (1993). Weight-related attitudes and behaviors of black women. *Journal of the American Dietetic Association, 93*(4), 416–422.

Kurth, C. L., Krahn, D. D., Nairn, K., & Drewnowski, A. (1995). The severity of dieting and bingeing behaviors in college women: Interview validation of survey data. *Journal of Psychiatric Research, 29*, 211–225.

Lerman, C., Audrain, J., Orleans, C. T., Boyd, R., Gold, K., Main, D., & Caporaso, N. (1996). Investigation of mechanisms linking depressed mood to nicotine dependence. *Addictive Behaviors, 21*, 9–19.

Marcus, B. H., Albrecht, A. E., Niaura, R. S., Abrams, D. B., & Thompson, P. D. (1991). Usefulness of physical exercise for maintaining smoking cessation in women. *American Journal of Cardiology, 68*, 406–407.

Marks, J. L., Hair, C. S., Klock, S. C., Ginsburg, B. E., & Pomerleau, C. S. (1994). Effects of menstrual phase on intake of nicotine, caffeine, and alcohol and nonprescribed drugs in women with Late Luteal Phase Dysphoric Disorder. *Journal of Substance Abuse, 6*, 235–244.

Midgette, A. S., & Baron, J. A. (1990). Cigarette smoking and the risk of natural menopause. *Epidemiology, 1*, 474–480.

Mullen, P. D., Quinn, V., & Ershoff, D. (1990). Maintenance of nonsmoking postpartum by women who stopped smoking during pregnancy. *American Journal of Public Health, 80*, 992–994.

Nides, M., Rand, C., Dolce, J., Murray, R., O'Hara, P., Voelker, H., & Connett, J. E. (1994). Weight gain as a function of smoking cessation and 2-mg nicotine gum use among middle-aged smokers with mild lung impairment in the first 2 years of the Lung Health Study. *Health Psychology, 13*, 354–361.

Norregaard, J., Tonnesen, P., & Petersen, L. (1993). Predictors and reasons for relapse in smoking cessation with nicotine and placebo patches. *Preventive Medicine, 22*, 261–271.

Novello, A. C. (1990). Surgeon General's report on the health benefits of smoking cessation. *Public Health Reports, 105*, 545–548.

Ockene, J. K. (1993). Smoking among women across the life span: Prevalence, interventions, and implications for cessation research. *Annals of Behavioral Medicine, 15*, 135–148.

O'Hara, P., Portser, S. A., & Anderson, B. P. (1989). The influence of menstrual cycle changes on the tobacco withdrawal syndrome in women. *Addictive Behaviors, 14*, 595–600.

Oncken, C. A. (1996). Nicotine replacement therapy during pregnancy. *American Journal of Health Behavior, 30*, 300–303.

Owen, N., & Davies, M. J. (1990). Smokers' preferences for assistance with cessation. *Preventive Medicine, 29*, 424–431.

Perkins, K. A. (1994). Issues in the prevention of weight gain after smoking cessation. *Annals of Behavioral Medicine, 16,* 46–52.

Pirie, P. L., McBride, C. M., Hellerstedt, W., Jeffery, R. W., Hatsukami, D., Allen, S., & Lando, H. A. (1992). Smoking cessation in women concerned about weight. *American Journal of Public Health, 82,* 1238–1243.

Pomerleau, C. S., Berman, B. A., Gritz, E. R., Marks, J. L., & Goeters, S. (1994). Why women smoke. In R. R. Watson (Ed.), *Drug and alcohol abuse reviews: Vol. 5. Addictive behaviors in women* (pp. 39–70). Totowa, NJ: Humana Press.

Pomerleau, C. S., Ehrlich, E., Tate, J. C., Marks, J. L., Flessland, K. A., & Pomerleau, O. F. (1993). The female weight-control smoker: A profile. *Journal of Substance Abuse, 5,* 391–400.

Pomerleau, C. S., Garcia, A. W., Pomerleau, O. F., & Cameron, O. G. (1992). The effects of menstrual phase and nicotine abstinence on nicotine intake and on biochemical and subjective measures in women smokers: A preliminary report. *Psychoneuroendocrinology, 17,* 627–638.

Pomerleau, C. S., & Krahn, D. D. (1993). Smoking and eating disorders: A connection? *Journal of Addictive Disorders, 12,* 169.

Pomerleau, C. S., & Kurth, C. L. (1996). Willingness of female smokers to tolerate postcessation weight gain. *Journal of Substance Abuse, 8,* 371–378.

Pomerleau, C. S., & Pomerleau, O. F. (1994). Gender differences in frequency of smoking withdrawal symptoms. *Annals of Behavioral Medicine, 16,* S118.

Pomerleau, C. S., Tate, J. C., Lumley, M. A., & Pomerleau, O. F. (1994). Gender differences in prospectively vs. retrospectively assessed smoking withdrawal symptoms. *Journal of Substance Abuse, 6,* 433–440.

Pomerleau, O. F. (1981). Underlying mechanisms in substance abuse: Examples from research on smoking. *Addictive Behaviors, 6,* 187–196.

Procopé, B. J., & Timonen, S. (1971). The premenstrual syndrome in relation to sport, gymnastics and smoking [abstract]. *Acta Obstetricia et Gynecologica Scandinavica, 50,* 77.

Rodin, J. (1987). Weight changes following smoking cessation: The role of food intake and exercise. *Addictive Behaviors, 12,* 303–317.

Shiffman, S. M. (1979). The tobacco withdrawal syndrome. In *Cigarette smoking as a dependence process* (NIDA Research Monograph Series No. 23, pp. 158–184). Washington, DC: Department of Health, Education, and Welfare.

Sloss, E. M., & Frerichs, R. R. (1983). Smoking and menstrual disorders. *International Journal of Epidemiology, 12*(1), 107–109.

Sorenson, G., & Pechacek, T. F. (1987). Attitudes toward smoking cessation among men and women. *Journal of Behavioral Medicine, 10,* 129–137.

Svikis, D. S., Hatsukami, D. K., Hughes, J. R., Carroll, K. M., & Pickens, R. W. (1986). Brief report: Sex differences in tobacco withdrawal syndrome. *Addictive Behaviors, 11,* 459–462.

Swan, G. E., Ward, M. M., Carmelli, D., & Jack, L. M. (1993). Differential rates of relapse in subgroups of male and female smokers. *Journal of Clinical Epidemiology, 46,* 1041–1053.

Talcott, G. W., Fiedler, E. R., Peterson, A. L., Pascale, R. W., Klesges, R. C., & Johnson, R. S. (1994). Is weight gain after smoking cessation inevitable? *Journal of Consulting Clinical Psychology, 63,* 313–316.

Tate, J. C., Pomerleau, O. F., & Pomerleau, C. S. (1993). Temporal stability and within-subject consistency of nicotine withdrawal symptoms. *Journal of Substance Abuse, 5,* 355–363.

U.S. Department of Health and Human Services. (1988). *The health consequences of smoking: Nicotine addiction. A report of the Surgeon General* (DHHS Publication No. [CDC] 88-8406). Rockville, MD: United States Department of Health and Human Services, Public Health Service, Office on Smoking and Health.

U.S. Department of Health and Human Services. (1994). *Preventing tobacco use among young people: A report of the Surgeon General.* Atlanta, GA: U.S. Department of Health and Human Services. Public Health Service, Centers for Disease Control and Prevention, National Center for Chronic Disease Prevention and Health Promotion, Office on Smoking and Health.

U.S. Public Health Service. (1964). *Smoking and health. Report of the advisory committee to the Surgeon General of the Public Health Service* (PHS Publication No. 1103). Atlanta, GA: U.S. Department of Health, Education, and Welfare, Public Health Service, Center for Disease Control.

Williamson, D. F., Madans, J., Anda, R. F., Kleinman, J. C., Giovino, G. A., & Byers, T. (1991). Smoking cessation and severity of weight gain in a national cohort. *New England Journal of Medicine, 324*, 739–745.

CHAPTER FIVE

Implementation of a Prenatal Smoking Cessation Program in Three Inner-City Communities

Michelle Drayton-Martin
Today's Child Communications, Inc.

Frances Trakis Manners
Consultant

Naomi Rock Novak
Community Outreach—St. Michael's Medical Center

Jill Shamban
Shamban Consulting

Healthy Start/NYC, a 5-year demonstration project initiated in 1991, seeks to reduce infant mortality by 50% in three inner-city health districts: Bedford, Central Harlem, and Mott Haven. The project is funded by the federal Health Resources and Services Administration (HRSA), Maternal and Child Health Bureau. Project principals include the Medical and Health Research Association of New York City (MHRA, the grantee), the New York City Department of Health, the Bronx Perinatal Consortium, the Brooklyn Perinatal Network, and the Northern Manhattan Perinatal Partnership.

The project uses a multidisciplinary, community-based, and comprehensive approach to address the multiple correlates of infant mortality. It has enlisted community support, by involving leaders, civic groups, churches, schools, service providers, and residents in the development of interventions that are locally perceived to be most likely to succeed in getting vital services to pregnant and parenting women and their families.

Nationwide, about 36,000 infants die annually in their first year. Low birth weight (infants born weighing under 5½ pounds) is a powerful predictor of infant mortality. In the United States, smoking is one of the most important, and preventable, determinants of low birth weight. Over the past three decades, numerous published reports have confirmed that cigarette smoking during pregnancy is dangerous to the health of the fetus and newborn infant, and adversely affects child development (Fingerhut & Kleinman, 1990). As examples of these findings, an Alameda County, California, low-birth-weight study group reported that quitting smoking during the first 3 months of pregnancy was associated with a lower relative risk for all categories of low birth weight in Whites and for two of three categories in Blacks (Alameda County Low-Birth-Weight Study Group, 1990). Further, the risk of having a low-birth-weight infant increases twofold among women who smoke (Floyd, Rimer, Giovino, Mullen, & Sullivan, 1993).

The 1990 U.S. Surgeon General's Report (U.S. Department of Health and Human Services, 1990) stated that smoking during pregnancy is associated with premature birth, increased respiratory problems among infants and young children, and sudden infant death syndrome (SIDS). Maternal smoking also increases the risk of abruptio placentae, placenta previa, and bleeding early or late in pregnancy, all of which increase the risk for perinatal loss (Missouri Department of Health, 1989).

Finally, an Institute of Medicine study (1985) strongly urges that efforts to help women stop or reduce smoking during pregnancy become a major concern of obstetric providers. Reviewing smoking cessation programs, the committee found that one-on-one sessions with a counselor or a physician are among the most effective prenatal smoking cessation strategies. They also found that although group counseling appears to be less effective, social support seems to be critical to reducing or eliminating pregnant women's smoking.

AN OVERVIEW

Given the enormous toll cigarette smoking is taking on pregnancy outcomes and child health, prenatal and postpartum smoking cessation is a critical priority. Unfortunately, few institutionalized smoking cessation initiatives exist within prenatal care programs.

In October 1994, with a grant from Project ASSIST, a New York State Department of Health tobacco control initiative funded by the National Cancer Institute, Healthy Start/NYC created a prenatal smoking cessation program (PSCP) targeted primarily at providers working in inner-city communities and serving diverse populations. The project seeks to help prenatal care providers implement smoking cessation programs in their facilities.

The Healthy Start/NYC PSCP's theoretical and clinical approach is based on several well-accepted, standard models. The first two are the Prochaska and DiClemente (1992) transtheoretical model for change, which addresses a smoker's level of readiness to quit, and Miller and Rollnick's motivational interviewing techniques (Miller & Rolnick, 1991). Additionally, the National Cancer Institute's Four As model guides our counseling and role play (Glynn

& Manley, 1990). Our approach is also consistent with the Agency for Health Care Policy and Research's Clinical Practice Guideline No. 18, Smoking Cessation (see Additional Resources).

The goal of our PSCP has been to train health care providers who work with pregnant and parenting smokers and/or nonsmokers who live with a smoker. We seek to (a) educate providers about the harmful effects of smoking during pregnancy and of secondhand smoke on the mother, baby, and family; (b) offer knowledge, resources, and techniques to help providers help clients reduce or eliminate smoking; and (c) help providers establish and/or sustain a PSCP, by training their staffs to train their colleagues and by integrating a PSCP into their prenatal care services.

To date, over 450 providers from Healthy Start/NYC's service areas have been trained, for a total of 41 facilities (22 prenatal care and 19 other health-related facilities). Twenty-one facilities (14 prenatal care and 7 other agencies) have implemented PSCPs or have enhanced existing ones. Moreover, the project has sponsored numerous information tables and demonstrations at community events such as health fairs.

Before describing our PSCP, it is helpful to review the demographics of Healthy Start/NYC's Project Area as well as some of our program's successes.

DEMOGRAPHICS AND SUCCESSES

This densely populated project area (PA) contains some of the nation's deepest poverty. In 1990, U.S. Census data showed 478,211 people, over half in families earning 200% or less of the federal poverty level. Almost one-third received public aid; 29% were women of childbearing age, 10–44 years.

In 1990, there were 11,254 reported live births: 67% to African Americans, 27% to Latinas, 4% to non-Hispanic Whites, and 1% to Asians. Of babies born alive, 230 died, for an average infant mortality rate of 20.4 per thousand live births (compared to 11.6 citywide and 9.8 nationwide) (New York City Department of Health, Office of Vital Statistics, 1994). Thus, nearly 1 in 50 infants died, more than double the U.S. average. Infant mortality was highest among Blacks, and alarmingly high among Latinas. In parts of this area, there was a 1 in 25 chance of losing a child at birth or in its first year.

A comprehensive Healthy Start/NYC needs assessment found many causes. Infants in our PA mainly were dying because they were born too soon or too small, or because their mothers had had too little medical care too late, or none at all. In 1990, 16.9% of PA babies were premature and 14.2% had low birth weights (compared to 12.1 and 9.4%, respectively, citywide) (New York City Department of Health, Office of Vital Statistics, 1994). Nearly 1 in 4 pregnant women did not see a doctor until at least their sixth month or never saw one, although prenatal care can prevent about one fourth of infant deaths.

Babies also were dying due to mothers' poor health and nutrition, which contribute to low birth weight. Short-staffed, overburdened, fragmented, and insufficient health care facilities, with limited hours as well as lack of access to and awareness on the parents' part of the need for prenatal/newborn care, also contribute to poor pregnancy outcomes. Compounding factors include teen pregnancy, drug abuse, AIDS, smoking, high school drop-out and unemployment rates, language and cultural barriers, unavailable child care, and domestic and community violence.

Between Healthy Start/NYC's inception in 1991 and 1995 (the last year with available figures), there have been substantial improvements in PA community-wide indicators of maternal and child health. Thus, the infant mortality rate dropped 40% (compared to 24% citywide), from 20.4 to 12.3 per 1,000 live births; the rate of late or no prenatal care fell 44%, from 24 to 13% of live births; low birth weight went from 14 to 13% of live births; the period between births for a woman declined 49%, from 12.4 to 6.3%; and the proportion of infants born to women with reported prenatal illicit drug use dropped 33%, from 6.3 to 4.2%. Healthy Start/NYC also has increased the availability of critical health and social services, by helping initiate and/or support 60-plus programs that promote a comprehensive, community-based approach to preventing infant mortality and improving maternal and child health.

THE RATIONALE

In 1994, smoking among pregnant women in our project area was reported on only 13.2% of birth certificates. This is known to be gross underreporting. For example, the University of California, Los Angeles, Center for Health Policy Research (1991) estimates that one in five women smokes during pregnancy, with the highest rates among underserved and poor women, 28%, and among women with less than a high school education, 33%. The center also reports that White and African-American women have higher smoking rates, 25%, than do Latinas, 15%, or Asians, 8%. Meanwhile, a 1994 Healthy Start/NYC survey of 13 primary health care facilities showed that only one had a smoking cessation program; all 13 asked for help to establish such programs.

PROVIDER DEMOGRAPHICS AND FACILITIES

The providers we have trained are predominately African American, Caribbean American, and Latin American. All speak English; some also speak Spanish or French. Most are nonmedical staff: case managers, social workers, health educators. About 30% are physicians, midwives, or nurses. They work largely in community-based maternal and child health care clinics and hospitals that offer such health care services as prenatal, pediatric, and family planning. All sites have a high patient census.

TRAINING PROVIDERS

Training Objectives

The training objectives for a PSCP, at the very least, should increase participants':

- Knowledge of the health affects of smoking and secondhand smoke on adults, pregnant women, fetuses, infants, and children.
- Counseling skills, in order to help women of diverse ethnic backgrounds quit smoking and/or reduce exposure to secondhand smoke.
- Awareness of strategies and resources needed to integrate smoking cessation education into a health care setting. For example, participants will be able to conduct waiting room education, piggyback secondhand smoke information into parenting skills workshops, and offer smoking cessation tips at health fairs.
- Ability to plan, develop, implement, and sustain a smoking cessation program for pregnant women. We discuss each site's existing program, as well as any barriers and possible ways to overcome them. This is very useful, as facilities learn from one another.

Cultural Considerations

Although well-documented differences exist among U.S. racial and ethnic groups regarding smoking patterns and quitting prevalence (Centers for Disease Control, 1997), our Healthy Start/NYC PSCP coordinator has found from experience that nicotine addiction, the desire to quit, and the process of quitting and staying quit are virtually identical for all racial and ethnic groups. Our PSCP trainer relies heavily on the providers' judgments and experiences to tailor interventions to their clients' needs. The providers are sensitive to individual differences and health beliefs that may influence treatment acceptance and success. Still, the trainer must be familiar with provider and client resources that are culturally specific. (For a more detailed discussion, see the Agency for Health Care Policy Clinical Practice Guideline No. 18, Smoking Cessation, listed in Additional Resources.)

GETTING STARTED

Publicity

Once a facility has expressed interest in a PSCP training, it is essential to do outreach in order to inform, recruit, and register providers. It is best to begin with a planning meeting wherein the coordinator/trainer can assess a facility's level of perinatal smoking cessation practice and commitment. Beforehand, you should prepare a needs assessment form (keep it to one page) and have the facility contact person complete it. It should contain such key questions as: "Do you have pamphlets and/or posters on smoking and secondhand smoke during and after pregnancy in waiting areas and/or in offices?" "Do you assess a patient's tobacco level at intake?" "Do you have a way to indicate on a patient's chart that (s)he uses tobacco (e.g., a sticker or stamp)?"

The Training Format

We have found that the training period must be flexible to meet diverse facilities' and providers' needs. Although the complete training is designed to last 6 hr, not all providers are willing or able to devote that much time, either on one day or over several days. For example, medical providers often want a 1- or 2-hr overview on how to motivate clients to quit smoking, conducted as part of their in-service training. Although not ideal for intensive patient counseling, this short period at least familiarizes providers with the major issues, techniques, and motivational strategies. It thus also can serve as a catalyst for intrafacility referrals to staff who have completed PSCP training and can counsel smokers. However, to reiterate, providers who counsel smokers and are responsible for implementing other educational activities will need to complete the full 6-hr training.

Because providers appreciate training that is customized to their needs in terms of both content and time, we have offered, when expressed, additional training sessions on counseling smokers and about secondhand smoke. Providers who work with smokers more frequently and intensively, and who have completed the 6-hr training, welcome these more in-depth sessions. The lesson is to take into account the interests, needs, and time constraints of facilities and providers when planning trainings.

The Trainer

To be truly effective, the trainer, as both teacher and coach, must know the subject and have basic presentation skills and experience. It helps to take a course in teaching methods. For instance, a train-the-trainer workshop teaches about adult learning styles, how to present, creative teaching skills, how to best use audiovisual resources, and so on. It also is important to be enthusiastic, in order to encourage and motivate, and to be sensitive to and respectful of trainees' opinions and feelings. Trainers can learn a lot from and about providers and their clients by following these precepts.

The PSCP Handbook and Client Education Materials

Each trainee receives a Healthy Start/NYC Prenatal Smoking Cessation Training Handbook and client education handouts. The handbook contains nearly 200 pages of instructional materials, reference articles, work sheets, and case studies. It also has an overview of the curriculum; information on nicotine addiction, hazards of cigarette smoking and secondhand smoke; quitting and counseling techniques; guidelines for program development and implementation; and information on resources. To train medical providers, we use as the core curriculum the Agency for Health Care Policy and Research's Quick Reference Guide for Smoking Cessation (see Additional Resources). As these providers also receive the latest product information on the pharmacological treatment of nicotine dependence, it is essential that trainers be informed and up to date.

THE TRAINING CURRICULUM/HEALTHY START/NYC

Our basic PSC training requires 6 hr. The training is divided into three parts.

Part I

- The Healthy Start/NYC PSCP, including provider training and education, PSC resources, and technical help in program planning, development, implementation, and sustainability.
- Health care providers' roles in PSCPs. We emphasize that because providers already have so much to discuss with patients, there must be shared responsibility among them if a PSCP is to succeed. Obviously, the specifics of each provider role will vary with the facility. It is expected that medical providers (physicians, midwives, medical assistants, nurses) will screen a patient at each visit about use of and exposure to tobacco, and will record the reply as part of a risk assessment.

Additionally, medical providers should refer the client to a colleague trained in PSC counseling. But first, the provider must provide a brief, personalized, positive intervention message, spoken in a firm but supportive tone. This is important because many patients are motivated by their provider's advice. A sample message is: "Joan, it's important for your high blood pressure and for your baby that you quit smoking. If you quit, you will help control your high blood pressure. Moreover, the risk that smoking has on your baby's health, such as respiratory problems, could be reduced. How do you feel about quitting? Are you ready?" If Joan is not ready, the provider can say: "Our health educator can help you when you want to try to quit. I'd like you to see her before you leave the clinic today. She can give you the support you need. We are here to help you."

• Who smokes in America, and the politics of the tobacco cartel, which spends $6 billion annually, much of it to target women, youth, and communities of color (U.S. Food and Drug Administration).

• What's in a cigarette: Some of the 4000 identified chemicals are described, as well as why nicotine, carbon monoxide, and tar are the three most dangerous. The query "Why is nicotine the easiest of drugs to take up and the hardest to give up?" is answered by examining nicotine's physical and psychological addictive powers, and the behavioral triggers and rituals associated with smoking.

• Smoking hazards and the risks and benefits of quitting: All known physiological effects are described, as well as general and disease-specific benefits of not smoking. (For a recent and comprehensive discussion of the health consequences of smoking, please see *Cigarettes, What the Warning Label Doesn't Tell You* [Napier, 1996] in Additional Resources.)

• Environmental tobacco smoke or secondhand smoke—hazards and risks: Mostly unaware of secondhand smoke's effects, providers are fascinated by a 12-min video, *Poisoning Our Children: The Perils of Secondhand Smoke* (Pyramid Film and Video), and often want to borrow it to use in their waiting rooms or in asthma education workshops.

Part II

• Strategies for managing nicotine dependency: We emphasize that smoking cessation is a complex process with three phases: (a) getting ready—motivations for and barriers to quitting; (b) quitting—Prochaska and DiClemente's stages of change model, and pharmacologic, behavioral, and treatment options; and (c) staying quit—relapse prevention.

As it is critical that providers understand the complex challenges of smoking cessation, particularly for pregnant and parenting women, this section emphasizes that a successful PSCP requires the interplay of four factors: (a) initial advice and support from medical providers and referral to a PSC-trained counselor, (b) selection of motivated clients, (c) psychological and behavioral treatment (e.g., education, counseling), and (d) nicotine replacement therapy (NRT), if not medically contraindicated. (Because nicotine gum and nicotine patches are now available over the counter, trainers must have current knowledge about each product. We suggest that for each NRT product a trainer both checks prices at two or more pharmacies and calls the manufacturer to get free samples and information available to health care providers.)

• Policy and program considerations: Here we review in detail the Agency for Health Care Policy and Research's (AHCPR) Smoking Cessation: Clinical Practice Guideline in Smoking Cessation (see Additional Resources). This exhaustive and systematic analysis of the scientific literature contains recommendations to help clinicians, smoking cessation specialists, and health care administrators identify tobacco users, and support and deliver effective interventions. The guideline lists six recommendations:

Every smoker should be offered cessation treatment at every office visit.

Clinicians should ask and record each patient's tobacco-use status.

Cessation treatments, even as brief as 3 minutes a visit, are effective.

More intensive treatment is more likely to yield long-term abstinence.

Nicotine replacement therapy (patches or gum), clinician-delivered social support, and skills training are especially effective treatment components.

Health care systems should make institutional changes that result in systematic identification of, and intervention with, all tobacco users at every visit.

• Practice guidelines for PSCPs: In addition to the AHCPR guidelines, we have developed minimal and ideal recommendations to guide facilities. These include: (a) how to identify prenatal active and passive smokers (those who breathe in others' smoke), (b) which providers should make referrals, and (c) the importance of follow-up care, especially for pregnant smokers, as relapse rates are very high in this group. (For instance, providers have said that a phone call is an effective form of follow-up. As some clients do not have a phone, but have access to one, leave a message asking the client to call.)

• Effective approaches to implement prenatal smoking cessation programs: During training, each provider is asked whether his or her facility has a formal PSC policy and/or program, how it works, and about successes and barriers. A common response is that group interventions fail, mainly because clients do not attend them at a hospital or clinic if that is the only reason for their visit. Waiting room education, one-on-one counseling when a client returns for prenatal or well-baby care visits, and integrating smoking cessation education into a workshop (e.g., describing, during a parenting skills workshop, how and why smoke should be kept away from infants and children) are more effective.

In *For You and Your Family: A Guide to Perinatal Trainers and Providers* (see Additional Resources), the California Department of Health Tobacco

Control Section identified the characteristics of a successful PSCP (defined as percentage of clients who quit):

One-on-one sessions.

Reinforcing sessions (the more the better) and varying the type of client contact: phone, mail, waiting room education.

Program duration and consistency (the longer the woman is in a program, the more likely she is to quit).

Use of various communication strategies (counseling supported by written and audiovisual materials).

In addition, we have found that the most effective way to assure that clients attend smoking cessation counseling sessions is to pair them with prenatal visits.

• Documentation: This is a key means of identifying smokers and passive smokers and of assessing smokers' quitting readiness. During training, we discuss the importance of asking about whether a client is a passive smoker—because nearly all facilities do not ask this at intake. We also give them forms that ask clients about passive smoking exposure, to increase the likelihood that providers will address this issue.

• Teachable moments: There are specific times during pregnancy and the postpartum period that offer the best opportunities for an intervention message to occur. Examples are in the first trimester when morning sickness is a concern or, for a client concerned about weight gain, during nutritional counseling. Moreover, because women fail to attend smoking cessation group sessions, educators must devise creative ways to reach such clients. One way is to incorporate the topic of smoking and secondhand smoke into discussions of prenatal care, parenting, or asthma education workshops. Also, try to incorporate smoking cessation information and counseling into breastfeeding education, stress management workshops, and substance abuse recovery clinics.

Part III

• Key counseling points: (a) Assess how ready each women is to quit, and tailor counseling accordingly; (b) help the client develop a quitting plan; (c) problem-solve with the client regarding her barriers to quitting; and (d) offer support. We have found that women who lack support or live with a smoker often have the most difficulty quitting; lack of information about the dangers of secondhand smoke also is a barrier to quitting.

• An important suggestion offered by our participants is that PSC counseling will be most effective within the context of a client's overall realities and needs. Thus, it is critical to assess all major client-related issues, before deciding whether its is best for a client to quit or to decrease the amount of smoking at a given time. This is especially true for substance-abusing women.

• Main provider concerns: Can providers who smoke or never have smoked counsel effectively? Providers who smoke may be less effective because they feel uncomfortable, or because smoking clients may not view them as a credible source of help. Such providers may be more confident doing educational activities, as in waiting rooms or at health fairs. Providers who believe they cannot succeed or who resent counseling about quitting smoking should not do so. Providers who never have smoked may fear failure because they do not understand a smoker's needs. They need reassurance that one can help a client to make an important health change without having had the same experience. Another concern is prior failure. The answer is for the provider to set realistic goals and for clients to know that smoking cessation is a process. For example, a desirable outcome would be a woman's beginning to think about quitting or cutting back.

• The *Ten Commandments of Clinical Communication* (Bass, 1995): This is an effective tool, especially when teaching physicians how to talk with patients. Examples of two commandments are: *Thou shalt communicate thy faith in thy patient's capacities, verbally and nonverbally*, and *Thou shalt be positive and patient with thy patient.*

• Counseling and education techniques: Those we recommend include: (a) determining a client's understanding of how smoking can harm her and her baby—although most smokers know smoking is a risk factor associated with lung cancer and heart disease, it cannot be assumed that they know the specific risks of maternal smoking and/or secondhand smoke; (b) personalizing the intervention message to meet the client's needs; (c) helping the client develop positive behavioral skills; (d) creating a mutually acceptable plan; (e) documenting information; and (f) following up. The counselor must be optimistic, supportive, and focused.

• Delivering a brief, effective intervention message: This is crucial. An effective way is to use the National Cancer Institute's Four A's: Assess/Ask, Advise, Assist, and Arrange. Each A should be addressed at every counseling session. During the Assess/Ask phase, the counselor gathers information to help assess the client's exposure to secondhand smoke; obtains a smoking history, including past attempts to quit and current smoking status; and determines the client's readiness to quit. In the Advise phase, the provider delivers a health message tailored to information gleaned in step one. (For example, for the passive smoker, the message should be about the health risks of secondhand smoke and strategies for reducing exposure.) In the Assist phase, the provider and the client agree on an action plan. The Arrange phase involves follow-up: an agreement about when and how follow-up contact will be made or that the provider will make an appropriate referral.

• Role play: We highly recommend allowing ample time for this. To practice counseling and problem solving, trainees take turns playing patient and provider. Provider attitudes about this vary, from shyness to believing initially that they do not need it. However, most state in evaluations that role play was invaluable. (For role-play ideas and how-to's, see *For You and Your Family: A Guide for Perinatal Trainers and Providers* [California Department of Health Services, 1991] in Additional Resources.)

ADDRESSING CLIENTS' MISBELIEFS

One of the hardest parts of counseling is knowing how to respond to clients who are in the precontemplative or denial stage. A common client statement is: *Don't talk to me about quitting. I have three other, healthy children, and I smoked during those pregnancies.* A possible response is: "Our experience tells us that you have been lucky. By smoking during pregnancy, a woman takes a big chance with her baby's health; the more she smokes, the greater the chance of harm. All pregnancies are different; it's hard to predict which baby will be affected or how." Also, the client's children may have one or more health problems the mother has not related to smoking or to secondhand smoke. Ask about her children: Do any have many incidents of colds, wheezing, asthma, ear infections, bronchitis, or pneumonia? Be careful to educate, not reprimand.

Another common client misbelief about smoking during pregnancy is: *A smaller baby means an easier delivery.* A twofold response could be, "Smaller babies often are sicker babies," and "As smoking diminishes breathing capacity, it is harder for a pregnant woman to breathe during delivery." Still another common client reason for not quitting is, *Smoking is my only pleasure; it's too much to ask me to give up cigarettes.* The response can be, "It sounds as though this may be a difficult time to quit smoking entirely. What do you think about cutting down on the number of cigarettes?" (This also is a good time to introduce stress management techniques.) (For a detailed discussion of how to handle difficult client questions or responses, order *A Guide for Helping Women Who Smoke: A Focus on Pregnancy and the Child-Bearing Years*, from Project ASSIST; see Additional Resources.)

LOCATING GOOD RESOURCES

Locating, evaluating, and ordering effective PSC resources, particularly culturally sensitive ones, is an ongoing, challenging process. Our experience shows that PSC materials need to be culturally and linguistically appropriate;

at a fourth- to sixth-grade reading level; presented in a pleasant, graphic style; and inexpensive or free.

INCENTIVES FOR PROGRAM IMPLEMENTATION

Healthy Start/NYC's PSCP gives health care professionals free continuing education opportunities, such as follow-up trainings, as well as diverse client resources. The most effective and popular provider incentives are:

1. Client resources: nearly 100 hand-outs (culturally neutral or culturally specific) that providers can copy for client education use.
2. Smoking Susie Smokes For Two: Perhaps the most dramatic, attention-getting visual aid, this is a doll head perched atop a 10-inch-high glass jar filled with water and a real-looking rubber fetus. When a lighted cigarette is placed in the doll's mouth and the jar lid is lifted, the fetus's mouth blows out puffs of smoke. The device has dramatic impact in ob/gyn areas, at health fairs, and during workshops.
3. Videos: The Massachusetts and California Health Departments have developed television public service announcements on tobacco control. Timely, upbeat and powerful, funny or poignant, they speak to all age groups and are culturally sensitive. Health care facilities can get these free, on a video. Two other videos popular with providers and clients are: *Poisoning Our Children: The Perils of Secondhand Smoke* (12 min) and *Feminine Mistake: the Next Generation* (32 min).

Other important incentives are:

4. Quitting survival kits: If your budget allows you to purchase these, they can be a powerful client incentive. These can contain, for example, an infant t-shirt and bib, water bottle, baseball cap, quitting tips, and air freshener. (The American Cancer Society, NYC Division, Inc., volunteered to assemble the kits and send them to our training sites.) Please note that only clients in the preparation or action stage of change should receive such kits.

5 Postcards: Artistically designed, they are used for follow-up contacts, especially for clients who have no phone. (See Additional Resources.)

6. Tote bags: Cloth bags, printed with an antismoking slogan and a provider's logo, are popular with clients and providers. The latter use them as an incentive tool during the client's quitting process.

7. Posters: On clinic and provider office walls, these effectively draw attention to health issues. It is important to rotate them regularly, to prevent them from becoming too familiar and thus virtually invisible.

DEVELOPING SYSTEMS TO IMPLEMENT A PRENATAL SMOKING CESSATION PROGRAM

Healthy Start/NYC's PSCP has helped some facilities develop PSC counseling efforts and others to pay more attention to, and thus improve or enhance, existing PSC practices (identification, referring, counseling, follow-up, and documentation). Before a PSCP can be implemented, each facility's administration must establish policy and practice guidelines for smoking cessation or, at least, for prenatal smoking cessation.

Barriers

There are several barriers to PSCP implementation. The most common are:

Lack of Administrative Support. There are many reasons a facility may not fully support the implementation of a PSCP, including lack of knowledge about its importance. To overcome this and other barriers, it is helpful to identify the agency's gatekeeper(s) and schedule a planning meeting. The goal is to discuss potential problems, explain the endeavor's importance, and gain strong support from one or more of the facility's top administrators.

We suggest that the planning meeting begin with a discussion of the importance of PSC efforts (to the provider's overall goals and clients' health); describe the PSCP and your role; learn whether prior PSC efforts have been made and assess the facility's PSC needs; determine possible barriers to a successful program and suggest possible solutions; describe other sites' experiences, including problems, solutions, successes, and lessons learned; work with the administrator(s) to identify which staff member(s) should be trained and why; and establish a training schedule. *For You and Your Family: A Guide for Perinatal Trainers and Providers* (California Department of Health Services; see Additional Resources) has a PSC needs assessment form that can help focus such discussions. Finally, try to get a sense of the administrator's commitment.

A note of caution: Because each site has unique ways of functioning, as well as strengths and weaknesses, try not to generalize about the likelihood of a PSCP success. For example, although a committed, organized administration provides the ideal environment, a PSCP can succeed even when the administration is not well organized and/or not totally committed. Two reasons are that motivated, well-trained, and confident providers often will do PSC counseling despite such barriers, and that even at sites lacking formalized PSCPs, much informal counseling occurs (e.g., in the waiting room, hallways, and, especially, outside the clinics where smokers congregate).

To best institutionalize a PSCP, it is advisable for a facility's administration to assign a coordinator to arrange trainings, train providers, set up waiting room education, obtain resources, and so on. Often, although a facility may send several providers for training, no one is made responsible for overseeing an actual initiative. (Even in such cases, it is hoped that at least those who have been trained will counsel clients.) To achieve effective implementation of a PSCP, the importance of a designated coordinator and a formalized program cannot be overemphasized.

We recommend that as many types and levels of staff as possible be trained. The more staff that are aware of the importance of PSC, the more support there will be for an effective program, and the more support all staff will be able to give patients.

Finally, when helping a facility develop and conduct a PSC training program, it is important to make sure there will be adequate room and necessary training equipment. For instance, at one of our trainings, the facility had been unable to schedule its conference room. So training was done in the ob/gyn waiting area (where the public address system was located); little was accomplished.

Assumption That Too Few Will Be Interested. Another major barrier to implementing successful PSCPs is whether a given provider knows how many clients smoke. Unless a site has a good client intake and tracking system, it usually cannot answer this, and thus may underestimate the number of smoking clients and the extent of outreach and education needed.

It is important to note that even if an intake assessment attempts to determine smoking status, smokers, especially pregnant women, often are reticent about divulging this. Reasons include embarrassment; fear of other questions the client may not want to answer (a notable exception is a pregnant drug-abuser who likely will admit smoking, because she views it as minor compared to other drug abuse); discomfort with and/or distrust of the provider; smoking during prior pregnancies with no evident ill effects on the children; unwillingness to recognize the dangers of smoking or the importance of quitting; and viewing smoking as a rare pleasure and/or as a stress reliever.

Another problem identifying smokers lies with how the query is made. Research has shown that in written self-assessment tools, a direct "Do you smoke?" question requiring a "yes" or "no" reply often is less effective than a multiple-choice format (Mullen, Carbonari, Tabak, & Glenday, 1991). Even if a client admits to smoking, underreporting of the number of cigarettes is common. A critical, but often omitted, question for intake and assessment is exposure to secondhand smoke.

Once an identification system is in place, a smoker's chart should be readily identifiable without upsetting the client. Because any sticker labeled "smoker" can often make clients feel stigmatized, it is preferable to use a colored dot outside or inside the chart. One site tried a red dot for heavy smokers, pink for light smokers, yellow for "in the process of quitting," and green for those who had quit. They soon abandoned this because it was cumbersome, and no one had been designated to monitor it. Therefore, keep it simple.

Staff Issues. Many facilities are plagued by staff shortage, rapid turnover, or burnout. The best approach to overcoming these barriers in relation to establishing a PSCP is to demonstrate to administrators that PSC counseling is not time-consuming, that it can be done in brief intervals, say of 1, 3, 5, and 10 min, and that it is a shared responsibility.

There also are two secondary barriers to implementation of PSCPs:

Priority. Many clients and some providers perceive smoking cessation to be a low priority for high-risk clients who are more concerned about such issues as housing, money, jobs, and general safety. To overcome this, it is necessary to educate providers and clients about the risks of smoking and the importance of PSC.

Provider Confidence. Once a provider completes PSC training, he or she usually feels more confident about working with smokers. However, to reinforce what they learned and to begin a successful PSCP, it is important that providers immediately begin using their new skills and reviewing all materials. By and large, providers who are former smokers are more confident than are current ones or those who never smoked.

Technical Assistance

The PSC trainer both provides training and offers technical assistance related to program planning, implementation, train-the-trainer endeavors, and resource development. For example, once a provider has completed the 6-hr PSC training, the provider may want to practice additional role playing. Moreover, the trainer works with administrators and/or designated PSC coordinators to implement a facilities PSCP and helps newly trained providers during their first training endeavor.

Follow-Up

Within a month after training, the trainer should arrange for a follow-up visit to help the facility institutionalize a PSCP. At this time, barriers and possible solutions are identified. This discussion should help the facility:

- Systematize identification of prenatal/postpartum smokers and passive smokers.

- Establish a referral system.
- Plan and conduct regularly scheduled education sessions on the risks of smoking and secondhand smoke, stress management techniques, and the latest quitting methods.

The last activity raises client awareness, indicates that the facility thinks this is an important health issue, and informs clients of PSC services and support. In our experience, multiple follow-up visits are essential, because a process is required to establish a PSCP. And just as smokers are in different stages of readiness to quit, facilities are in different stages or readiness to implement a PSCP.

EVALUATING TRAINING EFFECTIVENESS

An evaluation is essential to determine program effectiveness and how to improve it. At the end of our trainings, all participants complete an evaluation form. Ninety-nine percent have rated the training as good, very good, or excellent. Most say they have learned to understand pregnant smokers and the process of quitting and staying quit, and that the materials (written and audiovisual) will greatly help them plan culturally and linguistically sensitive and appropriate PSCPs. Overall, the results show that the training has increased provider confidence, helped them learn PSC counseling skills, motivated them to initiate PSCPs, and provided essential information on how to obtain culturally specific PSC resources.

Evaluation results also have provided feedback that has helped improve the training. For instance, providers who plan to do PSC counseling said that more role-play time was needed during their 6-hr session. Consequently, an in-depth workshop on counseling has been added, and has been well received.

It also was found that providers were most concerned about the time needed to counsel. Most providers want to learn how to motivate patients in a brief period of time. Again, such knowledge must be taught via role play, in a message that is positive and personalized.

Finally, respondents emphasized that for PSCPs to succeed, providers must share responsibility. Thus, although the provider can offer a brief motivational statement and make a referral, the staff person designated to do PSC counseling must work with the patient more intensively.

As for the evaluation form itself, two tips for developing an effective one are:

- If responses are to be coded in some quantifiable way (i.e., "Fifty percent of respondents felt . . ."), possible responses must be brief. Although open-ended questions yield helpful replies, they are not quantifiable. An example of an open-ended question is: "Which topic(s) would you have liked more or less of?" An example of a quantifiable question is: "Overall, how much did each of the following contribute to your learning: instructional materials, videos, role-play, group discussion?" (For each point, respondents should check: *a great deal*, *somewhat*, *very little*, or *not applicable*.)

- The form ideally should be one page, but not more than two. Make sure to allow time for participants to complete it.

SUPPLEMENTAL TRAININGS TO CONSIDER

Train the Trainer. Lack of adequate resources and lack of time, as well as lack of knowledge of how to sustain a program, always are major issues for any organization that is instituting a new initiative. Incorporating this component into a PSCP makes it possible to maintain the initiative indefinitely, by training providers to both work with clients and to train their colleagues. The train-the-trainer curriculum contains discussions on communication and teaching skills, adult learning styles, and trainer roles, and a section on how to teach a PSC curriculum. *For You and Your Family: A Guide for Prenatal Training and Provider* (California Department of Health Services; see Additional Resources) is a good resource.

Stress Management. Low-income pregnant and parenting women usually face multiple stressors. Because smoking often is used to relieve stress, Healthy Start/NYC, during a series of stress management sessions, has taught providers techniques to help them with their own stressful jobs and, in turn, to be able to teach brief, effective techniques to help clients manage stress while quitting smoking. Stress management is an extremely important component. With clients it can be used one-on-one or in a group setting.

CONCLUSION

1. Develop an ongoing, interactive relationship with your facility contact(s).

2. During training, be caring, encouraging, sensitive to participants' needs, learning styles, and interests, and be a good listener.

3. Be flexible in scheduling training sessions. We have found the ideal number of participants to be 15. We try to sign up 20, knowing that some will not appear.

4. Know your trainees and use culturally appropriate materials. During trainings, ask providers to choose which materials will best suit their clients.

5. When providers begin implementing PSCPs, be patient, but persevere. Remind them that they can call on you for help as much as necessary. Do not wait for their call. Make a schedule to call each facility monthly.

6. Remember that incentives work, for both clients and providers.

7. A sense of humor always relaxes people.

8. Be creative during role play. We schedule role play right after lunch. While the participants are out, we place on each chair a colored dot made of construction paper. On one color dot is written "client" and on another color dot "counselor." When role play begins, they pair up. Be sure to customize your role plays to reflect reality. Use real situations, and five different scenarios: One "client" is in the precontemplative stage, the second is in the contemplation stage, the third is in the preparation stage, the fourth is in relapse, and the fifth does not smoke but is a passive smoker. Have counselors practice using the Four A's to guide their work. Give each pair 5 min, and leave enough time for participants to process their role-play experiences. This is the time when participants gain the most confidence in their smoking cessation counseling skills.

9. After the role-play, offer refreshments. Participants really enjoy this. If possible, provide fresh fruit.

10. Keep in mind that if you are training providers who work with high-risk, medically underserved, low-income clients, quitting smoking may have a very low priority. If your client is pregnant, the goal may be to get her to reduce the number of cigarettes daily to five or fewer.

11. We have found that the better organized and prepared we are, the better the training. Be familiar with adult learning styles. For example, always provide auditory, visual, and experiential learning opportunities. If possible, invite guest speakers. It makes the training more interesting. If you show a video, choose one that is no longer than 15 min.

REFERENCES

Alameda County Low-Birth Weight Study Group. (1990). Epidemiology Resources, Inc.

Bass, F. (1995). *Ten commandments of clinical communication. BC doctor's stop smoking program.* Vancouver, British Columbia, Canada. Ordering: (604) 736-5551.

Centers for Disease Control. (1987). Cigarette smoking among blacks and other minority populations. *Morbidity and Mortality Weekly Report, 36*(25), 405–407.

Fingerhut, L., & Kleinman, J. (1990). Smoking before, during, and after pregnancy. *American Journal of Public Health, 80*, 541–544.

Floyd, L. R., Rimer, B. K., Giovino, G. A., Mullen, P. D., & Sullivan, S. E. (1993). A review of smoking in pregnancy: Affects on pregnancy outcomes and cessation efforts. *Annual Review Public Health, 14*, 379–411.

Glynn, T. J., & Manley, M. W. (1990). *How to help your patients stop smoking: A National Cancer Institute manual for physicians* (NIH Publication No. 90-3064). Bethesda, MD: U.S. Department of Health and Human Services, Public Health Service, National Institutes of Health, National Cancer Institute.

Institute of Medicine. (1985). *Preventing low birth weight.* Washington, DC: National Academy Press.

Miller, W., & Rollnick, S. (1991). *Motivational interviewing: Preparing people to change addictive behavior.* New York: Guilford Press.

Missouri Department of Health, Bureau of Health Promotion. (1989). *Baby and me smoke-free: Smoking cessation in pregnancy; Techniques for health professionals.* Columbia, MO: Author.

Mullen, P. D., Carbonari, J. P., Tabak, E. R., & Glenday, M. (1991). Improving disclosure of smoking by pregnant women. *American Journal of Obstetrics and Gynecology, 165,* 409–413.

Prochaska, J. O., & DiClemente, C. C. (1992). Stages of change in the modification of problem behaviors. In M. Hersen & R. M. Eisler (Eds.), *Progress in behavior modification* (pp.). Sycamore, IL: Sycamore Publishing.

University of California, Los Angeles, Center for Health Policy Research. (1991). *Women's health-related behaviors* [An Analysis of the 1991 National Health Interview Survey and its Supplements]. A report by the Commonwealth Fund Commission on Women's Health.

U.S. Department of Health and Human Services. (1990). *The health benefits of smoking cessation. A report of the Surgeon General* (DHHS Publication No. CDC 90-8416). Hyattsville, MD: U.S. Department of Health and Human Services, Public Health Service, Centers for Disease Control Center for Chronic Disease Prevention and Health Promotion, Office on Smoking and Health.

ADDITIONAL RESOURCES

Agency for Health Care Policy and Research, Centers for Disease Control and Prevention, U.S. Department of Health and Human Services Public Health Service. (1996). *Smoking cessation: Clinical practice guideline no. 18.* This presents recommendations for health care providers, with brief supporting information, tables and figures, and pertinent references. Ordering information: Call the Government Printing Office; ask for AHCPR Publication No. 96-0692; cost is $4.75. There is no other way to order this.

Agency for Health Care Policy and Research (AHCPR). Several versions of Guideline No. 18: *The quick reference guide for smoking cessation specialists*; *The quick reference guide for primary care clinicians* (a pocket guide for the busy clinician); *Smoking cessation: A systems approach guide for health care administrators, insurers, managed care organizations, and purchasers*; and the *Consumer version.* All are available in English and Spanish. Ordering information: For up to 100 free copies of each guideline, call the AHCPR Publications Clearinghouse: (800) 358-9295.

California Department of Health Services, Tobacco Control Section and Centers for Disease Control. (1991). *For you and your family: A guide for perinatal trainers and providers.* The interventions and support materials were developed for four ethnic groups: African Americans, American Indians, Asians, and Hispanics. They include a trainer's guide, a training video, ethnic-specific interventions, and educational materials. Ordering information: $20 each, but well worth it. Call Tobacco Education Clearinghouse of California: (408) 438-4822.

Missouri Department of Health, Bureau of Health Promotion. (1989). *Baby and me smoke-free: Smoking cessation in pregnancy; Techniques for health professionals.* Ordering information: Contact Katherine Binkley, (573) 751-6400.

Napier, K. (1996). *Cigarettes, what the warning label doesn't tell you.* New York: American Council of Science and Health. Ordering information: Call (212) 362-7044 and ask for a professional review copy; if they will not honor your request, the book will cost you $19.95 plus $5.00 shipping.

Project ASSIST (American Stop Smoking Intervention Study) Women's Health Subcommittee, North Carolina. (1995). *A guide for helping women who smoke: A focus on pregnancy and the childbearing years* [three-ring binder, 70 pages]. Ordering information: Although not yet available for sale outside of North Carolina, to obtain a single professional review copy contact Tracy Enright, Field Director for Project ASSIST, (919) 733-1881. This is an excellent provider guide on how to counsel pregnant/parenting women who smoke. It is culturally specific for the African American, American Indian, and Hispanic woman.

CHAPTER SIX

Intervening With Older Smokers

Neal Richard Boyd
Fox Chase Cancer Center, Philadelphia, Pennsylvania

C. Tracy Orleans
Robert Wood Johnson Foundation, Princeton, New Jersey

Many smoking cessation programs have been developed and targeted to various segments of the smoking population since the first *Surgeon General's Report on Smoking and Health* in 1964 (U.S. Department of Health, Education, and Welfare, 1964). Only recently, however, has attention been directed at the needs of midlife and older smokers, defined in this chapter as those aged 50 years and older. Smokers in this age group began smoking when smoking was considered a glamorous part of the American social culture and long before its health consequences were well known. The result is a generation of lifelong heavy smokers. With more baby boomers reaching midlife, the ranks of older smokers is on the rise. Older smokers not only experience significant adverse health consequences from continued smoking but derive many important health benefits by stopping smoking. However, after several decades of smoking, older smokers who attempt quitting encounter barriers somewhat different from those faced by smokers in younger age groups. This chapter reviews the smoking problem among midlife and older smokers by examining smoking prevalence, the health consequences of continued smoking, and the health benefits resulting from quitting smoking. In addition, programmatic strategies for successfully intervening with this population are discussed.

SMOKING PREVALENCE

Smoking prevalence data from the National Health Interview Survey (NHIS) (Centers for Disease Control, 1996a) and the Current Population Survey (CPS) (Shopland et al., 1996) indicate that smoking prevalence rates decrease as age increases. The most recent CPS showed that the overall smoking prevalence among men aged 50–59 years is 27.3%, whereas the rate among men aged 60–69 years is 20.5%. Among women aged 50–59 years, smoking prevalence is 22.9%, and 17.7% for women aged 60–69 years. The smoking rate for men over age 70 years is 11%, whereas the smoking rate for women in the same age category is 8.8%. Overall, more than 9 million people aged 50–64 years smoke cigarettes and over 4 million persons over age 65 years smoke (Centers for Disease Control, 1996a). The smoking prevalence rate among those over age 50 years constitutes about 27% of the U.S. smoking population (Centers for Disease Control, 1996a).

As has been observed in other age groups, smoking rates are higher among older smokers with less education than among older smokers with higher educational levels (Husten et al., 1997). Compared with younger smokers, older smokers show a tendency to sustain higher levels of nicotine dependence (Orleans, Jepson, Resch, & Rimer, 1994). In addition, older smokers are more likely than younger smokers to have smoked for longer periods of time (Orleans, Jepson, Resch, & Rimer, 1994). In most instances, older smokers have been smoking for many decades (Orleans et al., 1994). It is quite common to find smokers in their 60s who have smoked for over 50 years. When higher levels of nicotine addiction are combined with the length of time smoked, the quitting process can be an especially difficult task for the aged population. However, recent research has shown that older smokers respond well to smoking cessation programs, especially targeted interventions, and older smokers are as likely as younger smokers to achieve cessation (Orleans, 1997).

HEALTH CONSEQUENCES OF SMOKING

Smoking is estimated to kill over 400,000 Americans annually (Centers for Disease Control, 1996b). Of these smoking-related deaths, approximately 94% are among people aged 50 years and older and over 70% are among those aged 65 years and older (Centers for Disease Control, 1996b). Smoking is a risk factor in 7 of the top 14 causes of death for people age 65 years and older (Special Committee on Aging, United States Senate, 1986). Smoking significantly increases the likelihood of morbidity and mortality from cardiovascular, cerebrovascular, and respiratory diseases (Abrams et al., 1995; Frost et al., 1996; Howard, Toole, & Frye-Pierson, 1987; Larson, 1995; Menezes, Victora, & Rigatto, 1995; Tell et al., 1994; U.S. Department of Health and Human Services, 1984, 1989), as well as cancers of the lung, larynx, pharynx, bladder, kidney, pancreas, and cervix in women (Daniell, 1996; Shopland & Burns, 1993). In the over 65 age category, mortality from respiratory diseases attributable to smoking accounts for approximately one half and one third of the deaths in men and women, respectively (CDC, 1996b). In addition, mortality rates for chronic obstructive pulmonary disease (COPD) are about four times greater for older smokers than older nonsmokers (CDC, 1996b; U.S. Department of Health and Human Services, 1984). Compared to older nonsmokers, deaths from stroke are twice as likely in older men who smoke and one and one-half times more likely in older women who smoke (CDC, 1996b; Lee et al., 1995; Leonhardt & Diener, 1996; Shinton, 1997; U.S. Department of Health and Human Services, 1984).

Smoking also is associated with dental problems (Locker, 1992), especially periodontal disease (Dolan et al., 1997; Genco, 1996; Grossi et al., 1995). Recent research has shown active and passive tobacco smoke exposure to be related to a number of vision problems, including age-related maculopathy (Klein, Klein, Linton, & DeMets, 1993), age-related macular degeneration (Christen et al., 1996; Seddon, Willett, Speizer, & Hankinson, 1996), cataracts (Christen et al., 1992), lens opacities (Hirvela, Luukinen, & Lattikainen, 1995), and vision impairment. Other conditions associated with smoking in older adults include cognitive impairment (Ford, Mefrouche, Freidland, & Debanne, 1996; Letenneur et al., 1994) and gastrointestinal disorders (Cryer, Lee, & Feldman, 1992; Schoon, Mellstrom, Oden, & Ytterberg, 1991).

Smoking complicates many illnesses and conditions that are common among the elderly, including heart disease, hypertension, circulatory and vascular conditions, duodenal ulcers, osteoporosis, and diabetes (Achkar, 1985; Gamble, 1995; Moore, 1986; Rimm et al., 1995; Sima & Greene, 1996; Somerville, Faulkner, & Langman, 1986; Vogt et al., 1996). In fact, diabetics who smoke are more likely to suffer critical or fatal complications from diseases and conditions such as heart disease, blindness, and stroke (Schumacher & Smith, 1988). As smokers age, the likelihood rises of occurrence of problems with cough, phlegm, and chronic bronchitis (Burr, Phillips, & Hurst, 1985; Nejjari et al., 1996; U.S. Department of Health and Human Services, 1984). Recent survey research among midlife and older smokers showed that they are more likely than nonsmokers to report having trouble breathing, frequent coughing, tiring easily, being less physically active than nonsmokers in the same age group, and more likely to estimate their health as poor (Rimer et al., 1990). Research also documented that older smokers are less likely to have preventive health checks such as blood pressure screenings, PAP tests, physical examinations, electrocardiographs (EKGs), stool blood tests, and mammograms (U.S. Department of Health and Human Services, 1990).

Moreover, smoking interacts with and restricts the metabolism of many medications that are used to treat ailments common among the elderly (D'Arcy, 1984; Gundert-Remy, 1995; Lipman, 1985). Medications known to interact with smoking and be restricted in their efficacy in older smokers include antidepressants, lidocaine, pentazocine HCl, phenothiazines, and phenylbutazone (Hicks et al., 1981). Serum levels of theophylline, aminophylline, and oxtriphylline have been shown to be decreased in the presence of cigarette smoking (Talseth, Boye, Kongerud, & Bredesen, 1981). Research suggests that older diabetics who are heavier smokers may need 50% more insulin than diabetic nonsmokers (Todd, 1987). Consequently, drug dosage may be subtherapeutic or ineffective for older people who smoke (Greenblatt, Allen, Harmatz, & Shader, 1980).

BENEFITS OF QUITTING

The *Surgeon General's Report* of 1990 (U.S. Department of Health and Human Services, 1990) concluded from the existing medical and epidemiologic data that "it is never too late to stop smoking." Smoking cessation leads to significant health benefits regardless of the length of time one has smoked. Many older smokers, however, are unaware of the improvement in health that results from quitting smoking. Even for those who have smoked for 30–40 years or more, stopping smoking can prevent or reduce the likelihood of many diseases, including heart disease, cancer, and respiratory diseases (Paganini-Hill & Hsu, 1994; U.S. Department of Health and Human Services, 1989). Smoking cessation can also stabilize COPD and eventually lead to less disability and more independent functioning (Chang, Moran, Cugell, & Webster, 1995). The conclusion of a review of large clinical trials was that smoking cessation even during one's 60s increased longevity as well as independent functioning (Abramson, 1985).

Although considerable physical damage results from many years of smoking, the body responds almost immediately to quitting smoking (Gordon, Kannel, & McGee, 1974). Within 1 month of stopping smoking, benefits begin to accrue and increase with the length of time one is abstinent (Shopland & Burns, 1993). Research has shown smoking cessation at midlife and beyond to be associated with a reduction in mortality from coronary heart disease (Shopland & Burns, 1993). Data from the Coronary Artery Surgery Study (Hermanson, Omenn, Kronmal, Gersh, & Participants in the Coronary Artery Surgery Study, 1988) demonstrated that subjects who quit smoking at age 55 years or older immediately began to reduce their chances of a heart attack. In comparison with nonsmokers, smokers had a 70% higher risk of death. Other findings revealed that survival benefits were more pronounced in the moderately ill patients.

In addition to the physiological improvements that accompany quitting smoking, such as reduction in the risk of coronary heart disease and improved circulation and respiratory function, improvement in the quality of life is an aftermath of cessation that merits notice in the discussion of the benefits of quitting smoking for olders smokers (Hirdes & Maxwell, 1994). Fries, Green, and Levine (1989), for instance, argued that the most important outcome from stopping smoking may not be a longer life span but a longer *active* life span. This would manifest itself in the prevention or compression into a shorter time period of chronic diseases and illnesses in the later years. Another important outcome of stopping smoking is that quitters are more likely to maintain independent functioning for longer periods of time (Haug & Ory, 1987).

BELIEFS ABOUT SMOKING

Survey data have shown that older smokers have a different set of beliefs about smoking, compared with younger smokers. Orleans and colleagues (Orleans, Jepson, Resch, & Rimer, 1994) used data from the Adult Use of Tobacco Survey (AUTS) to compare beliefs about smoking among individuals aged 21–49 years and those 50–74 years. Smokers aged 50–74 years were not as likely as those aged 21–49 years to believe that smoking and illness were related. In addition, the older group was not as concerned about the health consequences of smoking, was more skeptical about the benefits of smoking cessation, and was more likely to view smoking as a stress coping mechanism and as a way to control weight. Furthermore, almost one-half of these older smokers believed that smoking did not pose as much of a health risk as being 20 pounds overweight.

The AUTS data also found a strong positive relationship between the beliefs about the health consequences of smoking and a physician's advice to quit (Orleans, Jepson, Resch, & Rimer, 1994). Among older smokers, those who reported having been advised to quit by a physician were more likely to believe they were at risk for smoking-related diseases than those who did not receive medical quitting advice. The investigators also found a positive relationship between older smokers' intentions to quit and a doctor's advice to quit (Orleans, Jepson, Resch, & Rimer, 1994). Of course these findings are only correlations, but they suggest that medical advice about smoking health risks and quitting methods represent a potentially powerful tool in interventions for older smokers. This is especially true given focus-group findings that older smokers underestimate not just the harms of smoking but the benefits of quitting (Rimer et al., 1994).

RATIONALE FOR INTERVENING WITH OLDER SMOKERS

In 1990 the Surgeon General (U.S. Department of Health and Human Services, 1990) reported that "it is never too late to quit smoking." At that time little was known of how immediate the benefits of smoking cessation for older smokers were (Orleans, 1997). A number of intervention studies among older smokers during the last 10 years has shown that older adults are as likely as, and possibly more likely than, smokers in younger age groups to quit when given appropriate assistance (Dale et al., 1997; Hill, Rigdon, & Johnson, 1993; Morgan et al., 1996; Orleans, 1997; Ossip-Klein, Carosella, & Krusch, 1997; Rimer et al., 1994; Vetter & Ford, 1990). These studies have also shown that the predictors of quitting success in older smokers are similar to those in younger age groups: lower nicotine dependence, higher quitting self-efficacy, prior quitting success, stronger quitting motivation, greater perceived health benefits, lower perceived quitting barriers, using a greater number of quitting strategies, having few acquaintances who smoke and/or a nonsmoking spouse, and, among older smokers quitting with transdermal nicotine, having more frequent contact with physicians or pharmacists, and less concomitant cigarette smoking (Orleans, 1997). These results suggest that older smokers are highly responsive to targeted smoking cessation programs.

In its comprehensive effort to improve the health of the nation, the U.S. Department of Health and Human Services (1991b) included a major tobacco control initiative as a part of *Healthy People 2000*. Among the tobacco control objectives are reducing overall adult smoking prevalence to 15% and increasing to 75% the proportion of physicians who routinely counsel their adult patients who smoke to quit. In April 1996, the Agency for Health Care Policy and Research (AHCPR) issued clinical guidelines for smoking cessation (Fiore et al., 1996) (Table 1). These guidelines, intended for physicians, smoking cessation specialists, health care administrators, insurers, and purchasers, were consistent with the National Cancer Institute (NCI) 4 A's model and were based on meta-analyses of controlled experimental studies demonstrating the effectiveness of office-based provider-initiated quit smoking interventions. The guidelines advocate the identification of tobacco users and means of delivery and support of effective smoking cessation interventions in clinical practice. Shortly after the publication of the AHCPR guidelines, the National Committee for Quality Assurance (NCQA) health plan added a measure of

TABLE 6.1
Smoking Cessation: Principal Recommendations of the AHCPR Panel

Every person who smokes should be offered smoking cessation treatment at every office visit.
Clinicians should ask and record the tobacco use status of every patient.
Cessation treatment even as brief as 3 min is effective.
The more intense the treatment, the more effective it is in producing long-term abstinence from tobacco.
Nicotine replacement therapy (e.g., patches, gum, nasal spray), clinician-delivered social support, and skills training are effective components of smoking cessation treatment.
Health care systems should be modified to routinely identify and intervene with all tobacco users at every visit.

Source: Agency for Health Care Policy and Research (AHCPR, 1996).

patient-reported provider advice to quit smoking in its standard Health Plan Employer Data and Information Set (HEDIS) 3.0 report card (NCQA, 1996). This means that the NCQA now requires participating health plans to survey their membership and report and be rated on the frequency of provider-delivered cessation advice. This provides health plans with a potentially powerful incentive to implement the new AHCPR guidelines and offering a range of state-of-the-art smoking cessation services to all enrolled smokers.

CLEAR HORIZONS: A SELF-HELP APPROACH FOR OLDER SMOKERS

Many smokers prefer quitting with self-help do-it-yourself smoking cessation methods (Fiore et al., 1990). Until relatively recent times, however, no self-help smoking cessation guides had been developed that specifically addressed the special needs of older smokers. To fill this void, the Fox Chase Cancer Center developed *Clear Horizons*, a self-help smoking cessation guide designed specifically to address the needs of older smokers (Orleans et al., 1989). *Clear Horizons* was developed by researchers from the Fox Chase Center and is based on data retrieved from focus groups, an extensive literature review, including the AUTS survey of older smokers' attitudes and beliefs about smoking, and on information gathered from focus groups of older smokers (Rimer et al., 1994). An early version of the guide was pretested through in-depth personal interviews with older smokers.

Clear Horizons is a four-color, 48-page guide specifically targeted to the smoking habits, quitting concerns, and lifestyle of older smokers (Orleans et al., 1989). To provide additional appeal, a magazine-style format, similar to the American Association of Retired Persons (AARP) publication *Modern Maturity*, was adopted. The guide's content blends entertainment and information, uses large, clear type, and was written at an eighth grade reading level. Multiracial smokers in their 50s, 60s, and 70s are depicted in photographs to provide information and inspiration to appeal to a wide audience of older smokers. Information on the specific health harms of smoking for older adults, and the health benefits of quitting, are highlighted. The guide also describes how smoking interacts with many common medications to restrict their efficacy. The Prochaska and DiClemente transtheoretical model (1983) is used to present relevant self-change methods that are appropriate for smokers in various stages of quitting. In 1995 *Clear Horizons* was revised to update information on the use of nicotine replacement (Orleans et al., 1995).

Clear Horizons has been tested in three large randomized trials, either alone or in combination with medical advice and treatment. In a community-based study (Rimer et al., 1994), 1,867 smokers aged 50–74 years were recruited through magazine advertisements appearing in publications targeting older smokers (e.g., *Modern Maturity*). Eligible respondents were randomly assigned to one of three study conditions. The control group received the National Cancer Institute's *Clearing the Air* (U.S. Department of Health and Human Services, 1991a), a 24-page nontargeted smoking cessation guide. Two intervention groups received the new *Clear Horizons* guide. One of these two groups received only the guide, and a second group received the guide plus two telephone counseling calls spaced 4–8 weeks and 16–20 weeks after the mailing of the guide. The second intervention group was also offered the Clear Horizons Quitline—a telephone helpline for further quitting assistance should subjects need more help. Telephone follow-up interviews were conducted at 3, 6, and 12 months. At the 3-month follow-up the three groups were asked to rate the quality and their overall satisfaction with their respective guides. Those who received *Clear Horizons* rated the guide higher than those who had used *Clearing the Air*. Quit rates at the 3-months follow-up were significantly higher for the *Clear Horizons* plus telephone counseling group (13%) than for the groups receiving either *Clear Horizons* alone (9%) or the *Clearing the Air* (7%). By the 12-month follow-up, however, the quit rate of the group receiving *Clear Horizons* guide alone (21%) had edged ahead of the quit rate of those who had received *Clear Horizons* plus telephone counseling (19%), and was significantly higher than the quit rate of the participants receiving the nontargeted *Clearing the Air* guide (14%). These findings indicated that a targeted self-help guide alone may benefit older smokers more than generic quitting guides.

The cessation rates in the *Clear Horizons* community trial increased over time. This is not unusual in self-help smoking cessation programs and is, in fact, one of the real highly attractive features of self-help quitting. A possible reason for this increase in quitting success over time is that many of those who did not succeed with their initial quitting attempt often put aside their self-help materials and then used them again in another quit attempt. Research in quitting success confirms that the more times those who fail try to quit, the more likely they are to eventually succeed.

THE PHYSICIAN'S ROLE

Although specific recommendations for clinic-based smoking cessation exist, not all physicians intervene with their patients who smoke. A survey among older smokers revealed that only about one-half reported that they had ever been asked by their doctor about their cigarette smoking habits (U.S. Department of Health and Human Services, 1990). In another survey, nearly two-thirds of smokers 50–74 years old reported that they were thinking about quitting in the next year (Rimer et al., 1990). With older adults making an average of 6.3 physician visits per year, there are approximately 1.5

million annual physician encounters with older smokers who have never been advised to quit (Rimer & Orleans, 1990). If only 10% of these smokers could be motivated to quit by their health care provider, more than 1 million adults aged 55 years and over would become ex-smokers annually. Thus, the physician is in an excellent position to play a key role in helping older smokers quit.

Patients consider their health care providers (e.g., physicians and dentists) as especially credible sources of health information and advice. Annual examinations (e.g., physical and dental) as well as other visits for acute and chronic ailments during the year yield a number of excellent "teachable moments" to promote smoking cessation. Providers should use these opportunities to recognize the age-related needs of their older patients who smoke. Symptoms like fatigue often are misattributed by smokers to be the result of aging and not smoking. Linking symptoms such as coughing, fatigue, periodontal disease, and gum problems to smoking or discussing how the patient's smoking interacts with and restricts the efficacy of their prescribed medication are excellent openings for a quit smoking discussion. Emphasis on the benefits of quitting, not just the harmful effects of smoking, is critical for smokers who may believe that the "damage already has been done" (Rimer et al., 1994). A provider's opinion that a patient's current condition is related to smoking and that quitting is beneficial can send a powerful message. Patients are likely to value this advice and be more likely to take action if the doctor provides the direction.

Two excellent tobacco cessation references for providers are the National Cancer Institute's manuals for physicians (Glynn & Manley, 1990) and dentists (Mecklenburg et al., 1990). These manuals describe the 4 A's model of *Ask* about smoking, *Advise* all smokers to quit, *Assist* patients by helping them devise a quit smoking plan and, if appropriate, the recommendation for nicotine replacement, and *Arrange* for follow-up to assess progress and provide support. Diligent use of this intervention results in significant cessation outcomes. In addition, Cummings, Rubin, and Oster (1988) estimated that provider advice to quit is as cost-effective as other preventive interventions, such as treating hypertension and hypercholesterolemia. Such cost-effectiveness is likely to be even greater in the presence of chronic disease. For instance, Krumholz and colleagues (1993) estimated that smoking cessation is 20–200 times more cost-effective than standard medical therapies post myocardial infarction.

A second randomized controlled trial of physician intervention that utilized *Clear Horizons* evaluated the efficacy of this self-help guide in conjunction with the tailored physician interventions for older smokers. Fox Chase researchers (Morgan et al., 1996) evaluated a brief physician-delivered quit smoking intervention consistent with the NCI 4 A's model and the recent AHCPR guidelines by comparing it with usual care for smokers aged 50–74 years. Forty-nine primary care practices affiliated with a large health maintenance organization (HMO) in Pennsylvania and New Jersey were recruited to participate in the trial. After randomization to either treatment or usual care conditions, all practices received a 45- to 60-min office-based training in quit smoking advice and assistance based on a pharmaceutical-detailing model (Avorn & Soumerai, 1983). Participating physicians were trained to administer a 3- to 10-min quit smoking intervention that included praising each patient's previous attempts to quit smoking, linking smoking to the individual patient's illness symptoms, discussing the health benefits of quitting smoking, and giving a clear message to quit smoking. Physicians in the usual care group were instructed not to modify in any way their style and methods for counseling older patients about smoking.

Patients aged 50–74 years who had smoked at least one cigarette in the previous 7 days and who were making a nonemergency visit to their physician were eligible for the study. To ensure that all smokers, not just those motivated to quit, enrolled in the study, potential subjects were assured that they did not have to quit smoking or even try to quit in order to participate. Of the 49 physician practices that were initially identified for the study, 39 practices were able to recruit five or more of their patients to participate in the study. The medical specialities included the following: family medicine ($n = 20$), internal medicine ($n = 17$), cardiology ($n = 1$), and obstetrics and gynecology ($n = 1$). During the office visit, older smokers were asked whether they smoked and would be willing to quit if given help to do so. Treatment subjects who declined help received counseling targeted toward their barriers to quitting, whereas those contemplating quitting received advice to quit, were given a copy of *Clear Horizons*, and were encouraged to set a quit date. When it was medically indicated, they also received a prescription for nicotine gum. Patients in the treatment group received a follow-up letter from their physician 1 week following their doctor's appointment, and a 5-min counseling telephone call from a member of the research staff 2 to 4 weeks after their office visit. Follow-up to assess smoking status was conducted by telephone interview at 6, 12, and 18 months postintervention. Quit rates were significantly higher for subjects receiving the *Clear Horizons* intervention than usual care at each follow-up observation point. At 6 months, the quit rate was 15.4% for the special physician intervention group and 8.2% for the usual care group. At 12 months the abstinence rate had increased to 19.5% among the group who received special physician intervention and to 12.9% in the usual care group. By the 18-month follow-up point, a further increase in abstinence was observed in both groups, with a 22.6% cessation rate in the special physician intervention group and a 15.8% cessation rate in the usual care group (Morgan et al., 1997).

Of course, not all smokers will be able to succeed with a minimal contact approach for a variety of reasons, including high nicotine addiction level, being medically at high risk, psychiatric comorbidity (see chap. 2, this volume), or a personal preference for more intensive treatment. Older smokers with those conditions and living alone often need more support than can be provided by a minimal quitting program; more intensive treatments, such as a group program, are indicated. However, providers attempting to successfully intervene with older smokers should begin initial treatment by offering the least intensive and least costly approach to the largest number of smokers, reserving the more costly and intensive treatments for those who do not succeed with the minimal methods. This approach is known as a stepped care model (Orleans, 1993; Abrams et al., 1996) and includes treatment and follow-up offered in the provider's practice and/or by referral. Although the model can be applied in a wide variety of inpatient and outpatient settings, it is also applicable to other segments of health care, such as dental practices and pharmacies, and to community and worksite establishments as well.

A COMPUTER-BASED TAILORED INTERVENTION FOR REACHING OLDER SMOKERS

The recent AHCPR guidelines for smoking cessation (Fiore et al., 1996) concluded that self-help materials when used alone (i.e., without additional counseling or therapeutic intervention) do not increase cessation rates, and that the success rates from minimal contact/self-help methods are disappointingly low when compared with outcomes of group or individualized counseling programs. A recent technological development in self-help methods that promises to improve quit rates of self-help methods is computer-based tailored messages. Computer-based tailoring offers the opportunity to efficiently deliver smoking cessation interventions "designed to exactly fit" the specific needs of the smoker who is making a quit attempt. Several seminal research studies (Campbell et al., 1994; Orleans et al., 1998; Skinner, Strecher, & Hospers, 1994; Strecher et al., 1994) have demonstrated that tailored interventions are more effective than generic approaches for important high-risk populations, including older smokers. In addition, a review in the *Journal of the American Medical Association* (personalized messages, 1994) concluded that tailored mailings may emerge as effective new weapons in cancer control. This review also concluded that this type of feedback is not intended to take the place of physician to patient consultation but rather to enhance it.

Computer-based tailored smoking cessation interventions vary by the frequency of feedback messages and by the number of variables used in the tailoring process. Information contained in each piece of feedback includes data collected directly from the smoker. This can include but not be limited to information on personal smoking history (number of cigarettes smoked per day, length of time smoked, level of nicotine addiction, etc.), stage of change, quitting desire, self-efficacy, beliefs of risk of smoking-related disease, scheduling of a quit date, barriers for quitting, reasons for quitting, temptations to smoke, previous quit attempts, and relapse circumstances.

Quitting feedback messages are written for various possible responses to the relevant smoking, demographic, and psychosocial information stimuli provided by the user. The feedback messages were guided by literature reviews and responses from smokers who were seen in interviews and surveys, pretested with members of the target population, and eventually assembled and arranged for presentation in a predetermined layout. Although the materials look similar, content is tailored to each person's individual needs. Once the feedback messages have been designed, algorithms specify how the messages will be placed in the feedback. The algorithms match the needs of the smokers with specific self-help messages.

Smokers who use individually tailored feedback receive a series of personalized mailings over a period of time. The mailings are designed to provide advice to help each individual with smoking behavior, quitting motives and barriers, and health profile. The individual feedback mailings change over time to coincide with the patient's progress through the stages of change described in the transtheoretical model (Prochaska et al., 1991). Each mailing conveys information designed to be useful to all subjects, regardless of where they are in the quitting process and whether they have quit.

The feedback mailings change over time in an orderly way. To assure that the information remains accurate and relevant, each mailing begins with brief self-staging directions and stage appropriate quit tips. Mailings further removed in time from the point where the data for tailoring was collected focus on variables that are less likely to change but are also formatted to cover the possibility that the specifics of the situation may have since changed. For example, tailored feedback concerning personal health benefits discussed a couple of months earlier when the tailoring data were taken might read, "Back in January, you stated you were bothered by shortness of breath. If you've quit smoking, you're breathing easier. If you haven't quit, remind yourself how much better you'll feel when you can breathe easier and walk further without resting."

As tailored mailings change over time they coincide with the natural sequences of self-change processes documented in longitudinal and cross-section studies testing the transtheoretical model (Prochaska et al., 1991; Prochaska, DiClemente, & Norcross, 1992). As Prochaska et al. (1992, p. 1110) indicated, "efficient self-change depends on doing the right thing (processes) at the right time (stages)." Each tailored mailing contains messages suitable for smokers who have and have not quit smoking. These messages concern and emphasize intrinsic quitting motives, quitting health benefits, overcoming quitting barriers, and the use of experiential processes of change that peak during the transition from precontemplation/contemplation stage to the preparation/action stage. Later, tailored mailings contain individualized advice to use behavioral processes associated with transitions from preparation to action to maintenance. Because self-efficacy increases linearly with progress from precontemplation to maintenance, tailored feedback messages in each mailing are designed to bolster self-efficacy (Velicer et al., 1993).

The Fox Chase Cancer Center has developed and tested a computer-based system to provide individualized tailored feedback to assist low-income older smokers (age 65 years and older) to successfully use the transdermal nicotine patch to quit smoking. The smokers in the study were identified through the Pennsylvania Pharmaceutical Assistance Contract for the Elderly (PACE), a prescription plan that delivers financial assistance to the low-income elderly for the purchase of medications (Orleans et al., 1996, 1998). Prescription and pharmacy management benefit plans are increasingly used by states to control pharmacy costs and improve drug use (Orleans et al., 1994). These organizations represent another important new channel for patient-focused interventions to improve medication compliance, especially among the elderly, who as a group constitute the nation's largest consumers of prescription drugs. This project tested two innovative approaches: identifying older smokers through PACE's computerized prescription plan database, and the delivery of a highly personalized, computer-generated smoking cessation approach for older smokers trying to quit with the patch.

A previous survey of PACE patch users found that 46% received no quitting materials or provider quitting advice and assistance when using the patch (Orleans et al., 1994). This survey also revealed that 40% of older smokers who quit via the patch and 75% of those older smokers who failed using the patch expressed considerable interest in personalized tailored mailings that would assist them in their efforts to quit smoking. To compensate for lacking medical and pharmaceutical advice and adjunctive treatment, this randomized controlled trial was designed to compare usual care with computer-based individually tailored print communications for older PACE smokers filling new nicotine patch prescriptions. A sample of 473 PACE patch users were recruited to evaluate the intervention innovation. Mailings included the targeted *Clear Horizons* self-help guide (Orleans et al., 1995) and a series of seven personalized computer-generated mailings tailored to each participant's quitting schedule, stage of change, patch dose/brand, quitting motives, and quitting barriers (Orleans et al., 1996, 1998). Follow-up to assess outcomes was conducted by mailed questionnaire at 3 months and by computer-assisted telephone interview at 6 and 12 months. These assessments showed that the vast majority of participants using the personalized tailored mailings rated them as very helpful, with most saying that they made using the patch easier. The majority of those receiving the tailored communications ($n = 236$) also reported that they had completely read the letters at least once. Ratings of the length, readability, and personalization were also favorable. Analysis of the 6 months quit rate of those subjects who successfully completed follow-up was 37.3% for usual care group and 47.5% for the tailored mailings group. The cessation rate difference was statistically significant (Orleans et al., 1998).

PHARMACOLOGIC INTERVENTIONS

Nicotine replacement therapy, either nicotine polacrilex (gum) or transdermal nicotine patches, is especially appropriate for older smokers who are highly addicted to nicotine, have had difficulty with nicotine withdrawal symptoms in previous quit attempts, and have no medical contraindications. Appropriately used nicotine gum helps alleviate nicotine withdrawal symptoms that are commonly cited by older smokers (Orleans et al., 1994), such as irritability, restlessness, anxiety, and difficulty concentrating. Successful use is dependent on proper chewing. The gum should be chewed slowly and then "parked" between the cheek and gum to release nicotine. This could be problematic for some older adults who have dentures or extensive bridgework, but it has been found that many older smokers can successfully use nicotine gum even in the presence of dentures or bridgework (Schneider, 1987).

Improperly chewed nicotine gum often causes unpleasant side effects such as a burning sensation in the throat, nausea, and gas, which deter adherence to recommended regimens (Fiore, Smith, Jorenby, & Baker, 1994; Silagy, Mant, Fowler, & Lodge, 1994). Some studies (Silagy et al., 1994) have shown that these effects were related to poor outcomes when used in the context of a brief medical advice intervention. Thus, practitioners who recommend the gum should spend some time giving the patient adequate instruction on how to use the gum correctly.

Research on transdermal nicotine (Fiore et al., 1994, 1996) indicates potentially more effective cessation outcomes in the context of routine physician intervention. This research suggests that the patch appears to benefit smokers at all levels of addiction. Appropriate use produces smoking cessation rates two to three times higher than for brief medical advice alone. Ease of adherence and fewer side effects were two reasons attributed to superior efficacy of the patch. A recent survey (Orleans, Resch, Noll, et al., 1994) of older patch users indicates that instruction in use is important for optimal benefit. Only about half of this study's patients reported that they had received any advice on patch use or quitting from their physician or pharmacist. This survey also revealed that the amount of provider instruction in use was significantly related to higher quit rates and lower rates of smoking while using the patch.

In July 1996, the FDA approved nicotine gum and nicotine patches for over-the-counter (OTC) sales. Although the OTC status of these medications will increase their availability, physicians and pharmacists must continue to intervene responsibly when recommending these aids. Doctors and pharmacists must deliver specific advice regarding proper utilization of these products. As OTC available medication, nicotine replacement is expensive. Its high price may lead some potential users to feel that either the gum or the patches are not affordable. This is especially true for older smokers on limited income. When the cost issue arises, the cost-effectiveness of using nicotine replacement versus the expense of continuing smoking should be emphasized. A pack-a-day smoker quitting via nicotine replacement will more than pay for the medication with money saved from not having to purchase cigarettes during the next year. Also, the cost of using nicotine replacement is not nearly as high as the cost of more frequent physician visits for the various smoking-associated ailments throughout the coming years.

Until the recent marketing of Zyban, whose major active ingredient is bupropion hydrochloride, an antidepressant medication, no other nonnicotine preparation had been demonstrated to be as consistently effective as nicotine replacement. Early results from trials of bupropion suggest that it rivals the transdermal nicotine patch in effectiveness (Hurt et al., 1997). What makes this medication so attractive is that it does not rely on nicotine for success. Bupropion hydrochloride triggers a brain response similar to that caused by nicotine without causing addiction. As promising as Zyban appears, it is unclear whether it is an appropriate pharmaceutical smoking cessation medication for older smokers. Pharmaceutical research has documented that the elderly metabolize drugs more slowly and are more sensitive to drug side effects (Lipman, 1985). It is not recommended if the smoker is already taking another medication that is known to interact with bupropion. With those over age 65 consuming the largest amount of prescription drugs, a careful evaluation of the medication regimen is essential before Zyban is recommended for an older smoker.

SUMMARY

Quitting smoking is a multistage process of change. The theoretical framework known as the transtheoretical model (Prochaska & DiClemente, 1983) is a helpful guide for the design of successful interventions. According to this model, smokers succeed at stopping smoking by advancing through a sequence of motivational and behavioral change stages. These stages are:

1. Precontemplation—not currently thinking about quitting smoking.
2. Contemplation—seriously considering quitting smoking in the next 6 months.
3. Preparation—planning on quitting smoking in the next 30 days, with at least one quit attempt in the last year.
4. Action—stopping smoking.
5. Maintenance—begins 6 months after quitting and includes working to stay smoke-free.

Often smokers find that they must recycle through the stages of change in repeated efforts to quit smoking.

Although older smokers are a vulnerable group and present a different set of circumstances compared with younger smokers, including being highly addicted, having smoked for decades, and having health problems that are complicated by smoking, research indicates they are as likely, or more likely, to quit, with standard treatments (Orleans, 1997). Nevertheless, successful intervention among older smokers is not without barriers. Older smokers are less likely to believe in the health hazards of smoking. They also are likely to express that they enjoy smoking and view quitting as giving up a pleasure that they have grown to love and look forward to. Moreover, they are likely to use smoking as a personal coping strategy for weight control and/or stress. Many do not see the need for quitting or want to quit. Convincing older smokers of the risk is important to motivating a quit attempt. Different motivational and behavioral self-change processes are important in the stages of quitting. Stage-matched treatments produce greater quitting outcomes than stage-mismatched treatments. Thus, it is important to assess the older smoker's stage of change and apply a treatment suited to that stage. Interventions that emphasize skills development, problem solving, effective and appropriate use of nicotine replacement, and social support are more likely to be most effective with this group. Appropriate application of these tested methods, as well as diligent follow-up, results in significant smoking cessation outcomes for older smokers.

REFERENCES

Abrams, D. B., Orleans, C. T., Niaura, R. S., Goldstein, M. G., Prochaska, J. O., & Velicer, W. W. (1996). Integrating individual and public health perspectives for treatment of tobacco dependence under managed care: A combined stepped-care and matching model. *Annals of Behavioral Medicine, 18,* 290–304.

Abrams, J., Vela, B. S., Coultas, D. B., Samaan, S. A., Malhotra, D., & Roche, R. J. (1995). Coronary risk factors and their modification: Lipids, smoking, hypertension, estrogen, and the elderly. *Current Problems Cardiology 20,* 533–610.

Abramson, J. H. (1985). Prevention of cardiovascular disease in the elderly. *Public Health Reviews, 13*(3–4), 165–223.

Achkar, E. (1985). Peptic ulcer disease: Current management in the elderly. *Geriatrics, 40*(77–79), 82–83.

Agency for Health Care Policy and Research. (1996). *Smoking cessation: Clinical practice guideline no. 18* (AHCPR Publication No. 96-0692). Rockville, MD: U.S. Department of Health and Human Services.

Avorn, J., & Soumerai, S. B. (1983). Improving drug-therapy decisions through educational outreach: A randomized controlled trial of academically based "detailing." *New England Journal of Medicine, 308*, 1457–1463.

Burr, M. L., Phillips, K. M., & Hurst, D. N. (1985). Lung function in the elderly. *Thorax, 40*, 54–59.

Campbell, M. K., DeVellis, B. M., Strecher, V. J., Ammerman, A. S., DeVellis, R. F., & Sander, R. S. (1994). The impact of message tailoring on dietary behavior change for disease prevention in primary care settings. *American Journal of Public Health, 84*, 783–787.

Centers for Disease Control. (1996a). Cigarette smoking among adults—United States, 1994. *Morbidity and Mortality Weekly Report, 43*, 588–590.

Centers for Disease Control. (1996b). Smoking-attributable mortality, morbidity and economic costs (SAMMEC) 3.0 [Computer software and documentation]. Atlanta, GA: Author.

Chang, J. T., Moran, M. B., Cugell, D. W., & Webster, J. R. (1995). COPD in the elderly. A reversible cause of functional impairment. *Chest, 108*, 736–740.

Christen, W. G., Glynn, R. J., Manson, J. F., Ajani, U. A., & Buring, J. E. (1996). A prospective study of cigarette smoking and risk of age-related macular degeneration in men. *JAMA, 276*, 1147–1151.

Christen, W. G., Manson, J. E., Seddon, J. M., Glynn, R. J., Buring, J. E., Rosner, V., & Hennekens, C. H. (1992). A prospective study of cigarette smoking and risk of cataract in men. *JAMA, 268*, 989–993.

Cryer, B., Lee, E., & Feldman, M. (1992). Factors influencing gastroduodenal mucosal prostaglandin concentrations: Roles of smoking and aging. *Annals of Internal Medicine, 116*, 636–640.

Cummings, S. R., Rubin, S. M., & Oster, G. (1988). The cost-effectiveness of counseling smokers to quit. *JAMA, 261*, 75–79.

Dale, L. C., Olsen, D. A., Patten, C. A., Schroeder, D. R., Croghan, I. T., Hurt, R. D., Offord, K. P., & Wolter, T. D. (1997). Predictors of smoking cessation among elderly smokers treated for nicotine dependence. *Tobacco Control, 6*, 181–187.

Daniell, H. W. (1996). A better prognosis for obese men with prostate cancer. *Journal of Urology, 155*(1), 220–225.

D'Arcy, P. F. (1984). Tobacco smoking and drugs: A clinically important interaction? *Drug Intelligence and Clinical Pharmacology, 18*(4), 302–307.

Dolan, T. A., Gilbert, G. H., Ringelberg, M. L., Legler, D. W., Antonson, D. E., Foerster, U., & Heft, M. W. (1997). Behavioral risk indicators of attachment loss in adult Floridians. *Journal of Clinical Periodontology, 24*, 223–232.

Fiore, M. C., Bailey, W. C., Cohen, S. J., Dorfman, S. F., Goldstein, M. G., Heyman, R. B., Holbrook, J., Kottke, T. E., Lando, H. A., Mecklenburg, R., Mullen, P. D., Nett, L. M., Robinson, L., Stitzer, M. L., Tommasello, A. C., Villejo, L., & Wewers, M. E. (1996). Smoking Cessation. Clinical Guideline No. 18 (AHCPR Publication No. 96-0692). Rockville, MD: U.S. Department of Health and Human Services, Public Health Service.

Fiore, M. C., Novotny, T. E., Pierce, J. P., Giovino, J. P., Hatziandreu, E. J., Newcomb, P. A., Surawicz, T. S., & Davis, R. M. (1990). Methods used to quit smoking in the United States: Do cessation programs help? *JAMA, 263*, 2760–2765.

Fiore, M. C., Smith, S. S., Jorenby, D. E., & Baker, T. B. (1994). The effectiveness of the nicotine patch for smoking cessation: A meta-analysis. *JAMA, 271*, 1940–1947.

Ford, A. B., Mefrouche, Z., Freidland, R. P., & Debanne, S. M. (1996). Smoking and cognitive impairment: A population-based study. *American Journal of Geriatric Sociology, 44*, 905–909.

Fries, J. F., Green, L. W., & Levine, S. (1989). Health promotion and the compression of morbidity. *Lancet,* 481–483.

Frost, P. H., Davis, B. R., Burlando, A. J., Curb, J. D., Guthrie, G. P., Isaacsohn, J. L., Wassertheil-Smaller, S., Wilson, A. C., & Stamler, J. (1996). Coronary heart disease risk factors in men and women aged 60 years and older: Findings from the systolic hypertension in the elderly program. *Circulation, 94,* 26–34.

Gamble, C. L. (1995). Osteoporosis: Making the diagnosis in patients at risk for fracture. *Geriatrics, 50,* 7, 24–26, 29–30, 33.

Genco, R. J. (1996). Current view of risk factors for periodontal diseases. *Journal of Periodontology, 67*(10 suppl.), 1041–1049.

Glynn, T. J., & Manley, M. W. (1990). *How to help your patients stop smoking: A National Cancer Institute Manual for physicians* (NIH Publication No. 92-3064). Washington, DC: National Institutes of Health.

Gordon, T., Kannel, W., & McGee, D. (1974). Death and coronary attacks in men giving up cigarette smoking. *Lancet, 2,* 1345–1348.

Greenblatt, D. J., Allen, M. D., Harmatz, J. S., & Shader, R. I. (1980). Diazepam disposition determinants. *Clinical Pharmacology and Therapy, 27*(3), 301–312.

Grossi, S. D., Genco, R. J., Machtei, E. E., Ho, A. W., Koch, G., Dunford, R., Zambon, J. J., & Hausman, E. (1995). Assessment of risk for periodontal disease. II. Risk indicators for alveolar bone loss. *Journal of Periodontology, 66,* 23–29.

Gundert-Remy, U. (1995). Age as a factor in dose-reponse relationship of drugs. *Zeitschrift fuer Gerontologie und Geriatrie, 28,* 408–414.

Haug, M., & Ory, M. (1987). Issues in elderly patient provider interactions. *Research on Aging, 9*(1), 3–44.

Hermanson, B., Omenn, G. S., Kronmal, R. A., Gersh, B. J., & Participants in the Coronary Artery Surgery Study. (1988). Beneficial six-year outcome of smoking cessation in older men and women with coronary artery disease. *New England Journal of Medicine, 319*(21), 1365–1369.

Hicks, R., Dysken, M. W., Davis, J. M., Lesser, J., Ripeckyj, A., & Lazarus, L. (1981). The pharmacokinetics of psychotropic medication in the elderly: A review. *Journal of Clinical Psychiatry, 42,* 374–385.

Hill, R., Rigdon, M., & Johnson, S. (1993). Behavioral smoking cessation treatment for older chronic smokers. *Behavioral Therapy, 24,* 321–329.

Hirdes, J. P., & Maxwell, C. J. (1994). Smoking cessation and quality of life outcomes among older adults in the Cambell's Survey on Well-Being. *Canadian Journal of Public Health, 85,* 99–102.

Hirvela, H., Luukinen, H., & Laatikainen, L. (1995). Prevalence and risk factors of lens opacities in the elderly in Finland—A population-based study. *Ophthalmology, 102,* 108–117.

Howard, G., Toole, J. F., & Frye-Pierson, J. (1987). Factors influencing the survival of 451 transient ischemic attack patients. *Stroke, 18,* 552–557.

Hurt, R. D., Sachs, D. P. L., Glover, E. D., Offord, K. P., Johnston, J. A., Dale, L. C., Khayrallah, M. A., Schroeder, D. R., Glover, P. N., Sullivan, C. R., Croghan, I. T., & Sullivan, P. M. (1997). A comparison of sustained-release bupropion and placebo for smoking cessation. *New England Journal of Medicine, 337,* 1195–1202.

Husten, C. G., Shelton, D. M., Chrismon, J. H., Lin, Y.-C. W., Mowery, P., & Powell, F. A. (1997). Cigarette smoking and smoking cessation among older adults: United States, 1965–94. *Tobacco Control, 6,* 175–180.

Klein, R., Klein, B. E. K., Linton, K. L. P., & DeMets, D. L. (1993). The Beaver Dam eye study: The relation of age-related maculopathy to smoking. *American Journal of Epidemiology, 137,* 190–200.

Krumholz, H. M., Cohen, B. J., Tsevar, J., Pasternak, R. C., & Weinstein, M. C. (1993). Cost-effectivness of a smoking cessation program after myocardial infarction. *American Journal of the College of Cardiology, 22,* 1697–1702.

Larson, M. G. (1995). Assessment of cardiovascular risk factors in the elderly: The Framingham heart study. *Statistics and Medicine, 14*, 1745–1756.

Lee, T. K., Huang, Z. S., Ng, S. K., Chan, K. W., Wang, Y. S., Liu, H. W., & Lee, J. J. (1995). Impact of alcohol consumption and cigarette smoking on stroke among the elderly in Taiwan. *Stroke, 26*, 790–794.

Leonhardt, G., & Diener, H. C. (1996). Epidemiology and risk factors in stroke. *Therapeutische Umschau, 53*, 512–518.

Letenneur, L., Dartigues, J. F., Commenges, D., Barberger-Gateau, P., Tessier, J. F., & Orgogozo, J. M. (1994). Tobacco consumption and cognitive impairment in elderly people—a population-based study. *Annals of Epidemiology, 4*, 449–454.

Lipman, A. G. (1985). How smoking interferes with drug therapy. *Modern Medicine, 53*, 141–142.

Locker, D. (1992). Smoking and oral health in older adults. *Canadian Journal of Public Health, 83*, 429–432.

Mecklenburg, R. E., Christen, A. G., Gerbert, B., Gift, H. C., Glynn, T. J., Jones, R. B., Lindsay, E. A., Manley, M. W., & Severson, H. H. (1990). How to Help Your Patients Stop Using Tobacco: A National Cancer Institute Manual for the Oral Health Team (NIH Publication No. 91-3191). Washington, DC: U.S. Department of Health and Human Services, National Cancer Institute.

Menezes, A. M. B., Victora, C. G., & Rigatto, M. (1995). Chronic bronchitis and the type of cigarette smoked. *International Journal of Epidemiology, 24*, 95–99.

Moore, S. R. (1986). Smoking and drug effects in geriatric patients. *Pharmacy International, 7*(1), 1–3.

Morgan, G. D., Noll, E. L., Boyd, N. R., Bonney, G., Amfoh, K., Orleans, C. T., & Rimer, B. K. (1997, April). *Smoking Cessation Interventions for Older Adults: Long Term Outcomes From a Randomized Trial.* Paper presented at the Society of Behavioral Medicine, San Francisco, CA.

Morgan, G. D., Noll, E. L., Orleans, C. T., Rimer, B. K., Amfoh, K., & Bonney, G. (1996). Reaching midlife and older smokers: Tailored intervention for routine medical care. *Preventive Medicine, 25*, 346–364.

National Committee for Quality Assurance. (1996, July). *Health plan employer data and information set 3.0.* http://www.ncqa.org.

Nejjari, C., Tessier, J. F., Letenneur, L., Lafant, S., Dartigues, J. F., & Salamon, R. (1996). Determinants of chronic bronchitis prevalence in an elderly sample from the southwest of France. *Monaldi Archives of Chest Diseases, 51*, 373–379.

Orleans, C. T. (1993). Treating nicotine addiction in medical care settings: A stepped care model. In C. T. Orleans & J. Slade (Eds.), *Nicotine addiction: Principles and management* (pp. 145–161). New York: Oxford University Press.

Orleans, C. T. (1997). Reducing tobacco harms among older adults: A critical agenda for tobacco control. *Tobacco Control, 6*, 161–163.

Orleans, C. T., Boyd, N. R., Noll, E. L., Crossette, L., & Glassman, B. (1996, March). *Intervening Through a Prescription Benefit Plan for Nicotine Patch Users.* Paper presented at the Society of Behavioral Medicine Annual Meeting, Washington, DC.

Orleans, C. T., Boyd, N. R., Noll, E. L., Crossette, L., & Glassmann, B. (1998, March). *Computer-generated Smoking Cessation Feedback for Older Smokers.* Paper presented at the Society of Behavioral Medicine Annual Meeting, New Orleans, Louisiana.

Orleans, C. T., Jepson, C., Resch, N., & Rimer, B. K. (1994). Quitting motives and barriers among older smokers: The 1986 adult use of tobacco survey revisited. *Cancer, 74*, 2055–2061.

Orleans, C. T., Resch, N., Noll, E. L., Keintz, M. K., Rimer, B. K., Brown, T., & Snedden, T. (1994). Use of transdermal nicotine in a state-wide prescription plan for the elderly. *JAMA, 271*, 601–607.

Orleans, C. T., Rimer, B., Fleisher, L., Keintz, M. K., Telepchak, J., & Robinson, R. (1989). *Clear Horizons: A Quit Smoking Guide Especially for Those 50 and Over.* Philadelphia: Fox Chase Cancer Center.

Orleans, C. T., Rimer, B. K., Telepchak, J., Fleisher, L., Keintz, M. K., Boyd, N. R., Noll, E. L., & Robinson, R. (1995). *Clear Horizons: A Quit Smoking Guide Especially for Those 50 and Over* (2nd ed.). Philadelphia: Fox Chase Cancer Center.

Ossip-Klein, D. J., Carosella, A. M., & Krusch, D. A. (1997). Self-help interventions for older smokers. *Tobacco Control, 6,* 188–193.

Paganini-Hill, A., & Hsu, G. (1994). Smoking and mortality among residents of a California retirement community. *American Journal of Public Health, 84,* 992–995.

Personalized messages invite more mammography. (1994). *JAMA, 721,* 733–734.

Prochaska, J. O., & DiClemente, C. C. (1983). Stages and processes of self change of smoking: Toward an integrative model of change. *Journal of Consulting Clinical Psychology, 51,* 390–395.

Prochaska, J. O., DiClemente, C. C., & Norcross, J. C. (1992). In search of how people change: Applications to addictive behaviors. *American Psychologist, 47,* 1102–1114.

Prochaska, J. O., Velicer, W. F., Guadanogli, E., Rossi, J. S., & DiClemente, C. C. (1991). Patterns of change: Dynamic typology applied to smoking cessation. *Multivariate Behavioral Research, 26,* 83–107.

Rimer, B. K., & Orleans, C. T. (1990). Family physicians should intervene with older smokers. *American Family Physician, 42*(4), 959–965.

Rimer, B. K., Orleans, C. T., Fleisher, L., Cristinzio, S., Resch, N., Telepchak, J., & Keintz, M. K. (1994). Does tailoring matter? The impact of a tailored guide on ratings and short-term smoking-related outcomes for older smokers. *Health Education Research, 9,* 69–84.

Rimer, B. K., Orleans, C. T., Keintz, M. K., Cristinzio, S., & Fleisher, L. (1990). The older smoker: Status, challenges and opportunities for intervention. *Chest, 97,* 547–553.

Rimm, E. B., Chan, J., Stampfer, M. J., Colditz, G. A., & Willett, W. C. (1995). Prospective study of cigarette smoking, alcohol use, and the risk of diabetes in men. *British Medical Journal, 310,* 555–559.

Schneider, N. G. (1987). Nicotine gum in smoking cessation: Rationale, efficacy, and proper use. *Comprehensive Therapy, 13*(3), 32–37.

Schoon, I., Mellstrom, D., Oden, A., & Ytterberg, B. (1991). Peptic ulcer disease in older age groups in Gothenburg in 1985: The association with smoking. *Age and Ageing, 20,* 371–376.

Schumacher, M., & Smith, K. (1988). Diabetes in Utah among adults. *American Journal of Public Health, 78,* 1195–1201.

Seddon, J. M., Willett, W. C., Speizer, F. E., & Hankinson, S. E. (1996). A prospective study of cigarette smoking and age-related macular degeneration in women. *JAMA, 276,* 1141–1146.

Shinton, R. (1997). Lifelong exposures and the potential for stroke prevention: The contribution of cigarette smoking, exercise, and body fat. *Journal of Epidemiology and Community Health, 51,* 138–143.

Shopland, D. R., & Burns, D. M. (1993). Medical and public health implications of tobacco addiction. In C. T. Orleans & J. Slade (Eds.), *Nicotine addiction: Principles and management* (pp. 105–128). New York: Oxford University Press.

Shopland, D. R., Hartman, A. M., Gibson, J. T., Mueller, M. D., Kessler, L. G., & Lynn, W. R. (1996). Cigarette smoking among U.S. adults by state and region: Estimates from the current population survey. *Journal of the National Cancer Institute, 88,* 1748–1758.

Silagy, C., Mant, D., Fowler, G., & Lodge, M. (1994). Meta-analysis on efficacy of nicotine replacement therapies in smoking cessation. *Lancet, 343,* 139–142.

Sima, A. A., & Greene, D. A. (1995). Diabetic neuropathy in the elderly. *Drugs and Aging, 6*(2), 125–135.

Skinner, C. S., Strecher, V. J., & Hospers, H. J. (1994). Physician recommendations for mammography: Do tailored messages make a difference? *American Journal of Public Health, 84,* 43–49.

Somerville, K., Faulkner, G., & Langman, M. (1986). Non-steroidal anti-inflammatory drugs and bleeding peptic ulcer. *Lancet, 1,* 462–464.

Special Committee on Aging, United States Senate. (1986). *Developments in aging* (vol. 3, p. 10). Washington, DC: U.S. Government Printing Office.

Strecher, V. J., Kreuter, M. W., DenBoer, D. J., Kabrin, S., Hospers, H. J., & Skinner, C. S. (1994). The effects of computer-tailored smoking cessation messages in family practice settings. *Journal of Family Practice, 39*, 262–270.

Talseth, T., Boye, N. P., Kongerud, J., & Bredesen, J. E. (1981). Aging, cigarette smoking and oral theophylline requirement. *European Journal of Clinical Pharmacology, 21*, 33–37.

Tell, G. S., Polak, J. F., Ward, B. J., Kittner, S. J., Savage, P. J., & Robbins, J. (1994). Relation of smoking with carotid artery wall thickness and stenosis in older adults—the cardiovascular health study (CHS) collaborative research group. *Circulation, 90*, 2905–2908.

Todd, B. (1987). Drugs and the elderly. Cigarettes and caffeine in drug interactions. *Geriatric Nursing, 8*, 97–98.

U.S. Department of Health, Education, and Welfare. (1964). *Smoking and health. Report of the Advisory Committee to the Surgeon General of the Public Health Service* (PHS Publication No. 1103). Atlanta, GA: U.S. Department of Health, Education, and Welfare, Public Health Service, Center for Disease Control.

U.S. Department of Health and Human Services. (1984). *The health consequences of smoking: Chronic obstructive lung disease: A report of the Surgeon General* (DHHS Publication No. (PHS) 84-50205). Atlanta, GA: U.S. Department of Health and Human Services, Public Health Service, Centers for Disease Control, Office on Smoking and Health.

U.S. Department of Health and Human Services. (1989). *Reducing the health consequences of smoking: 25 Years of progress. A report of the Surgeon General* (DHHS Publication No. (CDC) 89-8411, prepublication version). Atlanta, GA: U.S. Department of Health and Human Services, Public Health Service, Centers for Disease Control, Center for Health Promotion and Education, Office on Smoking and Health.

U.S. Department of Health and Human Services. (1990). Long-term psychological and behavioral consequences and correlates of smoking cessation. In *The health benefits of smoking cessation: A report of the Surgeon General* (DHHS Publication No. (CDC) 90-8416, pp. 532–555, 561–578). Atlanta, GA: U.S. Department of Health and Human Services, Public Health Service, Centers for Disease Control, Center for Health Promotion and Education, Office on Smoking and Health.

U.S. Department of Health and Human Services. (1991a). *Clearing the air* (PHS Publication No. 91-1647). Rockville, MD: U.S. Department of Health and Human Services, Public Health Service, National Institutes of Health, National Cancer Institute.

U.S. Department of Health and Human Services. (1991b). *Healthy people 2000: National health promotion and disease prevention objectives* (DHHS Publication No. (PHS) 91-50212). Bethesda, MD: Public Health Service.

Velicer, W. F., Prochaska, J. O., Bellis, J. M., DiClemente, C. C., Rossi, J. S., Fava, J. L., & Steiger, J. H. (1993). An expert system intervention for smoking cessation. *Addictive Behaviors, 18*, 269–290.

Vetter, N. J., & Ford, D. (1990). Smoking prevention among people aged 60 years and over: A randomized controlled trial. *Age and Ageing, 19*, 164–168.

Vogt, M. T., Cauley, J. A., Scott, J. C., Kuller, L. H., & Browner, W. S. (1996). Smoking and mortality among older women: The study of osteoporotic fractures. *Archives of Internal Medicine, 156*, 630–636.

Part IV

Treatment Approaches: Medical and Psychological

CHAPTER SEVEN

Current Issues in Nicotine Replacement

Thomas Eissenberg
Virginia Commonwealth University

Maxine L. Stitzer
Johns Hopkins University School of Medicine

Jack E. Henningfield
Pinney Associates, Bethesda, Maryland

Smoking cessation is a major health care issue: Cigarette smoking increases the risk for a variety of cancers, chronic bronchitis, myocardial infarction, angina, peripheral vascular disease, problem pregnancies, and stroke. Annual health care costs attributed to cigarette smoking have been estimated at $50 billion each year, with an additional estimated $50 billion in indirect costs related to premature death and disease (U.S. Department of Health and Human Services, 1994a). Smoking cessation decreases an individual's risk for smoking-related disease, and can be expected to produce subsequent decreases in smoking-related health care costs (Henningfield, Ramstrom, et al., 1994). Many cigarette smokers report that they want to stop smoking, and this self-reported desire is evident in their behavior: Approximately one-third of all cigarette smokers attempt to quit smoking each year (Hatziandreu et al., 1990). Unfortunately, it has been estimated that 1-year success rates among these self-quitters is between only 3 and 8% (Cohen, Lichtenstein, & Prochaska, 1989; Fiore et al., 1990). Many current smokers who have been unable to sustain abstinence cite tobacco withdrawal, characterized by anxiety, restlessness, irritability, and cigarette craving (e.g., Hughes & Hatsukami, 1986; Shiffman & Jarvik, 1976; Tiffany & Drobes, 1991), as a reason. Medications intended to aid smoking cessation efforts are designed, at least in part, to alleviate these nicotine withdrawal symptoms.

Nicotine replacement medications are the most widely used and studied smoking cessation medications. Therapeutic nicotine administration reduces tobacco withdrawal symptoms, can reduce the pleasurable effects of the nicotine delivered by concurrently administered cigarettes (e.g., Nemeth-Coslett, Henningfield, O'Keefe, & Griffith, 1987), and can provide some of the desired effects of smoking. Nicotine replacement medications include nicotine polacrilex (gum) transdermal nicotine (patch), intranasal nicotine (spray), and a nicotine inhaler (vapor). Importantly, these medications are not intended as the sole treatment for smokers attempting cigarette abstinence. Instead, each is intended to be used as part of a comprehensive program that also includes some form of concurrent behavioral or psychosocial treatment (Fiore et al., 1996; Hall, Tunstall, Rugg, Jones, & Benowitz, 1985; Henningfield & Singleton, 1994).

Despite the "nicotine replacement" descriptor, not one of the four medications previously listed is capable of "replacing" the high arterial concentrations of smoked tobacco. Indeed, under approved use conditions, no currently available nicotine delivery system even mimics the rapid rise in venous nicotine levels typically produced by tobacco use (e.g., Henningfield, 1995). In theory, mimicking the blood nicotine levels achieved during smoking might provide increased withdrawal relief and more effectively mimic the desired effects of cigarette-delivered nicotine. However, despite producing relatively low blood levels of nicotine, the efficacy of the four nicotine delivery systems has been demonstrated in many well-controlled clinical trials. In this review we discuss briefly the efficacy of the various nicotine replacement medications. For purposes of this discussion, efficacy is defined as cigarette abstinence, as verified by expired carbon monoxide levels. Following this discussion of efficacy we present a more detailed account of how a variety of pharmacotherapy combinations that include nicotine replacement may help patients to quit smoking. We also address recent data regarding the use of nicotine replacement in several patient subgroups, including pregnant women, adolescents, and smokers with concurrent cardiovascular disorders.

THE CLINICAL EFFICACY OF FOUR NICOTINE DELIVERY SYSTEMS

Each of the four nicotine medications previously described has demonstrable efficacy as an aid to smoking cessation, but a brief summary of their similarities and differences may be useful in making recommendations to patients. Nicotine gum is a transmucosal nicotine delivery system that was approved in a 2-mg dosage form by the Food and Drug Administration (FDA) in 1984 and in a 4-mg dosage form in 1992. Four nicotine patch systems, available in a variety of dosages for use over 16- or 24-hr periods, were approved from the end of 1991 to mid 1992. Nicotine nasal spray was approved by the FDA in late 1996 and was designed to allow patients to more quickly and easily administer controlled nicotine doses on demand. The vapor inhaler, approved by the FDA in mid 1997, was designed to simulate more closely the sensations and behaviors provided by a cigarette by delivering small amounts of nicotine to the mouth and throat when the system is "puffed" on. The pharmacokinetics of most of these medications have been discussed elsewhere (e.g., Balfour & Fagerström, 1996; Henningfield, 1995), and some basic data describing them are provided in Table 7.1. The clinical efficacy of each of these medications is briefly reviewed next.

Clinical Efficacy of Nicotine Gum

The efficacy of nicotine gum treatment has been reviewed extensively (e.g., Balfour & Fagerström, 1996; Henningfield, 1995; Jorenby, Keehn, & Fiore, 1995; Silagy, Mant, Fowler, & Lokge, 1994). In general, these reviews indicate that, compared to placebo gum, nicotine gum can approximately double the percent of patients who remain cigarette abstinent for 6 months when compared to placebo, and can increase cessation rates by three- to fivefold above those achieved by people attempting to "quit on their own" without structured intervention or medication. Moreover, recent studies have demonstrated the enhanced treatment efficacy of 4-mg over 2-mg nicotine gum in smokers with higher levels of nicotine dependence (e.g., Fagerström Tolerance Score >7 of 11; Herrera et al., 1995; Sachs, 1995). Successful treatment depends, in part, on appropriate use of the medication; patients should chew a piece slowly until they experience a peppery taste, and then "park" the gum between the cheek and teeth until that taste fades. Repeated use of the "chew and park" procedure maximizes buccal nicotine absorption (Sachs, 1989). Coffee, soft drinks, and most other beverages should be avoided while nicotine gum is in the mouth; absorption of nicotine is reduced when acidic beverages are consumed (Henningfield, Radzius, Cooper, & Clayton, 1990). Overall quitting rates are related to the level of ancillary care ("therapy") provided along with the medication. Simply dispensing nicotine gum to patients provided little benefit over placebo in one study (e.g., Schneider et al., 1983), but was significantly better than placebo in a general practice setting that provided minimal but structured guidance (e.g., Sachs, 1995). Intensive adjunctive therapy can lead to still better outcomes (e.g., Hall et al., 1985).

Clinical Efficacy of Nicotine Patch

The clinical efficacy of nicotine patch treatment has also been extensively reviewed (e.g., Balfour & Fagerström, 1996; Fagerström, Säwe, & Tønnesen, 1993; Fiore, Smith, Jorenby, & Baker, 1994; Jorenby, Keehn, & Fiore, 1995; Silagy et al., 1994). These reviews reveal the short-term (i.e., 2–3 month)

TABLE 7.1
Some Pharmacokinetic Characteristics of Various Nicotine Delivery Systems

Nicotine Delivery System (Available Doses)	*Duration of Administration*	*Delivery Control*	*Maximal Venous Plasma Concentration (µg/L)*	*Approximate Time to Maximal Concentration*
Cigarette (1–2 mg)[a]	10 min	Inhalation	15–30	5–10 min
Gum (2 and 4 mg)	30 min	Chewing	10 (4 mg gum)	30 min
Transdermal patch				
Habitrol (7, 14, and 21 mg), manufactured by Novartis	24 hr	Rate-limiting membrane	17 (21 mg patch)	6 hr
Nicoderm (7, 14, and 21 mg), manufactured by Alza	24 hr	Rate-controlling membrane	23 (21 mg patch)	4 hr
Nicotrol (5[b], 10[b], and 15 mg), manufactured by Cygnus	16 hr	Adhesive	13 (15 mg patch)	5–11 hr
Prostep (11 and 22 mg), manufactured by Elan	24 hr	Gel matrix	16 (22 mg patch)	9 hr
Nasal spray (0.5 mg/spray)	30 sec	Manual pump	12 (2 mg dose)	10–15 min
Vapor inhaler (13 µg/puff)	20 min	Inhalation	8 (80 puffs)	35 min

Note. Venous cigarette and gum data from Benowitz, Porchet, Scheiner, and Jacob (1988); spray data from Sutherland et al. (1992); inhaler data from Schneider et al. (1996); patch data from Medical Economics Company (1996).

[a]Henningfield, Benowitz, and Kozlowski (1994); Benowitz et al. (1988).

[b]Not currently available in the United States.

efficacy of nicotine patch treatment, but also indicate that there is substantial cross-study variability regarding long-term efficacy (i.e., ≥1 year). For example, 20 of 21 placebo-controlled trials of nicotine patch treatment demonstrated that active patch treatment significantly enhanced 6-week cigarette abstinence (Balfour & Fagerström, 1996). Some individual studies have also reported dramatic increases in long-term abstinence relative to placebo; active treatment has tripled or even quadrupled year-long cigarette abstinence (e.g., Sachs, Säwe, & Leischow, 1993; Tønnesen et al., 1991). However, the fact that only 6/11 studies report successful sustained abstinence (i.e., at 1-year follow-up) after treatment was discontinued (Balfour & Fagerström, 1996) indicates that this medication is also best used along with a structured therapeutic program to help successful quitters more effectively sustain long-term abstinence. Additionally, there is increasing evidence supporting the idea that sustained tobacco abstinence may require longer-term treatment with nicotine replacement medications (e.g., Sachs et al., 1993). The treatment efficacy of the nicotine patch might also be increased by increasing the treatment dose in smokers with a high level of nicotine dependence (Dale et al., 1995; discussed later), but results using higher patch doses are less reliable than those documented for nicotine gum at higher dose levels (e.g., 4 mg; Herrera et al., 1995).

Clinical Efficacy of Nicotine Spray

Intranasal nicotine spray was developed, in part, to provide patients with more rapid delivery of nicotine than either the gum or the patch (see Table 7.1). In principle, more rapid delivery may enhance treatment efficacy by providing the cigarette-abstinent patient with faster and more readily controllable relief of cigarette craving and other cigarette withdrawal symptoms. The nasal spray consists of a small bottle containing a 10-mg/ml nicotine solution; a 50-μl spray containing 0.5 mg nicotine can be conveniently delivered using an attached manual pump mechanism. As can be seen in Table 7.1, this delivery system can produce significant elevations in nicotine blood levels within approximately 10 min.

The nasal spray provides the most rapid therapeutic nicotine delivery system now on the market. In fact, the delivery is quick enough to produce an approximate twofold transient increase in arterial nicotine levels compared to venous levels (Gourlay & Benowitz, 1996). This arterial "bolus" effect is much less pronounced than the 10-fold increase in arterial to venous ratio possible with cigarettes, however. Such an effect would not be expected to be provided by any other currently available nicotine replacement medication.

Three studies have examined the clinical efficacy of intranasal nicotine spray relative to placebo, and all three have demonstrated the efficacy of the active medication (Hjalmarsom, Franzon, Westkind, & Wiklund, 1994; Schneider et al., 1995; Sutherland et al., 1992). Patients in these studies used the medication for a minimum of 3 (Hjalmarsom et al., 1994; Sutherland et al., 1992) or 6 (Schneider et al., 1995) months; in two studies patients could choose to continue administering the medication for up to a year (Hjalmarsom et al., 1994; Sutherland et al., 1992). Long-term (1 year) abstinence rates, relative to placebo-treated patients, were 1.8 to 2.6 times greater in patients receiving active medication, and these rates were significantly greater than 1.0 in all three studies. Thus the intranasal nicotine spray can be added to a clinician's armamentarium of effective smoking cessation aids.

Clinical Efficacy of Nicotine Vapor

The nicotine vapor inhaler became available by prescription in the Spring of 1998. The vapor inhaler consists of a plastic tube-like mouthpiece into which can be inserted a cartridge containing a flavored 10-mg nicotine-impregnated porous plug. Nicotine is administered by inhaling air through the tube. Dose is, in part, a function of temperature, with colder temperature resulting in less nicotine delivery. In some controlled settings each inhalation yields up to approximately 13 μg at room temperature, thus requiring over 70 "puffs" to obtain the level of nicotine provided by one piece of 2-mg nicotine gum (Henningfield, 1995). In practice, nicotine delivery levels might be lower (Schuh et al., 1997). As can be seen in Table 7.1, nicotine absorption when delivered via the inhaler is slow relative to cigarettes, and resembles the absorption profile of nicotine gum. Indeed, as with the gum, vapor absorption is primarily through the buccal mucosa rather than the lung alveoli (Bergström, Nordberg, Lunell, Antoni, & Långström, 1995). Thus, vapor-delivered nicotine cannot achieve the rapid and high venous blood levels of nicotine delivered by a cigarette.

The published results of three controlled studies have examined the clinical efficacy of the nicotine vapor inhaler relative to placebo, and all support the short-term efficacy of the active medication (Glover, Glover, Nilsson, & Säwe, 1992; Schneider et al., 1996; Tønnesen, Nørregard, Mikkelsen, Jørgensen, & Nilsson, 1993). Patients in these studies used the medication for a minimum of 3 months; all patients were instructed to wean themselves off the medications during 3 additional months. All three studies demonstrated that 3-month abstinence rates, relative to rates in placebo-treated patients, were 1.7 to 2.9 times greater in patients receiving active medication, and these rates were each significantly greater than 1.0. The two studies that reported long-term (1 year) abstinence data provided less clear evidence of efficacy. Schneider et al. (1996) reported no significant difference between active and placebo groups at 1 year, whereas Tønnesen et al. (1993) reported that the rate of abstinence was 3.0 times greater in the patients treated with the active inhaler relative to placebo-treated patients. Further study of the nicotine vapor inhaler will be important to determine if its demonstrable short-term value can yield more consistent long-term benefits. Moreover, the similarity of the vapor delivery system to actual cigarettes remains a controversial issue and may contribute to an increase in the medication's abuse liability (e.g., Leischow, 1993), although the nicotine vapor inhaler appears less likely to be abused than a cigarette (Schuh et al., 1997).

ENHANCING EFFICACY THROUGH COMBINED TREATMENT

The recent FDA approval of the nicotine gum and patch for over-the-counter use and the availability of the nicotine spray and vapor inhaler by prescription represent welcome and much-needed advances in the treatment of nicotine dependence. However, all of the clinical trials that demonstrate treatment efficacy of these various medications also demonstrate that further advances in effective smoking cessation treatment programs can be made. For example, a review of clinical trials examining the efficacy of the nicotine patch shows that, of 17 double-blind, placebo-controlled studies, 22% of patients assigned to active medication were cigarette abstinent after 6 months (vs. 9% for placebo; Fiore et al., 1994). Thus 78% of treatment-seeking smokers treated with active medication relapsed to smoking.

There are several strategies that might be used to enhance the efficacy of nicotine replacement treatment and thus reduce the relapse rate. For example, different types of nicotine medications might be combined to enhance efficacy. Part of the logic behind such combined treatment involves the increased efficacy that might be observed if smokers received therapeutic doses of nicotine that more closely matched the blood levels of nicotine obtained through smoking (Dale et al., 1995). Another strategy that might be used to further advance the treatment efficacy of nicotine replacement medications might be to combine them with nonnicotine pharmacotherapies. Data related to both of these approaches are discussed next.

Combining Nicotine Delivery Medications to Enhance Efficacy

One of the simplest strategies for enhancing the treatment efficacy of nicotine replacement medications might be to combine existing nicotine delivery systems into a single treatment program. For example, a "sequential" medication regimen might involve patients using the patch to achieve abstinence, and then intermittently using nicotine gum as needed to sustain long-term abstinence (Henningfield, 1995). Alternatively, a "simultaneous" regimen might involve patients using nicotine patch and gum together to achieve abstinence. Such combinations might improve efficacy by increasing blood levels of nicotine to pretreatment (i.e., smoking) levels, thus presumably further reducing the anxiety, restlessness, irritability, and urges to smoke normally associated with acute cigarette abstinence. Furthermore, combinations that involve the nicotine patch and one of the three other nicotine delivery systems may allow patients to maintain a relatively stable blood nicotine level, which they can then augment through gum, spray, or vapor. On-demand augmentation of blood nicotine levels when urges to smoke or other withdrawal symptoms are most intense may help patients to reduce environmentally elicited cigarette cravings. Several studies have examined the efficacy of combined nicotine replacement medication. These studies examined doubled patch doses and patch plus gum treatment. To date, no studies have examined the combined efficacy of the nicotine patch and the spray or vapor.

High-Dose Patch Treatment. Doubling nicotine patch doses is one potential method for increasing blood nicotine level, and thus potentially increasing patch treatment efficacy. The maximum daily nicotine dose delivered using a single FDA-approved patch is 22 mg; greater doses can be delivered by administering more than one patch per day. Two double-blind studies (Dale et al., 1995; Jorenby, Smith, et al., 1995) examining the safety and efficacy of high-dose nicotine patch treatment have been reported; both found that high doses increased side effects somewhat, but only one found evidence of reliably enhanced efficacy. One inpatient study of 71 smokers indicated that, at least for moderate and heavy smokers (>16 cigarettes/day), 44 mg/day transdermal nicotine is safe (Dale et al., 1995). The only signs of nicotine toxicity (nausea, vomiting, perspiration, dizziness, visual disturbance, and weakness) were reported by a 10-cigarette/day smoker assigned to 44 mg/day, and these symptoms resolved after patch removal. Results from this study also suggested that 44 mg/day nicotine may have provided at least 100% nicotine replacement, as assessed by comparing blood cotinine levels during patch treatment to the pretreatment period.

An outpatient phase of the same study assessed the clinical efficacy of high-dose transdermal nicotine treatment (Dale et al., 1995). At the end of the 8-week medication period, 100% of patients assigned to 44-mg/day treatment remained cigarette abstinent, compared to 62% and 59% for patients assigned to 22- and 11-mg/day conditions, respectively. Significant differences between dosing conditions were apparent at 8 weeks but not at 6 months or 1 year. Thus the results of this study suggest that, at least during the active medication period, doubling patch dose can dramatically enhance cigarette abstinence relative to single patch treatment.

A second study also evaluated the safety and efficacy of high-dose nicotine patch treatment (Jorenby, Smith, et al., 1995). The results provided little support for the efficacy of 44 mg/day transdermal nicotine, and raised the possibility of increased side effects. In this study, 44 mg/day nicotine patch treatment was associated with significantly more nausea and irritation at the patch site as compared to 22 mg/day. Moreover, three patients, all receiving 44 mg/day nicotine, each experienced a potentially treatment-related serious adverse event during the study. Treatment efficacy was negligible, with no significant benefits apparent at the end of the 8-week trial dosing period. Finally, an open-label crossover study examined the effects of double patch treatment on nicotine withdrawal symptoms and side effects in a small group of patients ($n = 18$; 42 mg/day; Leischow et al., 1997) relative to single patch and no nicotine replacement. Results from this study indicated that the double patch treatment resulted in significantly more insomnia than single patch treatment.

Patch Plus Gum Treatment. One disadvantage of simply doubling daily transdermal nicotine dose is that nicotine blood levels are constantly high; patients can neither decrease nicotine intake to respond to internal stimuli that indicate nicotine toxicity (e.g., nausea), nor increase nicotine intake to respond to external stimuli that might elicit or exacerbate nicotine withdrawal (e.g., stress). A potential solution to this disadvantage is to combine the relatively low and steady nicotine blood levels provided by a single patch with the somewhat quicker and more on-demand nicotine delivery provided by the nicotine gum (e.g., Fagerström, 1994; Henningfield, 1995). There have been four reports comparing patch plus gum treatment with patch treatment alone: One report presented the results of a well-controlled, nontreatment crossover experiment designed to assess safety and withdrawal suppression (Fagerström, Säwe, & Tønnesen, 1993), another was a double-blind, placebo-controlled clinical trial (Kornitzer, Boutsen, Dramaix, Thijs, & Gustavsson, 1995), and the third and fourth were less controlled, open-label studies examining safety (Leischow et al., 1997) and short-term efficacy (Bittoun & Petrie, 1994). These studies are described next.

Fagerström, Schneider, and Lunell (1993) reported the results of an elegant study in which 28 smokers participated in four controlled 3-day conditions. The study compared active patch (15 mg/day) and active gum (2 mg), active patch and placebo gum, placebo patch and active gum, or placebo patch and placebo gum. Patients were required to chew a minimum of 4 and a maximum of 20 pieces of gum each day. No signs of nicotine toxicity were evident in any condition. The combination (active patch and active gum) condition suppressed withdrawal symptoms to baseline (i.e., smoking) levels, and provided significantly greater withdrawal suppression relative to placebo and to gum alone (see Figure 7.1A). Moreover, the combination

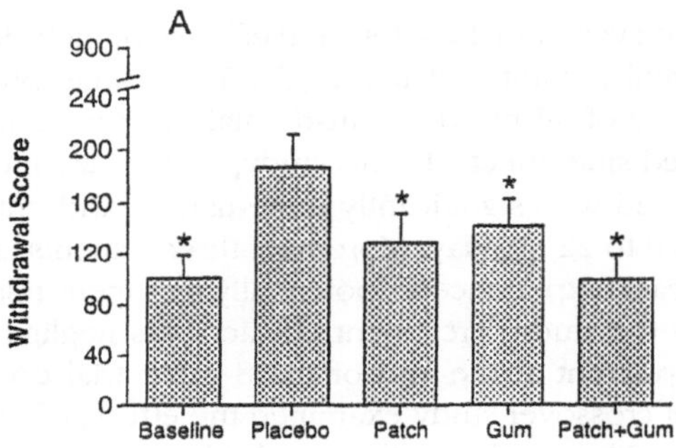

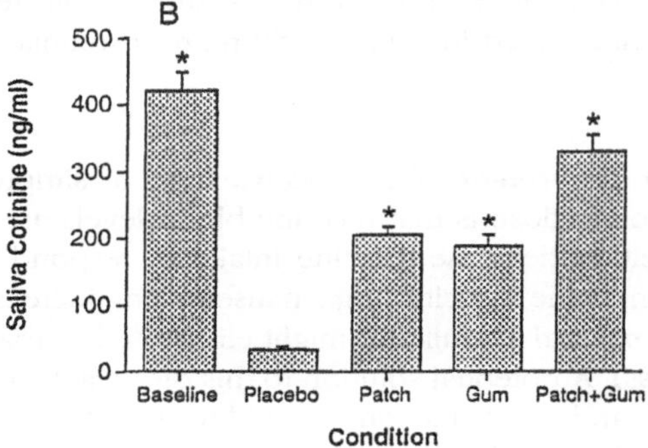

FIG. 7.1. (A) Subjective withdrawal and (B) blood cotinine levels from 28 smokers (10 female) who participated in four separate 3-day treatment conditions: smoking (baseline), placebo patch and placebo gum (placebo), active patch and placebo gum (patch), placebo patch and active gum (gum), and active patch and active gum (patch + gum). Asterisk indicates significant difference from placebo ($p < .05$). Data are from Fagerström, Schneider, and Lunnell (1993).

treatment produced saliva cotinine levels that were greater than in any other condition, and that were approximately 79% of baseline smoking levels (see Figure 7.1B). Thus, in this short-term, nontreatment study, combined nicotine patch and gum treatment was shown to be safe and completely effective at suppressing tobacco withdrawal.

The efficacy of the patch and gum combination has been tested in one placebo controlled clinical trial (Kornitzer et al., 1995). Patients ($n = 374$) in this study were moderate to heavy smokers (average of 24 cigarettes/day) who averaged two previous quit attempts. They were randomly assigned to one of three conditions: active patch and active gum (2 mg; $n = 149$), active patch and placebo gum ($n = 150$), or placebo patch and placebo gum ($n = 75$). All patients received patches for 24 weeks, and patients assigned to active patch treatment received 15 mg/day for 12 weeks, followed by 10 mg/day for 6 weeks and 5 mg/day for 6 weeks. No adverse events were reported. Significantly more patients assigned to the combination of active patch and gum remained cigarette abstinent at the end of the 24 week dosing period, relative to patients assigned to active patch and placebo gum (28% and 15%, respectively). However, this increased efficacy was not apparent at 52 weeks. Results from two open-label studies also support the safety (Bittoun & Petrie, 1994; Leischow et al., 1997) and short-term efficacy (Bittoun & Petrie, 1994) of the patch and gum combination.

The relatively few studies that have examined the efficacy of combined nicotine replacement therapy (either high-dose patch or patch and gum treatment) have produced somewhat equivocal results regarding long-term efficacy, and clearly more research is warranted. For example, 100% nicotine replacement, such as seen with the 44-mg patch treatment, may not necessarily lead to greater long-term efficacy. In an analysis of eight Phase III clinical trials of nicotine replacement products, only 1 of every 10 smokers required 100% or more nicotine replacement (based on pretreatment cotinine levels) to become cigarette abstinent (Li, Longmire, Kramer, & Wright, 1997). However, patients who attained 100% nicotine replacement had a significantly higher 1-year relapse rate relative to patients with less than 100% replacement (Li et al., 1997). A potential explanation for this higher relapse rate for multiple patch therapy is that excessive blood nicotine levels can make the patient sick and discontinue therapy. In comparison, patients who use gum plus patch can adjust their use of the gum if undesirable symptoms of nicotine exposure become apparent. Similar advantages seem likely with patch and spray or patch and vapor combinations.

Combining Nicotine Delivery With Nonnicotine Medications to Enhance Efficacy*

Another strategy that might be used to further advance the treatment efficacy of nicotine replacement medications might be to combine them with nonnicotine pharmacotherapies that also influence cigarette smoking. One of the most interesting of these nonnicotine pharmacotherapies is the nicotinic antagonist mecamylamine. Mecamylamine (Inversine) is an orally administered antihypertensive that acts peripherally and centrally as a noncompetitive nicotinic antagonist (e.g., Martin, Onaivi, & Martin, 1989). After acute administration, mecamylamine (10–20 mg) reduces the subjective and reinforcing effects of cigarettes and influences cigarette smoking behavior (Nemeth-Coslett, Henningfield, O'Keefe, & Griffiths, 1986; Pomerleau, Pomerleau, & Majchrzak, 1987; Rose, Sampson, Levin, & Henningfield, 1989;

**Editor's Note.* A recent clinical trial has demonstrated increased cessation rates when nicotine patch treatment is combined with bupropion, a nonnicotine aid for smokers who wish to stop. See chapter 8, pp. 168–170.

Stolerman, Goldfarb, Fink, & Jarvik, 1973) without adverse effect (Eissenberg, Griffiths, & Stitzer, 1996). Although the clinical efficacy of mecamylamine alone appears limited (Tennant, Tarver, & Rawson, 1984), theoretical and empirical support for nicotine patch plus mecamylamine treatment is growing (Rose & Levin, 1991; Rose et al., 1994b; Rose, Westman, & Behm, 1996b). We next review both the theory and data behind combined nicotine and mecamylamine treatment.

In theory, combined nicotine and mecamylamine treatment may lead to enhanced efficacy because the combination provides more complete nicotinic receptor blockade than would either medication if administered individually (Rose, 1996; Rose & Levin, 1991). More complete receptor blockade might enhance treatment efficacy by suppressing withdrawal and/or by decreasing the pleasurable effects of concurrently administered cigarettes (e.g., during a relapse episode). Side effects of mecamylamine, such as constipation, nausea, dry mouth, and dizziness, contributed to its negligible use as an antihypertensive medication and to its manufacturer discontinuing its marketing in 1996. However, supporters of the mecamylamine/nicotine combination argue that mecamylamine's side-effect profile might be reduced when used in combination with nicotine medications (e.g., Rose et al., 1996). Clearly, extensive work on these issues would be required if such a combination therapy were to be recommended for FDA approval and/or general use. Nonetheless, the concept of a combined nicotine antagonist/agonist therapy is intriguing and has received some empirical support, reviewed next.

There are four reports, all from the same laboratory, that support the idea of combined mecamylamine/nicotine smoking cessation therapy (Rose et al., 1994a, 1994b, 1996a; Rose et al., 1996b). In two experimental studies (Rose et al., 1994a, 1996a), combined nicotine patch and oral mecamylamine acted together to attenuate cigarette craving and subjective effects of concurrent smoking such as cigarette satisfaction, liking, and so on. There have been two double-blind placebo-controlled clinical trials of the nicotine patch plus oral mecamylamine combination (Rose et al., 1994b, 1996b). In the first of these (Rose et al., 1994b), 48 moderate to heavy smokers (average of 28 cigarettes/day) were randomized to nicotine patch (21 mg/day) plus mecamylamine (5 mg po, b.i.d.) or nicotine patch plus oral placebo. Patients were treated with the 21 mg patch for a maximum of 8 weeks, and then were given additional treatment with 14 mg (1 week) and then 7 mg (1 week) patches. Mecamylamine treatment overlapped with the 21 mg/day patch treatment, lasted for 5 weeks, and began with 2 days of 2.5 mg b.i.d. At 1 year follow-up, nine times as many patients treated with the patch plus mecamylamine combination remained cigarette abstinent, relative to those patients treated with the patch alone (37.5% vs. 4.2%, a statistically significant difference). Similar findings have been reported in a replication (Rose et al., 1996b). Thus the results of this trial demonstrate the potential benefit that might be gained through combined nicotine and mecamylamine treatment.

Besides mecamylamine, there have been many other nonnicotine medications that have been considered for use as smoking cessation aids (for a review, see Hughes, 1994). For example, the opioid antagonist naltrexone has been suggested as a medication that might increase cigarette abstinence, just as it increases alcohol abstinence (e.g., O'Malley et al., 1992; Volpicelli, Alterman, Hayashida, & O'Brien, 1992). However, few studies have demonstrated that opioid antagonists reliably influence smoking behavior (e.g., Karras & Kane, 1980; Nemeth-Coslett & Griffiths, 1986). Similarly, clonidine, an alpha-adrenergic agonist, has also been suggested as a nonnicotine smoking cessation medication (e.g., Covey & Glassman, 1991; Glassman et al., 1988; Gourlay & Benowitz, 1995; Niaura, Goldstein, Murphy, & Abrams, 1996; Prochazka et al., 1992). A meta-analysis of placebo-controlled trials using oral or transdermal clonidine as a smoking cessation medication revealed that active clonidine is more effective than placebo, at least in the short term (Covey & Glassman, 1991), although adverse effects such as sedation and dizziness may limit its clinical utility (Gourlay & Benowitz, 1995). There is also some evidence suggesting that clonidine's efficacy as a smoking cessation medication is greatest in women (Covey & Glassman, 1991; Gourlay & Benowitz, 1995). To date, there are no controlled studies evaluating these medications in combination with nicotine replacement.

One inventive approach that combines nicotine patch treatment with a nonnicotine treatment involves an inhaler that delivers no nicotine. Rather, the inhaler delivers a citric acid dose that provides smokers with an airway sensation similar to that of a smoked cigarette. Laboratory studies have demonstrated that this citric acid inhaler reduces cigarette craving (Levin, Rose, & Behm, 1990; Rose & Hickman, 1987) and enhances short-term (3 week) abstinence (Behm et al., 1993). In a large-scale placebo-controlled trial of moderate to heavy smokers (average of 31 cigarettes per day), this nonnicotine citric acid inhaler was combined with nicotine patch treatment (Westman, Behm, & Rose, 1995). All smokers were given 21-mg/day patches for 4 weeks, and then were given additional treatment with 14-mg (1 week) and then 7-mg (1 week) patches. No formal counseling was offered, although all patients received self-help manuals. Forty-one patients were randomized to active citric acid inhalers, and 59 were randomized to placebo (lactose) inhalers. Inhalers were provided for 10 weeks; thus, inhaler use was continued 4 weeks after patch treatment ceased. There were no differences in adverse effects between the two groups. At the end of the 10-week trial, a significantly higher proportion of patients assigned to active inhalers (19.5%) remained cigarette abstinent relative to those assigned to placebo (6.8%), although all patients had relapsed at 6-month follow-up. Despite poor long-term success rates, the citric acid inhaler represents an innovative method of therapeutically dissociating smoking-related cues (i.e., airway sensations that accompany smoke inhalation) from nicotine delivery. Dissociating smoking-related cues from nicotine delivery may be an important step in helping smokers to overcome cigarette cravings that have developed over years of repeated nicotine self-administration.

NICOTINE REPLACEMENT IN SPECIAL POPULATIONS

Many clinical trials of nicotine replacement pharmacotherapies include male and nonpregnant female patients who are over the age of 18 years and do not have a history of or active cardiovascular disease. Thus the safety and efficacy of these medications in pregnant women, adolescents, and patients with concurrent cardiovascular disorders is less well studied. Given that nicotine gum and patch are now available over the counter and thus readily available to all smokers, determining the safety and efficacy of these products in various patient subgroups is of increased importance. In this section we summarize recent research aimed at examining the safety and/or efficacy of nicotine replacement in pregnant women, adolescents, and patients with concurrent cardiovascular disorders.

Nicotine Replacement in Pregnant Smokers

An extensive literature demonstrates that smoking during pregnancy is associated with adverse reproductive effects such as prematurity, low birth weight, low Apgar scores, and increased fetal and neonatal mortality (e.g., Benowitz, 1991a; Garn, Johnston, Ridella, & Petzold, 1981; Haddow, Knight, Palomaki, Kloza, & Wald, 1987; Nieburg, Marks, McLaren, & Remington, 1985). Lack of oxygen to the fetus (i.e., fetal hypoxia) may underlie many of these adverse effects (Benowitz, 1991a). Fetal hypoxia may be due in part to cigarette-delivered nicotine, but is certainly also due to the carbon monoxide and several thousand other toxic chemicals that pregnant women inhale with each cigarette. The adverse reproductive effects of smoking can be avoided if pregnant smokers quit smoking early in their pregnancy (e.g., MacArthur, Newton, & Knox, 1987; Sexton & Hebel, 1984).

Nicotine may adversely alter uteroplacental circulation (Benowitz, 1991a); thus, the best way of avoiding smoking-related reproductive adverse effects is to cease all nicotine intake prior to or immediately after becoming pregnant. However, because nicotine replacement therapies typically produce blood nicotine levels well below those associated with smoking and do not involve the intake of carbon monoxide or other toxic chemicals, nicotine replacement poses fewer reproductive risks than does cigarette smoking (Benowitz, 1991a). A review of evidence supporting this statement can be found later in this section. Therefore, it has been suggested that pregnant women who have been unable to quit smoking in the past may experience better reproductive outcomes with nicotine replacement than without it. More controlled study of this topic is necessary before firm recommendations can be made.

Pregnancy is not a contraindication (i.e., Pregnancy Category X) for nicotine replacement therapy. Rather, nicotine gum carries a Pregnancy Category C warning, which means that "risk cannot be ruled out," whereas transdermal systems have been accorded Pregnancy Category D, which implies "positive evidence of risk." The more conservative warning for the patch is because patch treatment more readily provides nicotine doses equivalent to those that have adverse effects in studies of pregnant animals. Both of these warning levels imply that the medication may be used during pregnancy but that the risks and benefits should be evaluated against alternatives such as continued cigarette smoking, which poses a definite and substantial risk during pregnancy.

Few studies have explicitly examined the effects of nicotine replacement treatment on fetal development in the human. In studies that have examined single doses of nicotine gum, results indicate that, relative to smoking, nicotine gum produces smaller perturbations in fetal heart rate and breathing and uterine and umbilical blood flow (Lehtovirta, Forss, Rauramo, & Karniniemi, 1983; Lindblad, Marsal, & Andersson, 1988; Lindblad & Marsal, 1987). A recent study (Oncken et al., 1996) reported the results of a randomized safety trial of pregnant smokers who continued smoking or were treated for 5 consecutive days with 2-mg gum (minimum of 6 pieces/day). In that study, the first that has examined sustained use of nicotine replacement during pregnancy, gum use was associated with lower blood levels of nicotine and cotinine relative to smoking, with no significant differences in measures of maternal or fetal heart rate. Preliminary reports of a similar study of the nicotine patch suggest that nicotine levels are similar between patch and moderate smoking conditions, and that maternal blood pressure is increased during patch use relative to smoking (Hardardottir et al., 1997). Of course, when nicotine is delivered transdermally, neither the fetus nor the mother is exposed to the rapid and high nicotine dose level spikes produced by cigarettes.

Nicotine Replacement in Adolescent Smokers

Each day approximately 3,000 American adolescents begin to smoke on a regular basis (Glynn, Anderson, & Schwarz, 1991); one-third of these adolescent smokers may prematurely die, given current levels of cessation (FDA, 1996). Adolescent smokers who abstain from cigarettes experience tobacco withdrawal similar to that of adults (McNeil, West, Jarvis, Jackson, & Bryant, 1986; U.S. Department of Health and Human Services, 1994b). Over two-thirds of smokers regret having started smoking and nearly one-half of all adolescents smokers have tried to quit and failed by age 17 (FDA, 1996; U.S. Department of Health and Human Services, 1994b). Failed quit attempts in adolescent smokers may be at least partially due to a physical dependence on nicotine that leads to withdrawal during periods of cigarette abstinence (Prokhorov, Pallonen, Fava, Ding, & Niaura, 1996). If tobacco withdrawal during quit attempts leads to relapse in adolescents, than nicotine replacement may be useful in increasing abstinence rates in this population.

Only one study to date has examined nicotine replacement in adolescent smokers (Smith et al., 1997). In this open-label study, low rates of generally mild adverse events (e.g., skin reactions, headaches, nausea, and vomiting) were observed in 22 adolescent smokers assigned to 22-mg/day nicotine patch therapy, supporting the hypothesis that adolescent cigarette smokers generally respond like adult smokers to transdermal nicotine. These preliminary results suggest that more controlled safety and efficacy studies are warranted to evaluate the potential application of nicotine replacement therapy for adolescents.

NICOTINE REPLACEMENT IN SMOKERS WITH CONCURRENT CARDIOVASCULAR DISORDERS

Acute nicotine administration can increase heart rate and blood pressure and can cause coronary vasoconstriction. Such effects may increase the risk of using nicotine medications in smokers with concurrent cardiovascular disorders. However, the safety of these medications *relative to smoking* appear generally to outweigh the risks: Nicotine delivered by gum or patch leads to smaller cardiovascular effects than nicotine delivered by tobacco smoke (e.g., Benowitz, 1991b; U.S. Department of Health and Human Services, 1988). Thus use of these medications during a period of cigarette abstinence may actually decrease the likelihood of an acute cardiovascular event. In a recent randomized, double-blind, placebo-controlled clinical trial examining nicotine patch treatment in 584 patients with cardiovascular disease (576 males), 10 weeks of active treatment (21 mg for 6 weeks, 14 mg for 2 weeks, 7 mg for 2 weeks) did not lead to an increased incidence of cardiovascular events (Joseph et al., 1996). Short-term (14-week) efficacy of the active patch treatment relative to placebo was observed, but long-term (24-week) smoking cessation outcomes did not differ significantly between active and placebo conditions. Further research may be needed to help determine how nicotine replacement medications can be used in this population to maximize both safety and long-term efficacy.

CONCLUSIONS

Nicotine replacement therapy clearly can be an effective part of a comprehensive smoking cessation program. Across all of the four medications reviewed here, the odds of successful quitting approximately doubled (APA,

1996; Fiore et al., 1996; Silagy et al., 1994). Despite this demonstrable effectiveness of nicotine replacement medication over placebo, absolute abstinence rates show much room for improvement. In trials with long-term (i.e., 1 year) follow-up data, the portion of patients who remain abstinent is typically less than 30%. Future directions for research include how best to maximize treatment outcomes using nicotine replacement medications. Some of the possibilities reviewed here include combining nicotine replacement medications, either sequentially or simultaneously, and combining nicotine medications with other pharmacotherapies. Research already indicates that intensive concurrent psychosocial treatment enhances treatment outcomes (e.g., Hall et al., 1985).

The current literature is limited in that it applies largely to healthy, adult men and nonpregnant women. Smokers seeking help in achieving cigarette abstinence may suffer a variety of health problems, may be adolescents, and/or may be pregnant. The apparent safety and efficacy of nicotine replacement in the general population, as well as the clear risks of cigarette smoking, suggest that further study of nicotine replacement in these populations is appropriate and necessary.

REFERENCES

American Psychiatric Association. (1996). Practice guidelines for the treatment of patients with nicotine dependence. *American Journal of Psychiatry, 153*, 1–31.

Balfour, D. J. K., & Fagerström, K. O. (1996). Pharmacology of nicotine and its therapeutic use in smoking cessation and neurodegenerative disorders. *Pharmacology & Therapeutics, 72*, 51–81.

Behm, F. M., Schur, C., Levin, E. D., Tashkin, D. P., & Rose, J. E. (1993). Clinical evaluation of a citric acid inhaler for smoking cessation. *Drug and Alcohol Dependence, 31*, 131–138.

Benowitz, N. L. (1991a). Nicotine replacement therapy during pregnancy. *JAMA, 226*, 3174–3177.

Benowitz, N. L. (1991b). Nicotine and coronary heart disease. *Trends in Cardiovascular Medicine, 1*, 315–321.

Benowitz, N. L., Porchet, H., Sheiner, L., & Jacob, P. (1988). Nicotine absorption and cardiovascular effects with smokeless tobacco use: Comparison with cigarettes and nicotine gum. *Clinical Pharmacology and Therapeutics, 44*, 23–28.

Bergström, M., Nordberg, A., Lunell, E., Antoni, G., & Långström, B. (1995). Regional deposition of inhaled ^{11}C-nicotine vapor in the human airway as visualized by positron emission tomography. *Clinical Pharmacology and Therapeutics, 57*, 309–317.

Bittoun, R., & Petrie, J. (1994). Nicotine patch combined with nicotine gum in smoking cessation. *Journal of Smoking Related Disorders, 5*(suppl. 1), 314.

Cohen, S., Lichtenstein, E., & Prochaska, J. O. (1989). Debunking myths about self-quitting. *American Psychologist, 11*, 1355–1365.

Covey, L. S., & Glassman, A. H. (1991). A meta-analysis of double-blind placebo-controlled trials of clonidine for smoking cessation. *British Journal of Addiction, 86*, 991–998.

Dale, L. C., Hurt, R. D., Offord, K. P., Lawson, C. M., Schroeder, D. R., et al. (1995). High dose nicotine patch therapy. *JAMA, 274*, 1353–1358.

Eissenberg, T. E., Griffiths, R. R., & Stitzer, M. L. (1997). Mecamylamine does not precipitate withdrawal in cigarette smokers. *Psychopharmacology, 127*, 328–336.

Fagerström, K. O. (1994). Combined use of nicotine replacement products. *Health Values, 18*, 15–20.

Fagerström, K. O., Säwe, U., & Tønnesen, P. (1993). Therapeutic use of nicotine patches: Efficacy and safety. *Journal of Drug Development, 5*, 191–205.

Fagerström, K. O., Schneider, N. G., & Lunell, E. (1993). Effectiveness of nicotine patch and nicotine gum as individual versus combined treatments for tobacco withdrawal symptoms. *Psychopharmacology, 111*, 271–277.

Fiore, M. C., Bailey, W. C., Cohen, S. J., Dorfman, S. F., Goldstein, M. G., Gritz, E. R., Heyman, R. B., Holbrook, J., Jaen, C. R., Kottke, T. E., Lando, H. A., Mecklenburg, R., Mullen, P. D., Nett, L. M., Robinson, L., Stitzer, M. L., Tommasello, A. C., Villejo, L., & Wewers, M. E. (1996). *Smoking cessation. Clinical practice guideline no. 18* (AHCPR Publication No. 96-0692). Rockville, MD: U.S. Department of Health and Human Service, Agency for Health Care Policy and Research.

Fiore, M. C., Smith, S. S., Jorenby, D. E., & Baker, T. B. (1994). The effectiveness of nicotine patch for smoking cessation: A meta-analysis. *JAMA, 271*, 1940–1947.

Fiore, M. C., Novotny, T. E., Pierce, J. P., Giovino, G. A., Hatziandreu, E. J., Newcomb, P. A., Surawicz, T. S., Davis, R. M., et al. (1990). Methods used to quit smoking in the United States: do cessation programs help. *JAMA, 263*, 2760–2765.

Food and Drug Administration. (1996, August 28). 21 CFR Part 801, et al. Regulations restricting the sale and distribution of cigarettes and smokeless tobacco products to protect children and adolescents; Final rule. *Federal Register, 61*, 44396–45318.

Garn, S. M., Johnston, M., Ridella, S. A., & Petzold, A. S. (1981). Effect of maternal cigarette smoking on Apgar scores. *American Journal of Diseases of Children, 135*, 503–506.

Glassman, A. H., Stetner, F., Walsh, B. T., Raizman, P. S., Fleiss, J. L., Cooper, T. B., Covey, L. S., et al. (1988). Heavy smokers, smoking cessation, and clonidine. *JAMA, 259*, 2863–2866.

Glover, E. D., Glover, P. N., Nilsson, F., & Säwe, U. (1992, March). *Nicotine inhaler (nicohaler) versus placebo in smoking cessation: A clinical evaluation (preliminary results)*. Paper presented at the Society of Behavioral Medicine 13th Annual Scientific Sessions, New York.

Glynn, T. J., Anderson, D. M., & Schwarz, L. (1991). Tobacco use reduction among high-risk youth. *Preventive Medicine, 20*, 279–291.

Gourlay, S. G., & Benowitz, N. L. (1996, March). *Arterio-venous differences in plasma nicotine concentrations with nicotine nasal spray*. Paper presented at the Society for Research on Nicotine and Tobacco, Second Annual Scientific Conference, Washington, DC.

Gourlay, S. G., & Benowitz, N. L. (1995). Is clonidine an effective smoking cessation therapy? *Drugs, 50*, 197–207.

Haddow, J. E., Knight, G. J., Palomaki, G. E., Kloza, E. M., & Wald, N. J. (1987). Cigarette consumption and serum cotinine in relation to birthweight. *British Journal of Obstetrics and Gynaecology, 94*, 678–681.

Hall, S. M., Tunstall, C. D., Rugg, D., Jones, R. T., & Benowitz, N. (1985). Nicotine gum and behavioral treatment in smoking cessation. *Journal of Consulting Clinical Psychology, 2*, 256–258.

Hardardottir, H., Oncken, C., Lupo, V. R., Daragjati, L., Chang, R., & Smeltzer, J. S. (1997). Maternal and fetal cardiovascular effects of a nicotine-patch versus maternal smoking. *American Journal of Obstetrics and Gynecology, 174*, 367.

Hatziandreu, E. J., Pierce, J. P., Lefkopoulou, M., Fiore, M. C., Mills, S. L., Novotny, T. E., Giovino, G. A., & Davis, R. M. (1990). Quitting smoking in the United States in 1986. *JNCI, 82*, 1402–1406.

Henningfield, J. E. (1995). Nicotine medications for smoking cessation. *New England Journal of Medicine, 333*, 1196–1203.

Henningfield, J. E., Benowitz, N. E., & Kozlowski, L. T. (1994). A proposal to develop meaningful labeling for cigarettes. *JAMA, 272,* 312–314.

Henningfield, J. E., Ramstrom, L. M., Husten, C. G., Giovino, G. A., Zhu, B. P., Barling, J., Weber, C., Kelloway, E. K., Strecher, V. J., Jarvis, M. J., & Weiss, J. (1994). Smoking and the workplace: Realities and solutions. *Journal of Smoking-Related Diseases, 5*(suppl. 1), 261–270.

Henningfield, J. E., & Singleton, E. G. (1994). Managing drug dependence: Psychotherapy or pharmacotherapy? *CNS Drugs, 1,* 317–322.

Henningfield, J. E., Radzius, A., Cooper, T. M., & Clayton, R. R. (1990). Drinking coffee and carbonated beverages blocks absorption of nicotine from nicotine polacrilex gum. *JAMA, 264,* 1560–1564.

Herrera, N., Franco, R., Herrera, L., Partidas, A., Rolando, R., Fagerström, K. O., et al. (1995). Nicotine gum, 2 and 4 mg, for nicotine dependence: A double-blind placebo controlled trial within a behavior modification support program. *Chest, 106,* 447–461.

Hjalmarson, A., Franzon, M., Westin, A., & Wiklund, O. (1994). Effect of nicotine nasal spray on smoking cessation: A randomized, placebo-controlled, double-blind study. *Archives of Internal Medicine, 154,* 2567–2672.

Hughes, J. R. (1994). Non-nicotine pharmacotherapies for smoking cessation. *Journal of Drug Development, 6,* 197–203.

Hughes, J. R., & Hatsukami, D. K. (1986). Signs and symptoms of tobacco withdrawal. *Archives of General Psychiatry, 43,* 289–294.

Jorenby, D. E., Keehn, D. S., & Fiore, M. C. (1995). Comparative efficacy and tolerability of nicotine replacement therapies. *CNS Drugs, 3,* 227–236.

Jorenby, D. E., Smith, S. S., Fiore, M. C., Hurt, R. D., Offord, K. P., Croghan, I. T., Hays, J. T., Lewis, S. F., & Baker, T. B. (1995). Varying nicotine patch dose and type of smoking cessation counseling. *JAMA, 274,* 1347–1352.

Joseph, A. M., Norman, S. M., Ferry, L. H., Prochazka, A. V., Westman, E. C., Steele, B. G., Sherman, S. E., Cleveland, M., Antonnucio, D. O., Hartman, N., & McGovern, P. G. (1996). The safety of transdermal nicotine as an aid to smoking cessation in patients with cardiac disease. *New England Journal of Medicine, 335,* 1792–1798.

Karras, A., & Kane, J. (1980). Naloxone reduces cigarette smoking. *Life Sciences, 27,* 1541–1545.

Kornitzer, M., Boutsen, M., Dramaix, M., Thijs, J., & Gustavsson, G. (1995). Combined use of nicotine patch and gum in smoking cessation: A placebo-controlled clinical trial. *Preventive Medicine, 24,* 41–47.

Lehtovirta, P., Forss, M., Rauramo, I., & Karniniemi, V. (1983). Acute effects of nicotine on fetal heart rate variability. *British Journal of Obstetrics and Gynaecology, 90,* 710–715.

Leischow, S. J. (1994). The nicotine vaporizer. *Health Values, 18,* 4–9.

Leischow, S. J., Valente, S. N., Hill, A. L., Otte, P. S., Aickin, M., Holden, T., Kligman, E., & Cook, G. (1997). Effects of nicotine dose and administration method on withdrawal symptoms and side effects during short-term smoking abstinence. *Experimental and Clinical Psychopharmacology, 18,* 4–9.

Levin, E. D., Rose, J. E., & Behm, F. M. (1990). Development of a citric acid aerosol as a smoking cessation aid. *Drug and Alcohol Dependence, 31,* 131–138.

Li, C. Q., Longmire, A. W., Kramer, E. D., & Wright, C. (1997, March). *Doses of nicotine replacement therapy (NRT).* Paper presented at the American Society of Clinical Pharmacology and Experimental Therapeutics 98th Annual Meeting, San Diego.

Lindblad, A., & Marsal, K. (1987). Influence of nicotine chewing gum on fetal blood flow. *Journal of Perinatal Medicine, 15,* 13–19.

Lindblad, A., Marsal, K., & Andersson, K. E. (1988). Effect of nicotine on human fetal blood flow. *Obstetrics and Gynecology, 72,* 371–382.

MacArthur, C., Newton, J. R., & Knox, E. G. (1987). Effect of anti-smoking health education on infant size at birth: A randomized controlled trial. *British Journal of Obstetrics and Gynaecology, 94,* 295–300.

Martin, B. R., Onaivi, E. S., & Martin, T. J. (1989). What is the nature of mecamylamine's antagonism of the central effects of nicotine? *Biochemical Pharmacology, 38*, 3391–3397.

McNeil, A. D., West, R. J., Jarvis, M. J., Jackson, P., & Bryant, A. (1986). Cigarette withdrawal symptoms in adolescent smokers. *Psychopharmacology, 90*, 533–536.

Medical Economics Company. (1996). *Physicians' desk reference.* Montvale, NJ: Author.

Nemeth-Coslett, R., & Griffiths, R. R. (1986). Naloxone does not affect cigarette smoking. *Psychopharmacology, 89*, 261–264.

Nemeth-Coslett, R., Henningfield, J. E., O'Keefe, M. K., & Griffiths, R. R. (1986). Effects of mecamylamine on human cigarette smoking and subjective ratings. *Psychopharmacology, 88*, 420–425.

Nemeth-Coslett, R., Henningfield, J. E., O'Keefe, M. K., & Griffiths, R. R. (1987). Nicotine gum: Dose-related effects on cigarette smoking and subjective ratings. *Psychopharmacology, 92*, 424–430.

Niaura, R. S., Brown, R. A., Goldstein, M. G., Murphy, J. K., & Abrams, D. B. (1996). Transdermal clonidine for smoking cessation: A double-blind randomized dose-response study. *Experimental Clinical Psychopharmacology, 4*, 285–291.

Nieburg, P., Marks, J. S., McLaren, N. M., & Remington, P. L. (1985). The fetal tobacco syndrome. *JAMA, 253*, 2998–2999.

Oncken, C. A., Hatsukami, D. K., Lupo, V. R., Lando, H. A., Gibeau, L. M., & Hansen, R. J. (1996). Effects of short-term use of nicotine gum in pregnant smokers. *Clinical Pharmacology and Therapeutics, 59*, 654–661.

O'Malley, S. S., Jaffe, A., Chang, G., Schottenfeld, R. S., Meyer, R. E., & Rounsaville, B. J. (1992). Naltrexone and coping skills therapy for alcohol dependence: A controlled study. *Archives of General Psychiatry, 49*, 881–887.

Pomerleau, C. S., Pomerleau, O. F., & Majchrzak, M. J. (1987). Mecamylamine pretreatment increases subsequent nicotine self-administration as indicated by changes in plasma nicotine level. *Psychopharmacology, 91*, 391–393.

Prochazka, A. V., Petty, T. L., Nett, L. M., Silvers, G. W., Sachs, D. P., Rennard, S. I., Daughton, D. M., Grimm, R. H., Jr., & Heim, C. (1992). Transdermal clonidine reduced some withdrawal symptoms but did not increase smoking cessation. *Archives of Internal Medicine, 152*, 2065–2069.

Prokhorov, A. V., Pallonen, U. E., Fava, J. L., Ding, L., & Niaura, R. S. (1996). Measuring nicotine dependence among high-risk adolescent smokers. *Addictive Behaviors, 21*, 117–127.

Rose, J. E. (1996). Nicotine addiction and treatment. *Annual Review of Medicine, 47*, 493–507.

Rose, J. E., Behm, F. M., & Westman, E. C. (1996a). Interactive effects of nicotine and mecamylamine. Poster presented at the 2nd annual meeting of the Society for Research on Nicotine and Tobacco, Washington, DC.

Rose, J. E., Westman, E. C., & Behm, F. M. (1996b). Nicotine/mecamylamine combination treatment for smoking cessation. *Drug Development and Research, 38*, 243–256.

Rose, J. E., Behm, F. M., Westman, E. C., Levin, E. D., Stein, R. M., Lane, J. D., & Ripka, G. V. (1994a). Combined effects of nicotine and mecamylamine in attenuating smoking satisfaction. *Experimental Clinical Psychopharmacology, 2*, 328–344.

Rose, J. E., Behm, F. M., Westman, E. C., Levin, E. D., Stein, R. M., & Ripka, G. V. (1994b). Mecamylamine combined with nicotine skin patch facilitates smoking cessation beyond nicotine patch treatment alone. *Clinical Pharmacology and Therapeutics, 56*, 86–99.

Rose, J. E., & Levin, E. D. (1991). Concurrent agonist-antagonist administration for the analysis and treatment of drug dependence. *Pharmacology, Biochemistry, and Behavior, 41*, 219–226.

Rose, J. E., Sampson, A., Levin, E. D., & Henningfield, J. E. (1989). Mecamylamine increases nicotine preference and attenuates nicotine discrimination. *Pharmacology, Biochemistry, and Behavior, 32*, 933–938.

Rose, J. E., & Hickman, C. S. (1987). Citric acid aerosol as a potential smoking cessation aid. *Chest, 92,* 1005–1008.

Sachs, D. P. L. (1989). Nicotine polacrilex: Practical use requirements. *Current Pulmonology, 10,* 141–148.

Sachs, D. P. L. (1995). Effectiveness of 4 mg nicotine polacrilex for the initial treatment of high-dependent smokers. *Archives of Internal Medicine, 155,* 1973–1980.

Sachs, D. P. L., Säwe, U., & Leischow, S. J. (1993). Effectiveness of a 16-hour transdermal nicotine patch in a medical practice setting, without intensive group counseling. *Archives of Internal Medicine, 153,* 1881–1890.

Schneider, N. G., Olmstead, R. E., Nilsson, F., Mody, F. V., Franzon, M., & Doan, K. (1996). Efficacy of a nicotine nasal inhaler in smoking cessation: A double-blind, placebo-controlled trial. *Addiction, 90,* 1671–1682.

Schneider, N. G., Olmstead, R., Mody, F. V., Doan, K., Franzon, M., Jarvik, M. E., & Steinberg, C. (1995). Efficacy of a nicotine nasal spray in smoking cessation: A placebo-controlled, double-blind trial. *Addiction, 91,* 1293–1306.

Schneider, N. G., Jarvik, M. E., Forsythe, A. B., Read, L. L., Elliott, M. L., & Schweiger, A. (1983). Nicotine gum in smoking cessation: A placebo-controlled, double-blind trial. *Addictive Behaviors, 8,* 253–261.

Schuh, K. J., Schuh, L. M., Henningfield, J. E., & Stitzer, M. L. (1997). Nicotine nasal spray and vapor inhaler: abuse liability assessment. *Psychopharmacology, 130,* 352–361.

Sexton, M., & Hebel, R. (1984). A clinical trial of change in maternal smoking and its effect on birth weight. *JAMA, 251,* 911–915.

Shiffman, S. M., & Jarvik, M. E. (1976). Smoking withdrawal symptoms in two weeks of abstinence. *Psychopharmacology, 50,* 35–39.

Silagy, C., Mant, D., Fowler, G., & Lokge, M. (1994). Meta-analysis on efficacy of nicotine replacement therapies in smoking cessation. *Lancet, 343,* 139–142.

Smith, T. A., House, R. F., Croghan, I. T., Gauvin, T. R., Colligan, R. C., Offord, K. P., Gomez-Dahl, L. C., & Hurt, R. D. (1996). Nicotine patch therapy in adolescent smokers. *Pediatrics, 98,* 659–667.

Stolerman, I. P., Goldfarb, T., Fink, R., & Jarvik, M. E. (1973). Influencing cigarette smoking with nicotine antagonists. *Psychopharmacologia, 28,* 247–259.

Sutherland, G., Stapleton, J., Russell, M. A. H., Jarvis, M. J., Hajek, P., Belcher, M., & Feyerabend, C. (1992). Randomized controlled trial of nasal nicotine spray in smoking cessation. *Lancet, 340,* 324–329.

Tennant, F. S., Jr., Tarver, A. L., & Rawson, R. A. (1984). Clinical evaluation of mecamylamine for withdrawal from nicotine dependence. *NIDA Research Monographs, 49,* 239–246.

Tiffany, S. T., & Drobes, D. J. (1991). The development and initial validation of a questionnaire on smoking urges. *British Journal of Addiction, 86,* 1467–1476.

Tønnesen, P., Nørregaard, J., Mikkelsen, K., Jørgensen, S., & Nilsson, F. (1993). A double-blind trial of a nicotine inhaler for smoking cessation. *JAMA, 269,* 1268–1271.

Tønnesen, P., Nørregaard, J., Simonsen, K., & Säwe, U. (1991). A double-blind trial of a 16-hour transdermal nicotine patch in smoking cessation. *New England Journal of Medicine, 325,* 311–315.

U.S. Department of Health and Human Services. (1988). *The health consequences of smoking: Nicotine addiction: A report of the Surgeon General* (DHHS Publication No. [CDC] 88-8406). Washington, DC: Government Printing Office.

U.S. Department of Health and Human Services, Public Health Service. (1994a). Medical-care expenditures attributable to cigarette smoking—United States, 1993. *Morbidity and Mortality Weekly Report, 43,* 469–471.

U.S. Department of Health and Human Services, Public Health Service. (1994b). Reasons for tobacco use and symptoms of nicotine withdrawal among adolescent and young adult tobacco users—United States, 1993. *Morbidity and Mortality Weekly Report, 43,* 745–750.

Volpicelli, J. R., Alterman, A. I., Hayashida, M., & O'Brien, C. P. (1992). Naltrexone in the treatment of alcohol dependence. *Archives of General Psychiatry, 49*, 876–880.

Westman, E. C., Behm, F. M., & Rose, J. E. (1995). Airway sensory replacement combined with nicotine replacement for smoking cessation: A randomized, placebo-controlled trial using a citric acid inhaler. *Chest, 107*, 1358–1364.

CHAPTER EIGHT

Nonnicotine Medications for Smoking Cessation

Andrew Johnston
Glaxo Wellcome, Inc.,
Research Triangle Park, North Carolina

Mark D. Robinson
David P. Adams
Cabarrus Family Medicine Residency Program,
North Concord, North Carolina

Alexander H. Glassman
Lirio S. Covey
New York State Psychiatric Institute,
and Columbia University

Modern interest in smoking cessation began in the late 1950s and the early 1960s with the growing awareness of the risks of cigarette smoking, culminating in the first Surgeon General's Report on the health consequences of smoking (U.S. Department of Health, Education, and Welfare, 1964). The initial emphasis on cessation methods was not on drug treatments, but on psychological interventions. As the need to help some smokers in their efforts to stop became recognized, various group and individual counseling methods were developed by organizations such as the American Lung Association, the American Cancer Society, and the American Heart Association, as well as private groups such as Smokenders (Schwartz, 1987). The actual birth of drug treatment for smoking cessation began not with smoking cessation, but with the successful use of methadone for the treatment of opiate addiction in the early 1960s. Methadone treatment popularized the concept that one drug of abuse, administered by a different route, could diminish craving and propensity to relapse to the initial drug of abuse.

This led to the development and initial introduction of nicotine gum in the early 1980s. Nicotine replacement therapy (NRT), initially with nicotine gum, subsequently with the nicotine patch, and later with the nicotine inhaler and nasal spray, has consistently proven efficacious when compared with placebo, as discussed in detail in this book by Eissenberg and colleagues.

Although NRTs have consistently been better than placebos, the proportions of quitters among NRT users observed in multiple studies have been relatively low, with long-term success rates hovering around the 20–25% mark (Fiore, Smith, Jorenby, & Baker, 1994). Although twice higher than the success rates among smokers treated with the placebo, the overall NRT success rate still leaves approximately 75% of its users continuing to smoke. The major impetus to the development of nonnicotine drugs as smoking cessation aids is undoubtedly related, at least in part, to the unsatisfactory success rates achieved by the nicotine replacement therapies.

Another issue influencing the effort to develop alternative treatment is the general concern that nicotine, by alternative routes of administration, is only substituting one form of addiction for another. There did seem to be a certain amount of long-term continuing use of the nicotine gum, although there never was any evidence that such use was harmful. In fact, occasional use of nicotine replacements over the long term might even be a useful way of preventing relapse, but many smokers and therapists as well perceive this continued use of nicotine to be unacceptable.

One of the earliest nonnicotine drugs to be tested for smoking cessation was lobeline, a drug that shows cross-tolerance with nicotine and has been the active ingredient in a number of over-the-counter smoking remedies. Lobeline, however, has not been demonstrated to be effective in a controlled trial. This chapter focuses on the nonnicotine pharmacotherapies for smoking cessation that have been tested in a number of trials: buspirone, clonidine, and bupropion. Promising results found for mecamylamine when combined with the nicotine patch, are also described by Eissenberg and colleagues in chapter 7.

CLONIDINE

Clonidine is an alpha$_2$-noradrenergic agonist that was initially used for the treatment of hypertension, and subsequently found to diminish symptoms of both opiate and alcohol withdrawal syndromes. In 1986, Glassman and colleagues demonstrated its efficacy for diminishing craving and withdrawal symptoms among heavy cigarette smokers who had been abstinent for 24 hours (Glassman et al., 1986). These encouraging results led to a randomized trial for smoking cessation in which 71 smokers were randomly assigned to receive either clonidine or placebo for 4 weeks with adjunctive individual behavior therapy. In this study, dosage began at 0.5 mg on the first day, increasing by 0.5 mg daily until reaching the therapeutic level of 0.15 mg mg per day taken in divided doses. The patient was told to stop smoking upon reaching .15 mg/day. Thereafter, dosage was adjusted according to the appearance of side effects or severe withdrawal discomfort up to an upper limit of .40 mg/day. This study found a success rate among clonidine-treated subjects that was more than twice that in the placebo-treated group, showing for the first time an ability to improve cessation by a nonnicotine drug (Glassman et al., 1988). There have been more than a dozen trials comparing clonidine against placebo for smoking cessation. Although some of those studies failed to find a statistically significant difference between drug and placebo, the majority of studies did. The first meta-analysis of clonidine studies (nine trials) found significantly higher rates among clonidine-treated subjects. Although no differences in clonidine efficacy by dosage or duration of use were observed, greater clonidine efficacy was observed among studies that used adjunctive behavioral therapy compared with trials without adjunctive clinical support. A superior clonidine effect was also observed among studies where clonidine was delivered transdermally compared with oral administration (Covey & Glassman, 1991). Another meta-analysis of clonidine found it to be efficacious in the short term, particularly for alleviating withdrawal symptoms, but concluded that clonidine had limited effects on long-term abstinence (Gourlay & Benowitz, 1995). Although it does appear that clonidine is different from a placebo, the story remains obscure. Typically, clonidine's effect has not been as robust or as easy to demonstrate as has been seen with nicotine substitution products. Slightly more than half of the studies have found a statistically significant effect, in contrast with the nicotine replacement therapies, for which efficacy relative to placebo is almost universally observed.

An interesting trend in the clonidine results was its greater efficacy for female smokers than males as observed in a review of several trials (Covey & Glassman, 1991). In a study published subsequently, which was conducted on 300 smokers, the drug effect was again seen among females but not males (Glassman et al., 1993). Furthermore, clonidine's effect in the latter study was greatest among females with a history of recurrent major depression, the subgroup that showed the poorest response to the placebo. This finding was unexpected, because there had been concern earlier that clonidine might actually increase depression. In addition to demonstrating modest clinical efficacy, clonidine has side effects such as drowsiness, fatigue, and dry mouth, which make it more difficult to use than the nicotine substitution therapies. This combination relegates clonidine to a second-tier role in smoking cessation.

ANXYIOLITICS

Among the persistent theories about smoking is that for many smokers it is a form of self-medication. Smoking has long been seen as a form of "stress management" or a way of reducing anxiety. Such theories would naturally lead to considering the antianxiety drugs as a means of helping smokers stop. This speculation led to a number of efforts to examine antianxiety drugs. In one of the large-scale randomized trials of clonidine, a benzodiazepine, in addition to placebo, was used. The cessation rate among subjects who received benzodiazepine was not different from those who received placebo (Wei & Young, 1988).

Buspirone

In addition to the traditional sedatives, barbiturates, and benzodiazepines, there have been trials of other sedative-like drugs including both beta blockers and certain specific serotonin receptor drugs. The most widely tested of these compounds is buspirone, a nonsedating, nonaddicting compound that became available in the 1980s for the treatment of anxiety. Buspirone is pharmacologically unrelated to benzodiazepines, barbiturates, or other potentially habituating sedative-hypnotic agents. Recent research has suggested that buspirone is a selective agonist for the serotonin 5-HT1A receptor with lesser dopamine D2 receptor activity (Lucki, 1996; Rijnders & Slangen, 1993).

Buspirone is presently indicated for the management of anxiety disorders or the short-term relief of anxiety symptoms. Investigators observed no withdrawal syndrome among patients who had received buspirone for an extended period of time (Lader, 1991; Sussman, 1993). No well-controlled studies of buspirone have been performed among pregnant women. Individuals who have taken busipirone report dizziness (12%), nausea (8%), headache (6%), nervousness (5%), and lightheadedness (3%) as the most common side effects (Cada, 1996). Overall, buspirone has an excellent safety profile (Cada, 1996; Gelenberg, 1994).

Researchers have studied buspirone for the treatment of nicotine dependence since the late 1980s. Early studies typically involved small, uncontrolled pilot studies that identified buspirone as a promising therapy to relieve tobacco withdrawal symptoms and to aid smoking cessation (Gawin, Compton, & Byck, 1989; Robinson, Smith, Cederstrom, & Sutherland, 1991). Gawin et al. (1989) reported decreased withdrawal symptoms and reduced smoking in an exploratory study with eight smokers who used up to 60 mg/day of buspirone. Robinson and colleagues (Robinson et al., 1991) also reported promising reductions in nicotine withdrawal and decreased urges to smoke in 13 heavy smokers who received 30 mg/day of buspirone.

Effect of Buspirone on Smoking Cessation

There have been five placebo-controlled trials of buspirone as a cessation aid (Cinciripini et al., 1995; Hilleman, Mohiuddin, Delcore, & Sketch, 1992; Robinson, Pettice, Smith, Cederstrom, & Sutherland, 1992; Schneider et al., 1996; West, Hajek, & McNeill, 1991). Each employed generally healthy subjects who lacked underlying active mood disorders. In these unselected cohorts of smokers, buspirone therapy yielded contradictory effects on smoking cessation. Differences in methodology and dosage have complicated interstudy comparisons and could account for some of the conflicting results.

Cinciripini and colleagues (1995) were the first investigators to stratify smokers into high-anxiety and low-anxiety groups with the anxiety/tension scale from the Profile of Moods Inventory (POMS). Their study randomized 101 healthy community volunteer. Smokers with serious psychopathology, as defined by a symptom checklist (SCL-90R) greater than 65 t-score (Derogatis, 1977) were excluded. Tension-anxiety scale scores averaged 51 in the high-anxiety groups and 39 in the low-anxiety group. In double-blind fashion, investigators randomly assigned smokers in each anxiety level either to placebo or buspirone. Cinciripini and colleagues observed no significant relief of nicotine withdrawal symptoms with buspirone, but they did find significant group effects on cessation. The buspirone-treated smokers with high baseline anxiety had an 88% 4-week abstinence rate, compared to 61% of the placebo group ($p < .01$). Interestingly, in low-anxiety smokers, a negative effect of buspirone on cessation was noted, with a 60% abstinence rate in the buspirone group compared to 89% in the placebo group ($p < .01$). The explanation for the lower cessation rates with buspirone in low-anxiety smokers is unclear but may reflect increased withdrawal symptom as described later. Cinciripini et al. (1995) concluded that buspirone enhanced short-term cessation rates only in those smokers who were already generally anxious—and only for as long as they remained on treatment. One-year cessation rates did not differ significantly between buspirone and placebo groups.

The most recently published randomized controlled trial by Schneider and colleagues (1996) showed no cessation or nicotine withdrawal benefit from buspirone in a general sample of smokers. Post hoc analysis of the data stratified by baseline anxiety levels showed no cessation benefit in "high-anxiety" (POMS anxiety/tension score ≥19) versus "low-anxiety"

(POMS anxiety/tension score ≤18) smokers. Differences in the levels of baseline anxiety between the smokers studied by Schneider against those of Cinciripini could possibly explain the discrepant results between the studies; that is, Schneider's high-anxiety smokers had lower anxiety ratings than those in the Cinciripini study.

Effects of Buspirone on Nicotine Withdrawal Symptoms

Despite the proven efficacy of buspirone as an anxyliotic (Cada, 1996), four out of five placebo-controlled trials failed to show any significant relief of nicotine withdrawal over placebo (Robinson et al., 1992; Cinciripini et al., 1995; West et al., 1991; Schneider et al., 1996). Some preliminary evidence, however, suggests that nonanxious smokers who received buspirone may experience worse nicotine withdrawal symptoms compared to placebo. Schneider et al. (1996) actually found increased "craving" in buspirone-treated subjects who met strict abstinence criteria. West and his colleagues (1991) also observed that after the second or third week of cessation, the abstinent subjects in the buspirone group reported significantly stronger urges to smoke compared to placebo. Similarly, Robinson et al. (1992) observed a trend toward increased withdrawal discomfort and state-anxiety after cessation in buspirone-treated compared to placebo, but this did not achieve statistical signficance.

At the present time, anxiety reduction in characteristically anxious smokers appears to be the only known benefit of usual doses of buspirone (15–60 mg/day). A pragmatic approach currently used by one of the authors (MDR) at the Cabarrus Nicotine Dependence Center is to screen all smokers for generalized anxiety using the Spielberger Trait Anxiety Scale (Spielberger, Gorsuch, Lushene, Vagg, & Jacobs, 1983). Those with scores greater than one standard deviation over normal who also report symptoms of generalized anxiety are offered anxiolytic therapy with buspirone. Therapy is initiated with 7.5 mg oral buspirone twice daily for 1 week and then 15 mg twice daily for at least 3 weeks prior to the target quit date. On the quit date, NRT with either patch, spray, or gum monotherapy or combination NRT with patch and gum is started. Buspirone therapy is continued indefinitely (usually at 30 mg/day) unless side effects develop or the patient desires to discontinue or no longer needs anxiolytic pharmacotherapy.

In summary, available evidence suggests that there is no robust effect of buspirone on smoking cessation for all smokers. Short-term studies in small samples of "healthy" smokers have yielded modest results at best with no benefit on nicotine withdrawal symptoms. However, it does remain to be determined whether buspirone will be helpful for smokers for whom high levels of anxiety comprise a serious impediment to their ability to stop smoking. As noted in chapter 2 of this volume, findings from a few community based studies have suggested that certain forms of anxiety diagnoses have significant associations with nicotine dependence (Breslau, Kilbey, & Andreski, 1991) and the ability to stop smoking (Covey, Hughes, Glassman, et al., 1993). One reason that research has been limited is the fact that, although anxious mood (along with depression) has long been implicated as a predictor of continued smoking, smokers with high levels of anxiety have been rarely seen in controlled smoking cessation trials. Future studies of buspirone or other anxyliotic medications that focus on smokers selected for generalized anxiety or cessation-related anxiety are needed. Other unanswered questions include: (a) whether combination therapy with NRT is beneficial, (b) the ideal dose and duration of buspirone that would be most helpful to smokers, and (c) the best method to identify anxious smokers.

ANTIDEPRESSANTS

Even though clonidine itself did not prove to be enormously successful, post hoc analyses of data collected from the clinical trials on this drug did have unexpected findings that influenced investigations into the use of antidepressants as cessation aids. In the course of the first clonidine smoking cessation study (Glassman et al., 1988), the researchers decided that because it was difficult enough to stop smoking without being depressed, schizophrenic, or addicted to some other drug, a structured psychiatric examination would be administered to exclude smokers with any evidence of schizophrenia, drug abuse, alcoholism, or present depressive illness. This study procedure enabled the researchers to observe the proportion of smokers with a past history of major depression, and those with "present depressive illness" who were then excluded. *Present illness* was defined as meeting diagnostic criteria for major depression in the last 6 months or taking antidepressant drugs to avoid recurrence of affective disorder at any time during the prior 6 months. As a result, everyone who entered the study had been free of any depressive symptoms for at least 6 months; on the average, they had actually been free of any depressive illness for more than 4 years.

The first surprising observation was the very high proportion of smokers (60%) with a past history of major depression who entered the trial. This figure was several times greater than expected based on depression rates of 10% to 20% observed in studies of the general population (Baldesarrini, 1984). Given this observation, the data were further examined to determine if smoking cessation was influenced by this history of depression. It was found that those people who had such a history were half as likely to succeed in their smoking cessation efforts as smokers free of a history of depression. This finding has been replicated in other smoking cessation studies (Hall et al., 1994), and in data gathered from the general population (Glassman et al., 1990).

A second finding from the initial clonidine smoking cessation data further suggested the usefulness of antidepressant treatment. Examining only those subjects who received the placebo to control for confounding effects due to the medication, the researchers observed that among the symptoms reported by quitters during the first week, depressed mood most strongly and significantly predicted who would return to smoking by the end of the 4-week study (Covey, Glassman, & Stetner, 1990). The study also found that smokers with the history of major depression were more likely to report depressed mood during the abstinence period, thus suggesting a mechanism, that is, a greater propensity to become depressed, for the higher failure rate among smokers with past major depression.

These findings about the effects of depression occurring before and after cessation led to the speculation that antidepressant drugs might be useful in smoking cessation. Actually, the effects of antidepressants on smoking cessation had been examined earlier by Sellers in a study of the effect of selective serotonin reuptake inhibitors (SSRIs; citalopram and zimelodine) on spontaneous alcohol consumption (Sellers, Naranjo, & Kadlec, 1987). No marked effect of the SSRIs on smoking cessation was seen, although it should be noted that the purpose of those trials was to examine the effects of SSRIs on alcohol consumption and no efforts at promoting nicotine abstinence were involved.

Bupropion (Zyban)

There is one antidepressant preparation for which extensive testing has been completed, with very favorable results. On the strength of positive findings from considerable data, bupropion hydrochloride, originally marketed for the treatment of depression as Wellbutrin, has been approved by the federal Food and Drug Administration as a treatment for nicotine dependence.

Bupropion sustained release (SR) represents the first robust nonnicotine pharmacologic treatment for tobacco dependence. This drug has been shown to be efficacious as a smoking cessation treatment and is marketed under the trade name Zyban by Glaxo Wellcome, Inc. The mechanism by which bupropion assists patients to stop smoking is not clear, but it is thought to be related to both noradrenergic and dopaminergic activity. In animals, bupropion administration results in decreased neuronal firing rates in the locus ceruleus; in humans it results in decreased whole-body norepinephrine turnover (Ascher et al., 1995). It is hypothesized that the dopaminergic activity of bupropion affects the reward pathways, and that the noradrenergic activity of bupropion affects the withdrawal pathways, of nicotine addiction. Bupropion and its metabolites have no affinity for nicotine receptors (Glaxo Wellcome data). Bupropion is a Pregnancy Category B medication; however, well-controlled studies of bupropion safety efficacy related to pregnancy have yet to be conducted.

In 1991, Dr. Linda Ferry at the Jerry L. Pettis Veterans Memorial Center in Loma Linda, CA, who became aware of the association between depression and cigarette smoking as a result of the findings from the clonidine study, decided to test an antidepressant drug for smoking cessation. She reasoned that, among the antidepressants on the market, bupropion had the most clear-cut activity on the dopamine system. Given dopamine's importance both to nicotine and to addictive drugs in general, she elected to use bupropion in a placebo-controlled trial with group counseling for all subjects. The outcome for bupropion in that study was strikingly positive and was particularly impressive because it was observed in a Veterans Administration (VA) patient population heavily populated with addicted smokers with various co-occurring psychiatric conditions, including depression and alcoholism (Ferry et al., 1992). Initial response to these observations, however, was unenthusiastic. Critics of the study reasoned that bupropion's reputation as an antidepressant drug might have caused an enhanced response in a patient population that was heavily comorbid with depressive illness, as the veterans were likely to be. If bupropion was to be marketed for smoking cessation, it would require some evidence that it worked not only in depressed smokers, but in smokers without any history of depression. In a second study where smokers with a history of depression were excluded, Ferry was able to demonstrate that bupropion continued to exert a beneficial effect on cessation effort (Ferry & Burchette, 1994).

In addition to the early trials conducted by Ferry, bupropion was evaluated in two large multisite placebo-controlled trials, both of which also demonstrated efficacy. These trials, a dose-response study and a nicotine patch-comparison study, evaluated the sustained release (SR) formulation in conjunction with brief individual counseling. The dose-response study was conducted at three centers and consisted of a 7-week treatment phase with follow-up to 1 year. Self-report of smoking cessation was confirmed using exhaled carbon monoxide levels. Three doses were evaluated: 100 mg/day (50 mg b.i.d.), 150 mg/day (150 mg q. am), and 300 mg/day (150 mg b.i.d.). The primary efficacy variable was continuous quitting for the last 4 weeks of treatment (weeks 4–7). This timeline allowed 1 week, prior to quitting, to reach steady-state plasma concentrations and 2 weeks for patients to stop smoking. As seen in Fig. 8.1, a clear dose response was demonstrated with the two higher dose groups reaching statistical superiority over placebo. At

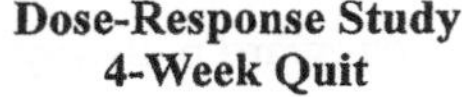

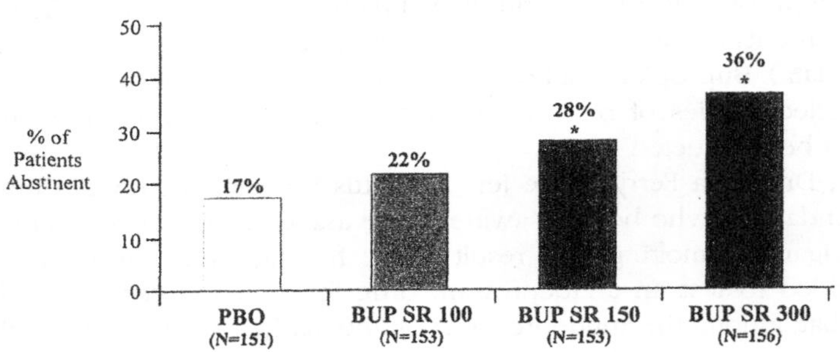

*p< .05 versus PBO

FIG. 8.1. Percent of subjects abstinent during the last 4 weeks of treatment across groups who received placebo and varying doses of bupropion daily (100 mg, 150 mg, 300 mg).

1-year follow-up, significantly more patients in the two highest dose groups reported smoking cessation than in the placebo group (300 mg = 23.1%, 150 mg = 22.9%, placebo = 12.4%) (Johnston & Ascher, 1996; Hurt et al., 1997).

The patch-comparison study was conducted at four centers and evaluated bupropion SR 300 mg/day (150 mg b.i.d.), nicotine patch 21 mg/day (Habitrol), combination bupropion SR 300 mg/day and nicotine patch 21 mg/day, and placebo. The design was similar to the dose-response study with the exception that 2 weeks were added to the treatment phase (9 weeks total) to allow for tapering of the patch: 14 mg during week 8 and 7 mg during week 9. Bupropion SR was not tapered. All patients took tablets, active or placebo, and applied patches, active or placebo, to ensure the blind. The primary efficacy variable was continuous quit for weeks 4–7. Results are presented in Fig. 8.2. All three active treatment groups were statistically superior to placebo. Bupropion SR was statistically superior to nicotine patch. Lastly, the combination of bupropion SR and nicotine patch produced the highest quit rates and was statistically superior to the nicotine patch. The difference between combination treatment and bupropion SR approached significance ($p = .06$) (Hurt et al., 1997; Johnston & Ascher, 1996).

In clinical trials, bupropion SR attenuated the craving or urge to smoke, as well as the withdrawal associated with smoking cessation. Withdrawal symptom reduction was most pronounced for the following: irritability, frustration, or anger; anxiety; difficulty concentrating; restlessness; and depressed mood or negative affect. In the dose-response study, an analysis of quitters revealed a dose-related attenuation of weight gain; once treatment was

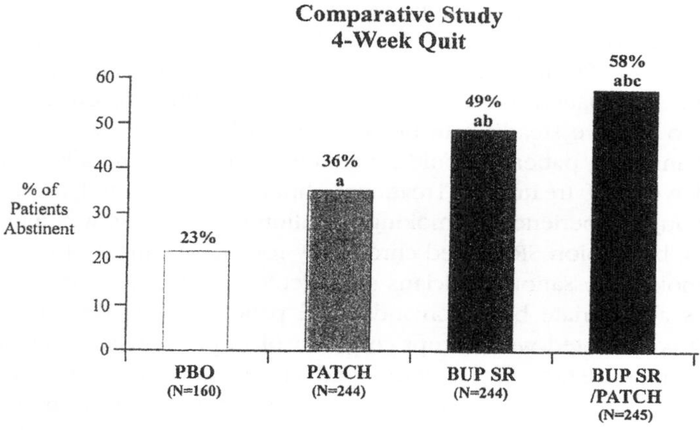

FIG. 8.2. Percent of subjects abstinent during the last 4 weeks of treatment across groups who received placebo, nicotine patch only, bupropion SR only, or nicotine patch/bupropion SR.

stopped, however, differences between the active and placebo groups were not maintained (Hurt et al., 1997). However, bupropion should not be used in patients with anorexia and bulimia because of an increased risk of seizures.

Bupropion SR was well tolerated in the smoking cessation studies. Only two adverse events, insomnia and dry mouth, were observed at an incidence 5% higher than that of placebo. Insomnia can be managed by avoiding bedtime dosing. Dry mouth is usually mild and rarely requires intervention. Both insomnia and dry mouth generally improve with continued treatment. The incidence of premature discontinuation due to an adverse event was also low, 8% across studies. The most common adverse events leading to premature discontinuation were tremor and rash. Bupropion SR combined with the nicotine patch was also well tolerated. Blood pressure elevation was noted in a few patients receiving combination treatment; most had preexisting hypertension. Patients receiving combination treatment should have their blood pressure monitored. In trials evaluating bupropion SR for depression, seizure was rarely reported as an adverse event (less than 1/1,000 patients); no seizures were reported in the smoking cessation clinical trials involving approximately 2,000 bupropion-treated patients. Nevertheless, patients with a history of or a predisposition to seizure should not be treated with bupropion.

Dosing for bupropion SR as an aid to smoking cessation should begin at 150 mg/day for 3 days and increase, for most patients, to the recommended maximum dose of 300 mg/day given as 150 mg b.i.d. Treatment should be initiated while the patient is still smoking, because approximately 1 week is required to achieve steady-state blood levels of bupropion. At the time treatment is initiated, patients should set a target quit date, generally during the second week of treatment. Treatment should be continued for 7–12 weeks. Although experience in smoking cessation clinical trials was limited to 12 weeks, bupropion SR is used chronically for the treatment of depression. For smoking cessation, clinicians must determine if treatment beyond 12 weeks is appropriate based on individual patient needs. No rebound phenomena were noted with abrupt cessation of bupropion SR in clinical trials. Therefore, dose tapering is not required when discontinuing treatment. As with other pharmacologic treatments for smoking cessation, bupropion SR should be used in conjunction with behavioral support. The manufacturer provides a patient support program with the product (Johnston & Ascher, 1996).

In summary, bupropion SR is the first nonnicotine treatment marketed in the United States as a treatment for tobacco dependence. It is an oral tablet formulation and, in contrast to nicotine replacement therapy, is initiated prior to smoking discontinuation. For efficacy, a clear pharmacologic dose-response exists. Attenuation of both craving and withdrawal symptoms has been demonstrated. The quit rates for bupropion SR are greater than those seen with a nicotine patch, and combined with a nicotine patch the quit rates are greater than those seen with either treatment alone.

Other Antidepressant Drugs

To our knowledge, several trials of other antidepressant drugs for smoking cessation have now been conducted. Edwards and his group (Edwards et al., 1988) were the first to test an antidepressant in a controlled smoking cessation study. Although their initial study of 20 smokers found encouraging results for doxepin, a tricylic antidepressant, on the reduction of the number of cigarettes smoked, no definitive study has been published with that drug. A large multisite study of the selective serotonin reuptake inhibitor (SSRI) fluoxetine appears to have yielded generally negative results (Mizes et al., 1996). However, a post hoc stratified analysis by researchers at Brown University who examined the data by high or low depression scores at baseline found a positive fluoxetine effect at the higher dose of 60 mg/day among smokers with high depression mood scores (Hamilton Depression Scale) at baseline (Niaura et al., 1994). In 1995, a clinical trial of 88 smokers found that the monoamine oxidase inhibitor moclobemide, also an antidepressant, facilitated quitting among highly dependent smokers (Berlin et al., 1995). At the Veterans Hospital in San Francisco, Sharon Hall completed a trial of nortriptyline and found it to be superior to placebo regardless of a history of major depression (Hall et al., 1998). These findings from a number of nonnicotine medications are likely to be developed in future work, providing smokers and clinicians further and much needed help in the treatment of nicotine addiction.

REFERENCES

Ascher, J. A., Cole, J. O., Colin, J. C., Feighner, J. P., Ferris, R. M., Fibiger, H. C., Golden, R., Martin, P., Potter, W. Z., Richelson, E., & Sulser, F. (1995). Bupropion: A review of its mechanism of antidepressant activity. *Journal of Clinical Psychiatry, 56*, 395–401.

Baldesarrini, R. J. (1984). Risk rates for depression. *Archives of General Psychiatry, 41*, 103.

Berlin, I., Said, S., Spreux-Varoquaux, O., Launay, J., Olivares, R., Millet, V., Lecrubier, Y., & Puech, A. J. (1995). A reversible monoamine oxidase A inhibitor (moclobemide) facilitates smoking cessation and abstinence in heavy dependent smokers. *Clinical Trial and Therapeutics, 58*, 444–452.

Breslau, N., Kilbey, M., & Andreski, P. (1991). Nicotine dependence, major depression and anxiety in young adults. *Archives of General Psychiatry, 48*, 1069–1074.

Cada, D. J. (Ed.). (1996). Buspirone HCL. In *Drug facts and comparisons* (pp. 1453–1456). St. Louis, MO: Facts and Comparisons.

Cinciripini, P. M., Laptizky, L., Seay, S., Wallfisch, A., Meyer, W. J. III, & van Vanakis, H. (1995). A placebo-controlled evaluation of the effects of buspirone on smoking cessation: Differences between high- and low-anxiety smokers. *Journal of Clinical Psychopharmacology, 15*, 182–191.

Covey, L. S., & Glassman, A. H. (1991). A meta-analysis of double-blind placebo-controlled trials of clonidine for smoking cessation *British Journal of Addiction, 86*, 991–998.

Covey, L. S., Glassman, A. H., & Stetner, F. (1990). Depression and depressive symptoms in smoking cessation. *Comprehensive Psychiatry, 31*, 350–354.

Covey, L. S., Hughes, D. C., Glassman, A. H., Blazer, D. G., & George, L. K. (1993). Ever-smoking, quitting, and psychiatric disorders: Evidence from the Durham, North Carolina, Epidemiologic Catchment Area. *Tobacco Control, 3*, 222–227.

Derogatis, L. R. (1977). *SCL-90 administration, scoring, procedures manual.* Baltimore: Johns Hopkins University Press.

Edwards, N. B., Simmins, R. C., Rosenthal, T. L., et al. (1988). Doxepin in the treatment of nicotine withdrawal. *Psychosomatics, 29*, 203–206.

Ferry, L. H., & Burchette, R. J. (1994). Efficacy of bupropion for smoking cessation in non-depressed smokers. *Journal of Addictive Diseases, Abstract 9A*, 13:249.

Ferry, L. H., Robbins, A. S., Scariati, P. D., Masterson, A., Abbey, D. E., & Burchette, R. J. (1992). Enhancement of smoking cessation using the antidepressant, bupropion hydrochloride [abstract]. *Circulation, 86*(4), I–671.

Fiore, M. C., Smith, S. S., Jorenby, D. E., & Baker, T. B. (1994). The effectiveness of nicotine path for smoking cessation: A meta-analysis. *JAMA, 263*, 2760–2765.

Gawin, F., Compton, M., & Byck, R. (1989). Buspirone reduces smoking. *Archives of General Psychiatry, 46*, 288–289.

Gelenberg, A. J. (1994). Buspirone: Seven year update. *Journal of Clinical Psychiatry, 55,* 222–229.

Glassman, A. H., Covey, L. S., Dalack, G. W., Stetner, F., Rivelli, S. K., Fleiss, J. L., & Cooper, T. B. (1993). Smoking cessation, clonidine, and the vulnerability to nicotine among dependent smokers. *Clinical Pharmacology and Therapeutics, 54*(6), 670–679.

Glassman, A. H., Helzer, J. E., Covey, L. S., Cottler, L. B., Stetner, F., Tipp, J. E., & Johnson, J. (1990). Smoking, smoking cessation, and major depression. *JAMA, 264,* 1546–1549.

Glassman, A. H., Jackson, W. K., Walsh, B. T., Roose, S. P., & Rosenfeld, R. (1984). Cigarette craving, smoking withdrawal, and clonidine. *Science, 226,* 864–866.

Glassman, A. H., Stetner, F., Walsh, B. T., Raizman, P. S., Fleiss, J. L., Cooper, T. B., & Covey, L. S. (1988). Heavy smokers, smoking cessation, and clonidine: Results of a double-blind, randomized trial. *JAMA, 259,* 2863–2866.

Gourlay, S. G., & Benowitz, N. L. (1995). Is clonidine an effective smoking cessation therapy? *Drugs, 50,* 197–207.

Hall, S. M., Munoz, R. F., & Reus, V. I. (1994). Cognitive-behavioral intervention increases abstinence rates for depressive-history smokers. *J Consult Clinical Psychology, 62,* 141–146.

Hall, S. M., Reus, V. I., Munoz, R. F., Sees, K. L., Humfleet, G., Hartz, D. T., Frederick, S., & Triffleman, E. (1998). *Archives of General Psychiatry, 55,* 683–690.

Hilleman, D. E., Mohiuddin, S. M., Delcore, M. G., & Sketch, M. H., Sr. (1992). Effect of buspirone on withdrawal symptoms associated with smoking cessation. *Archives of Internal Medicine, 152,* 350–352.

Hurt, R. D., Sachs, D. L., Glover, E. D., Offord, K. P., Johnston, J. A., Dale, L. C., Khayrallah, M. A., Schroeder, D. R., Glover, P. N., Sullivan, C. R., Croghan, I. T., & Sullivan, P. M. (1997). A comparison of sustained-release bupropion and placebo for smoking cessation. *New England Journal of Medicine, 337,* 1195–1202.

Johnston, J. A., & Ascher, J. A. (1996, December). *Bupropion SR for smoking cessation.* Paper presented at the FDA Drug Abuse Advisory Committee Meeting, Washington, DC.

Lader, M. (1991). Can buspirone induce rebound, dependence or abuse? *British Journal of Psychiatry Supplement, 12,* 45–51.

Lucki, I. (1996). Serotonin receptor specificity in anxiety disorders. *Journal of Clinical Psychiatry, 57* (suppl. 6), 5–10.

Mizes, J. S., Sloan, D. M., Segraves, K., Spring, B., Pingatore, R., & Kristeller, J. (1996, May). *Fluoxetine and weight gain in smoking cessation: Examination of actual weight gain and fear of weight gain.* Presented at the New Clinical Drug Evaluation Unit Program, 36th Annual Meeting, Boca Raton, FL.

Niaura, R., Goldstein, M. G., Depne, J., Keuthen, N., Kristeller, J., & Abrams, D. (1995). Fluoxetine. Symptoms of depression, and smoking cessation (Abstract). *Annals of Behavioral Medicine, 17,* Suppl: 5061.

Rijnders, H. J., & Slangen, J. L. (1993). The discriminative stimulus properties of buspirone involve dopamine-2 receptor antagonist activity. *Psychopharmacology, 111,* 55–61.

Robinson, M. D., Pettice, Y. L., Smith, W. A., Cederstrom, E. A., & Sutherland, D. E. (1992). Buspirone effect on tobacco withdrawal symptoms: A randomized placebo-controlled trial. *Journal of the American Board of Family Practices, 5,* 1–9.

Robinson, M. D., Smith, W. A., Cederstrom, E. A., & Sutherland, D. E. (1991). Buspirone effect on tobacco withdrawal symptoms: A pilot study. *Journal of the American Board of Family Practice, 4,* 89–94.

Schneider, N. G., Olmstead, R. E., Steinberg, C., Sloan, K., Daims, R. M., & Brown, H. V. (1996). Efficacy of buspirone in smoking cessation: A placebo-controlled trial. *Clinical Pharmacology and Therapeutics, 60,* 568–575.

Schwartz, J. (1987). *Review and evaluation of smoking cessation methods: The United States and Canada, 1978–1985* (NIH Publ. No. 87-2940). Bethesda, MD: U.S. Department of Health and Human Services.

Sellers, E. M., Naranjo, C. A., & Kadlec, K. (1987). Do serotonin uptake inhibitors decrease smoking? Observations in a group of heavy drinkers. *Journal of Clinical Psychopharmacology 7*(6), 417–420.

Settle, E. C. (1993). Bupropion: Update. *International Drug Therapy Newsletter, 28*, 29–36.

Spielberger, C. D., Gorsuch, R. L., Lushene, R., Vagg, P. R., & Jacobs, G. A. (1983). *Manual for the state-trait anxiety inventory (STAI form Y)*. Palo Alto, CA: Consulting Psychologists Press.

Sussman, N. (1993). Treating anxiety while minimizing abuse and dependence. *Journal of Clinical Psychiatry, 54*(suppl.), 44–51.

U.S. Department of Health, Education, and Welfare. (1964). *Smoking and health: Report of the Advisory Committee to the Surgeon General of the Public Health Service* (PHS Publ. No. 1103). Washington, DC: U.S. Government Printing Office.

Wei, H., & Young, D. (1988). Effect of clonidine on cigarette cessation and in the alleviation of withdrawal symptoms *British Journal of Addiction, 83*, 1221–1226.

West, R. J., Hajek, P., & McNeill, A. (1991). Effect of buspirone on cigarette withdrawal symptoms and short-term abstinence rates in a smokers clinic. *Psychopharmacology, 104*, 91–96.

CHAPTER NINE

A Psychotherapeutic Approach for Smoking Cessation Counseling

Lirio S. Covey
New York State Psychiatric Institute, and Columbia University

Motivated by health concerns, spurred on by social pressure, and aided by efficacious treatments, many smokers have managed to stop smoking. For a certain group of smokers, however, this outcome has been short-lived, as within months, weeks, or even days for some, a relapse to smoking occurs. Indeed, it has been documented that 1 year after a quit attempt, about 90% of would-be ex-smokers will have gone back to smoking (Fiore et al., 1990). Numerous studies have shown that negative affects such as anxiety, depression, and anger are the most frequent precipitants of smoking relapse (see Carmody, 1989, for an extensive review). In support of those findings, it has also been shown that smokers who suffer from concomitant psychological or psychiatric problems, including depressive disorders and anxiety, have markedly lower rates of quitting than other smokers (Covey, Hughes, Glassman, Blazer, & George, 1994; Glassman, 1993; Hall, Munoz, & Reus, 1994). This evidence indicates that smoking cessation treatments need to address the apparent dynamic association between negative emotional states and a return to smoking.

This chapter describes a counseling approach for *emotionally dependent smokers*, broadly defined as that subset of smokers whose inability to stop smoking is determined by emotional factors. Despite their strong wish to stop smoking and multiple attempts to do so, their efforts are stymied by the emergence of distressful and painful feelings that they attempt to alleviate through smoking cigarettes.

THE EMOTIONALLY DEPENDENT SMOKER

Emotionally dependent smokers are identifiable by these criteria: They smoke heavily, often 20 or more cigarettes daily; they are unable to abstain from cigarettes for a an extended period, usually not more than 2 to 4 weeks; and the return to smoking is associated with a negative emotion or stressful event. Although they may deny dysphoric feelings when first seen for treatment, their responses to a psychological inventory will indicate characteristically high levels of depression, anger, or anxiety. Often, but not always, they will recall a period of severe depression, when they felt depressed mood and loss of pleasure accompanied by physical symptoms such as sleep difficulties and appetite changes that lasted for several days.

THEORETICAL BACKGROUND

The theoretical underpinning of a psychotherapeutic approach to nicotine dependence treatment begins with a phenomenological view of nicotine dependence, derived from ample clinical observations, as a disorder comprised of physiological, behavioral, and emotional factors. Additionally, in a psychometric test of this concept, my colleagues and I observed that these factors were conceptually separable yet sufficiently intercorrelated that in a higher order factor analysis they clustered together to form a single principal factor (Covey et al., 1997). This evidence for a multidimensional quality of nicotine dependence implies that full recovery requires a comprehensive and specialized therapeutic attention to each of those domains. A similar view was recently expressed in a recent article by Dr. Alan Leshner, the Director of the National Institute of Drug Abuse (NIDA), who pointed to the importance of addressing the nonphysical aspects of addictive disorders and lamented the superficial treatment of nonphysical features in current models of addiction (Leshner, 1997).

The idea that emotional factors are involved in persistent cigarette smoking is not new. As early as the 1960s Tomkins, in his affect-regulation theory to explain smoking behavior, had proposed that positive and negative affective states, in addition to a pure addictive construct, determined smoking behavior (Tomkins, 1968). Positive affect smokers (PAS) smoke because they enjoy smoking; negative affect smokers (NAS) do so to avoid painful feelngs. Tomkins also suggested that it was negative affect, not positive affect, tendencies that impeded the ability to sustain nicotine abstinence. Many later investigations subsequently obtained data confirming the deleterious influence of negative psychological states. Of those studies, frequently cited are Shiffman's (1986) paper which reported that of six factors related to a relapse episode, the "upset" factor most strongly predicted a relapse, accounting for as many as two thirds of relapse events, and the finding by Covey, Glassman, and Stetner (1990) that depressed mood during the first week of a quit attempt was the withdrawal symptom most predictive of eventual treatment failure.

Compatible with the negative affect theory is the recent growing literature that has shown substantial comorbidity between nicotine dependence and psychiatric illness. Much of this evidence has concerned major depressive disorder (MDD), but more and more data are emerging that show a strong association between cigarette smoking and other psychiatric conditions including anxiety disorders, attention deficit disorders, schizophrenia, and, not surprisingly, alcohol and drug dependence (Breslau, Kilbey, & Andreski, 1991; Covey et al., 1994; Glassman, 1993; Hughes, Hatsukami, Mitchell, & Dahlgren, 1986; Pomerleau, 1997). Clearly, what was also pointed out with regard to drug addiction by Leshner (1997) is also true of nicotine dependence—"Comorbidity is reality!" The effect of psychiatric comorbidity on the ability to stop smoking is less clear; nevertheless, there have been demonstrations that a high level of depressed mood (Anda et al., 1990), major depression (Glassman et al., 1988, 1990; Hall, Munoz, & Reus, 1994), generalized anxiety disorder (Covey et al., 1992), and active alcoholism (Breslau, Peterson, Schultz, Andreski, & Chilcoat, 1996) are associated with a decreased ability to quit smoking.

A corollary of a dimensional view of nicotine dependence is the notion that smokers vary in nicotine dependence profile, according to the component dimensions. Thus, one smoker may be low on all dimensions—for example, the "chipper," who may smoke regularly, in small amounts, and does not have great difficulty stopping smoking (Shiffman, 1989). Another smoker may be high in physiological and behavioral dependence but low in emotional dependence, conceivably Tomkins's (1968) "addictive smoker," who will experience extreme difficulty stopping, but having done so, stands a good chance of sustaining the abstinence state. Another smoker may be low on both physiological and behavioral factors but high on emotional factors; although able to stop smoking in the short term, say with low-dose nicotine replacement and low-intensity behavioral therapy, this smoker may have a hard time sustaining abstinence if the emotional factor is not addressed. Although still other patterns are possible, there might also be the smoker who is high on all three dimensions; this smoker, one would suspect, will have the greatest difficulty in stopping and in avoiding a relapse, and will require high-dose nicotine replacement therapy (NRT), considerable smoking cessation skills training, and psychotherapy-oriented counseling.

HISTORICAL BACKGROUND

Since the beginning of smoking cessation treatments shortly after the 1964 Surgeon General's Report (SGR) report on the health consequences of tobacco (U.S. Department of Health, Education, and Welfare, 1964), the armamentarium of smoking cessation treatments has included strategies that have addressed mainly the behavioral and physiological elements of nicotine dependence. Noticeably lacking are treatments that address the emotional component. From my own clinical experience and reading of the literature, I have come to believe that this failure to recognize and address the emotional dimension of nicotine dependence accounts, to a large degree, for the intractibility of cigarette smoking among many smokers who wish to but are unable to stop smoking.

It is generally accepted that advances in treatment are linked to the progress of science on the disorder. The history of smoking cessation treatments exemplifies that association. The earliest perception about persistent tobacco usage was about its repetitive, conditioned, and habit-like character. This view gave rise to the development and use of behavioral change methods that marked smoking cessation treatment efforts shortly after the 1964 SGR until the 1970s (Schwartz, 1987). These treatments helped the smoker employ specific behaviors for managing tobacco withdrawal symptoms, coping with smoking cues, and developing new "habits" to take the place of smoking. This manner of psychological treatment, however, produced success rates that were consistently no better than 30%, thus leaving the majority of would-be quitters thwarted in their efforts (Schwartz, 1987).

After the 1964 Surgeon General's Report, the physiological and addictive character of regular tobacco became increasingly better understood. This recognition started with the scientific community, moved on to government and to the lay public as more information about nicotine, the main pharmacological ingredient in tobacco, and its effects on the central nervous system became known. The 1988 Surgeon General's Report marked another milestone for tobacco research in its compilation of available scientific evidence on the addictive nature of nicotine and tobacco use (U.S. Department of Health and Human Services, 1988). To a large degree because of this increased knowledge, and in part due to the poor outcomes of the early behavior therapies, attention shifted to pharmacological agents as smoking cessation aids. An early candidate drug was lobeline, but the evidence for that drug was not encouraging. Subsequently, the early 1980s saw the introduction of the nicotine replacement therapies (NRT), beginning with the nicotine gum and, some years later, the nicotine patch. Both preparations, and later nicotine delivered by nasal spray or inhaler, were found in controlled trials to be significantly more efficacious than were placebo preparations in their ability to aid would-be quitters (Henningfield, 1995).

As discussed in chapter 8, other medications, including several antidepressants, have been tested as smoking cessation aids. In the light of scientific scrutiny that followed the studies of these various pharmacotherapies for quitting smoking, what became apparent was a beneficial effect of adjunctive clinical support. In several review papers, it was reported that the efficacy of medication aids (NRT or clonidine) increased to near double rates when delivered with concomittant behavioral counseling compared to medication alone (Covey & Glassman, 1991; Hughes, 1994; Lam, Sacks, Sze, Chalmers, 1987). This finding contributed to a renewed interest in psychological treatments for nicotine dependence. It is important to note, however, that in spite of the ability of psychological treatments to increase the efficacy of pharmacotherapy, combined psychological and pharmacological behavioral treatments resulted in response rates no better than 40% at the end of treatment and 20% six months later (Hughes, 1994). Thus, failure rather than success remained the more frequent outcome. This treatment gap points toward new directions for smoking cessation treatment research.

RATIONALE FOR A PSYCHOTHERAPEUTIC APPROACH

Traditional models of psychological support for smoking cessation such as those developed by the American Lung Association (Lerner & Schneider, 1984) have featured mainly cognitive and behavioral methods designed to help the smoker move toward a quit day, and to practice specific behaviors to cope with withdrawal symptoms and external triggers of cravings to smoke. These methods have comprised the bread-and-butter strategy of groups such as the FreshStart Smoking Cessation Program of the American Cancer Society (ACS). A recent meeting of ACS group facilitators brought home for me the urgency of a different level of treatment. I was deeply touched by the plaintive note among the attendees. They spoke of seeing different clients from those of several years ago. Now, they find that about 8 out of 10 report serious psychological problems as well, and that the program was producing very few successes. (According to data I obtained from their clients, they were right!) More importantly, they were feeling helpless, without the tools to truly help these smokers. Where can we send them, they asked? What can we offer them? From reading the literature, I have little doubt that these sentiments are felt by other smoking cessation practitioners.

The truth is, there is little to offer the smoker with concurrent psychological problems, whether the problem is as serious as a diagnosed psychiatric condition such as major depression, bipolar disorder, or schizophrenia, or a less severe yet more prevalent form such as low-grade dysthymia. Underlying the treatment drought is a lack of knowledge about the active ingredients that might help the smoker who is emotionally vulnerable. However, data provided by two recent studies offer some clues.

Hall and colleagues (1994) conducted a trial where they used either a mood-management (MM) counseling protocol or a health education (HE) treatment for smokers with or without a history of major depressive disorder (MDD), then examined differential effects of these treatments for the two types of smokers. The investigators found that smokers with MDD responded better to the mood-regulation therapy than to the standard health education treatment, whereas smokers without MDD responded better to the HE treatment but did not do well when they received the MM intervention. Thus, that study not only confirmed the greater cessation problems of smokers with MDD history, but importantly, it signaled a possible advantage of mood-oriented treatments for smokers whose smoking is associated with an emotional factor, in this case, major depressive disorder.

A second, related study was conducted by Zelman and colleagues (1992). This study classified subjects on two dimensions, depression proneness and level of nicotine dependence, and assigned them in random fashion to psychological counseling that focused on delivering either skills training or supportive counseling. The researchers found that depression-prone smokers benefited more (i.e., higher smoking cessation success rates) from supportive counseling than from skills training, whereas the highly dependent–low depression subjects benefitted more from the skills training. Furthermore, those treatment-specific benefits extended to the subjects' ability to sustain abstinence 6 months later.

Taken together, the two studies suggest that smokers who are prone to depression are at high risk of cessation failure when given non-mood-oriented counseling; when treated with a more psychological approach, they stand a greater chance of succeeding. Hall's data suggested that a helpful technique is to help the patient learn to manage and improve a characteristic depressive condition. Zelman's data suggested that a supportive technique exerted a beneficial effect. Although the two studies describe different treatment ingredients, they both demonstrated a positive effect of a mood-regulating psychological intervention.

MECHANISMS OF ACTION FOR SMOKING CESSATION PSYCHOTHERAPY

This section describes the principles, techniques, and sequencing of a time-limited psychotherapeutic approach for smoking cessation, based on approximately 10 years of my work with many "emotionally dependent" patients. The reader will recognize that elements of the treatment are similar to those described in published psychotherapies including Supportive-Expressive Therapy (Luborsky, 1984) and Interpersonal Behavior Therapy (Klerman, Weissman, Rounsaville, & Chevron, 1984).

Principles

The organizing principle of this therapeutic approach is the assumption that cigarette smoking is maintained by the (emotionally dependent) patient's tendency to use cigarettes in the service of denying painful feelings. The consequence of this self-medicating tendency, which is sustained by the psychoactive nature of nicotine (Corrigall, 1991), is a learned and practiced inability to recognize feelings and to respond adaptively to the stressful, emotionally arousing events, large or small, of everyday life. The emotionally dependent smoker will often be emotionally unaware, constricted in emotional experience, and lacking in appropriate coping mechanisms.

A key concept underlying this psychotherapeutic approach for the hardcore emotionally dependent smoker is the notion that it is not negative affect itself but rather the inability to cope with negative affect that presents an impediment to sustained abstinence. This explanatory model is rooted in the emotionally dependent smoker's history of conveniently using cigarette smoking as a "psychological tool" with which to self-medicate painful feelings. Although the long-term benefit of using smoking to cope with negative feelings is questionable, the pharmacology of nicotine, a drug with multiple psychoactive effects (Balfour, 1982), and the pharmacokinetics of smoked nicotine (Henningfield, 1985) do make it plausible that feelings of anxiety, depression, or anger are attenuated at the time the cigarette is smoked. Although short-lived, this balming quality of smoking behavior is reinforcing, leading to its repetition whenever such negative affects are experienced, and ultimately to a state of emotional dependence on smoking. It is possible that this process begins early in the persons's smoking career, as suggested by the evidence that the relationship between being a regular smoker and depression starts as early as during the adolescent years (Covey & Tam, 1990; Fergusson, Lynskey, & Horwood, 1996; Patton et al., 1996).

An important psychological consequence of the smoker's emotional dependence on cigarette smoking (or nicotine) is an estrangement from the smoker's own painful feelings. (A severe form of this condition is referred to in the medical literature as alexithymia [Thomas, 1993], and also referred to in chap. 12 of this book.) The estrangement occurs on several levels: cognitive, in an inability to identify and label those negative emotional states; experiential, an inability to accept, experience, and tolerate them; and behavioral, an impoverished coping repertoire for resolving the source of painful feelings. Clinically, I have seen this estrangement to be associated with negative self-esteem, feelings of inadequacy, and a tendency toward persistent depressive mood.

Following this line of thinking, the therapeutic challenge presented by the emotionally dependent smoker can be conceptualized on multiple levels. The presenting complaint is persistent, compulsive smoking, with an inability to sustain abstinence. (With a high level of motivation, a pharmacological agent, and behavioral counseling, the person may actually be able to stop on a given quit day). The underlying dysfunctionality that precipitates a return to smoking is an inability to cope with (recognize, accept, and act on) feelings that are uncomfortable, unpleasant, or unwanted. The propensity to relapse and continue to self-medicate by smoking has internal (low feelings of self-efficacy, poor self-esteem, depression), and external (the upsetting problem is not resolved) consequences.

This analysis suggests the required elements of treatment. Because nicotine has been used to perpetuate a maladaptive problem-solving style (e.g., the inclination to suppress or inhibit painful feelings), the first therapeutic goal is to help the patient stop smoking. Every available means—pharmacological agent, behavioral instructions for quitting and coping with withdrawal, enhancement of motivation to stop smoking—should be used toward that end. The next level of therapeutic action is to strengthen the patient's affect management skills by encouraging the patient to express negative affects. The fact that craving and psychological symptoms such as irritability, restlessness, and anxiety regularly follow quitting smoking presents the therapist with a natural setting for helping the patient begin to express and discuss the emergence of negative emotions. By helping the patient to clarify, name, and accept those psychological symptoms during nicotine withdrawal, and to relate them to external life events, the therapist offers the patient a model for managing affect that can be used outside the smoking cessation therapy relationship. As the therapy progresses, the focus of affect expression extends to emotions that may not be precipitated by the physiological disequilibrium resulting from nicotine withdrawal, but by a larger emotional disequilibrium resulting from the absence of a favored tool for coping with general life concerns. Subsequently, in later sessions, the focus of therapy is to help the patient develop adaptive cognitive and behavioral strategies that will fulfill the comforting and medicating effects formerly attributed to smoking. The therapist helps the patient consider new or alternative behaviors or attitudes that are productive, ego-compatible, self-fulfilling, and ultimately, enjoyable. Finally, the orientation and challenge to change that pervades the psychotherapeutic approach requires that the therapist, beginning at the screening visit, communicate a constant, reassuring, and supportive stance.

Especially when the nicotine-dependent patient begins to present more complex problems, there is a tendency for the therapy to take on the general mental health problem of the patient. When this occurs, it is important to cast treatment content within the context of nicotine dependence—for example, by elucidating, whenever appropriate, the part played by cigarette smoking in hindering the patient's particular approach to resolving conflict. This may clarify a need for more in-depth and prolonged psychotherapy.

Techniques

A psychotherapeutic approach for smoking cessation (PSC) uses cognitive, supportive, and expressive therapeutic techniques that are generally delivered in an active, directive therapeutic style. The therapy is change oriented, sequenced, and time limited.

Education About Nicotine Dependence. During an early session, a conceptual view of nicotine dependence, for example, the presence of physiological–behavioral–emotional features, will be explained to the patient. The ability to conceptualize what until then has been a bewildering and intractible compulsion gives the patient a sense of mastery over the process of quitting. It is also useful to describe the withdrawal syndrome and present it as an event that, albeit very difficult and inevitable, is time limited and surmountable.

Supportive. Recovery from nicotine dependence requires changes on several levels: physiological (nicotine withdrawal), behavioral (termination of smoking and other behaviors previously linked with smoking), and emotional (experiencing rather than inhibiting painful feelings). These changes are uncomfortable, provoke anxiety, and tend to weaken the patient's customary psychological defenses. By presenting an accepting, nonjudgmental posture, the therapist fosters the therapeutic alliance, and provides a supportive relationship to help wean the patient from dependence on cigarettes as the patient begins new patterns of behaviors and feelings.

Encouragement of Affect. The therapist's effort to promote the patient's capacities of self-expression even during the prequit sessions collects its payoff during the period after quit day when the behavioral and emotional void brought about by nicotine abstinence begins to be experienced. It may begin with a simple question—"How have you been feeling since you stopped smoking?" or "Have you noticed any changes in the way you feel since you stopped smoking?" The therapist will help the patient distinguish between psychological states that may be attributable to physiological effects of nicotine withdrawal or feeling states that are revealed because of the absence of smoking as a self-medicating tool.

Clarification. Because of a smoking-career history of repressing painful feelings by smoking, the patient may be emotionally constricted and unable to recognize or acknowledge the tendency to use smoking as a psychological tool. Using a directive approach, the therapist helps the patient gain more insight into the psychological features of the smoker's dependence on smoking.

Change Oriented. The patient's ability to acknowledge, experience, and tolerate negative affect is a necessary step that mediates the essential therapeutic goal of relinquishing old smoking-related patterns of behavior, cognitions, and emotional style. The most evident behavior relinquished is cigarette smoking. Other behaviors known to trigger smoking urges will also need to be changed and replaced with behaviors that are not conditioned to provoke urges to smoke. Cognitions that require changing are maladaptative beliefs about the unchangeable, essential quality of smoking, or the patient's belief of possessing inadequate resources to maintain current functioning in the absence of cigarettes (I'm a writer, I won't be able to write if I stop smoking). Emotional changes involve a transformation from repression, inhibition, or fears about negative feelings to an attitude of acceptance, tolerance, and a mastery of those negative feelings.

Sequenced and Short Term. Recovery in nicotine dependence involves multiple stages and the content of psychological treatment unfolds in response to those stages. Often occurring in chronological order, the major phases of nicotine dependence recovery involve beginning treatment; preparing to quit; learning how to quit; reaching quit day; managing acute withdrawal; and preparing for long-term abstinence. The latter phase includes lessons on extinguishing smoking-conditioned behaviors; dealing with emotional changes; establishing substitute behaviors for coping with painful, distressful feelings; and managing life events without smoking.

Thus, the phases of treatment may include a screening visit, 1–3 weeks of preparing for quit day (depending on whether the pharmacological adjunct is nicotine replacement, in which case it could be 1 week, or 2 to 3 weeks if the pharmacotherapy is an antidepressant), 2 weeks of acute withdrawal management, and 4 to 6 weeks of examining and exploring abstinence-related affects, problem solving, and development of substitute behaviors and new beliefs. Following these sessions (possibly up to nine), which make up the acute treatment phase, is the maintenance segment, which takes place during the next 3 months. The rationale for an extended, that is, 6-month, treatment lies in previous empirical data from our clinic and also reported by others showing that the relapse rate is most precipitous during the first 6 months and levels off thereafter. Furthermore, I have repeatedly heard patients in our clinical trials express strong disappointment at the brief duration of our treatments, which are usually of 8 to 12 weeks duration. Treatment session length may vary from 30 to 45 min.

A CASE EXAMPLE

To illustrate the application of this psychological treatment, the case of Ms. G with a description of the prescribed treatment tasks and patient response is given here.

Visit 1—Assessment

Screening procedures include a personal and social history, tobacco use history, a psychiatric diagnostic interview, and psychological ratings.

Ms. G was 28 years old when I first saw her. During that first session, the screening assessment measures had determined that she had a history of recurrent episodes of major depression and alcohol dependence. She smoked 30 cigarettes a day and had made multiple attempts to stop smoking, which never lasted for more than three days. For the past 6 years, she had been working evenings as a waitress and during the day made the rounds of talent agencies auditioning for work on Broadway and TV. She had a boyfriend (a nonsmoker) with whom she had been living for 3 years. In spite of that longevity, G did not feel secure about the permanence of her relationship with the boyfriend. G did not appear to be depressed at the time of screening and scored within the normal range on clinical measures of psychological well-being. G was clearly highly motivated to stop smoking but was also unsure about her ability to do it. G attended AA meetings regularly and was seeing a therapist weekly.

Visit 2—Week 2, Smoking History

Assessment continues as the therapist begins by asking the patient to describe his or her cigarette smoking history and current pattern of cigarette smoking. Following this, the therapist describes the multidimensional concept of nicotine dependence, pointing out through this exposition how the patient's given self-description coincides with the model. This session ends with the therapist giving out a homework assignment: The patient is to pay attention to his or her pattern of smoking during the next week, with particular attention to those cigarettes that he or she considers most pleasurable and the ones most difficult to give up.

Visit 3—Preparing for Quit Day

The objective of this visit is to enhance the patient's motivation to quit and to provide instrumental information on how to prepare for quit day (QD). The therapist gives instructions for performing prequit and early postcessation techniques designed to alleviate craving and nicotine withdrawal symptoms. The therapist will elicit the patient's feelings about stopping. Ambivalence will be recognized. Attention will be paid to the patient's positive feelings about smoking, which the therapist will acknowledge as natural and acceptable. Reasons for wanting to stop will also be elicited and supported. It should be made clear at this session that the patient should stop smoking completely on QD and that under no circumstances should the patient yield to an urge to smoke even a puff. Instructions on how to use nicotine replacement medication (or other pharmacotherapy) are also given.

Visit 4—Post-QD Visit

If this visit does not take place on the day after QD, arrangements should be made for the patient to call either at the end of QD or early the next day. The patient who has not smoked at all on the targeted quit day should be strongly commended. Many patients will be feeling very uncomfortable at this time. They should be encouraged to describe any adverse reactions, to which the therapist will respond by pointing out that the patient is entering the peak period of nicotine withdrawal and that the coming week will likely be the most difficult in terms of experiencing the typical nicotine withdrawal symptoms. The therapist will offer hope by describing the time-limited nature of the nicotine withdrawal syndrome. The patient will be asked to call the therapist the following day and again 2 or 3 days later to report on his or her progress. During these calls, the therapist will inquire about the presence and severity of withdrawal symptoms and about adverse experiences that may be induced by the NRT. The therapist will make suggestions on how to alleviate symptoms or side effects. If the patient does not make these calls, the therapist will do it.

If substantial smoking, such as more than five cigarettes, has taken place on QD, the patient's motivation and resolve about stopping smoking at this time should be reviewed. If the patient's resolve seems to be genuine, a second QD may be assigned. If fewer than five cigarettes have been smoked, the patient should be told to stop smoking the next day. Failure to do this would also signal a need to reevaluate the patient's resolve. In this case as well, a second QD may be selected. In either case, if complete abstinence is not reached by the second QD, treatment should be terminated and, particularly in cases where the patient expresses a continued desire to stop, referral may be made to other treatment resources.

> The post quit day session found G ebullient with strong though mixed emotions. She had not been smoking for 24 hours, she felt "great" yet she also felt scared. I felt that the most important messages she needed to hear at this time were a commendation for a goal accomplished, a view of the road ahead (the rise and gradual ebb of nicotine withdrawal symptoms), and an exhortation to continue to be vigilant against the next smoke because, as was her history, she was highly vulnerable to smoking again, and finally, to view me as a source of emotional support during this time. Her week's assignment was to phone me at least twice during the coming week.

Week 5—1 Week After QD, Early Withdrawal

The patient will usually have been nicotine abstinent for 1 week at this visit. For most patients, withdrawal symptoms and craving may be continuing to a noticeable degree. In addition to repeating the congratulations, the emphasis at this session will be to call the patient's attention to the substitute behaviors he or she performed during those times that a cigarette would have been customarily smoked. The therapist will also encourage the patient to talk about his or her feelings about nicotine abstinence at this time.

Visit 6 (Week 6)—2 Weeks After QD, Withdrawal Period

For patients who have been consistently abstinent, this period is a transition between the decline of withdrawal symptoms and the beginning of relapse prevention counseling. More so than at week 5, the therapist will ask about new, unusual, or impressive events or feelings that have occurred. If the patient is unable to recount any such event, the therapist will foster the patient's self-expression by explicit questioning. For example, "What did you do this morning immediately after waking up (instead of smoking)?" "Was there any moment in the past week (today, yesterday) that you felt an urge to smoke? What was going on at that time? Was your reaction (behavior/feeling) different from what usually happened in the past?"

I have found a range in the reporting of new events (behaviors, feelings, even beliefs about the self) and found myself responding alternatively with encouragement, listening, directive clarification, or explicit words of congratulations, according to the content of the patient's responses.

> G saw me each week for the next 2 weeks, and after that in biweekly meetings. During the first of the biweekly sessions, G's mood had begun to take a downturn. Instead of the euphoria that she had come with in the earlier sessions, she was quiet and listless. In response to my questioning, she said she was feeling disappointed. She had anticipated feeling better now that she had met the long-sought after goal of not smoking, but she was not. I asked G to talk more about this new feeling. She continued by talking about her dissatisfaction with her career progress. She was realizing she had been working so hard yet not achieving her goal of a substantial role in a Broadway play or a television show. I then related these new feelings to the absence of cigarette smoking, and to the possibility that she may have contained long-standing negative emotions by smoking; when the smoking stopped, it became impossible to hold them down. G agreed with this interpretation.
>
> At this same session, G continued to express more negative feelings. She felt angry and resentful at her mother who was an alcoholic, at her father who was unable to make up for the mother's absence, and at theater bosses who were unable to appreciate her talent. She was also angry that she was not feeling better. (Was she also angry with me?) In fact, although she still detested the idea of herself as a smoker, her urges to smoke were as strong as ever. I responded to G's expressions by listening attentively and without judgment. Again, I suggested that her feelings of anger reflected how in the past cigarette smoking may have masked such strong negative feelings. Pointing out that it had been about 2 weeks since her quit day and that her body's

withdrawal from nicotine was likely to be at its end, I suggested that the strong urges to smoke were reminders of how she had in the past smoked as a way of coping with negative feelings. Therefore, she should begin to interpret those urges as a signal to the presence of negative feelings that in the past she had repressed or inhibited. I then recommended a strategy of paying attention to those negative feelings, devoting time to recognizing them and then allowing herself to feel them. I also told her that I would like her to call me if she felt that my help was needed.

Visits 7–9 (Weeks 8–12)—Managing Changes

These latter sessions continue the process of clarifying feelings, identification of the patient's emotional response patterns, and discussion of new and alternative coping patterns to replace cigarette smoking. Physically and psychologically, most patients' emotional state will be close to if not better than how they were at baseline. Urges to smoke will have decreased in frequency and intensity. The situation is different, however, for the emotionally vulnerable patient, who is likely to still report intense cravings to smoke, even if they are less frequent than during the early weeks of abstinence. The absence of negative feelings is a good sign; however, continued feelings of depression, anxiety, restlessness, and irritability portend more serious emotional sequelae of nicotine abstinence. These will need to be addressed to prevent a severe psychiatric episode.

It had become clear after some discussion that the main issue for G at this time of her life centered on her unfulfilled ambition for a career in the theater. She recognized her good fortune in being involved in a stable relationship with a caring and loving man, and she felt that the major negative elements of her childhood had been and were continuing to be addressed in long-term psychotherapy. That she had continued to smoke had also been a source of frustration, but she was genuinely pleased with herself that even smoking now appeared to be under control. But the unfulfilled career was still a source of emotional pain.

I asked G if, given what to me was her obvious wealth of talents, she had ever considered any other occupation. After a moment of deliberating on whether to express it or not, G responded with much anger to my question. There had been too much affirmation from others in the past, she said, regarding her great talent for the acting world, to question the fitness of her ambition. She was and, despite these years of setbacks, remained resolute in her desire for a career in acting. I took pains to communicate that I admired her determination, and acknowledged her anger but did not respond to her anger in a deeper way. Instead I returned to my perception of her as a highly competent person. I also said that I thought any employer she worked for, including the restaurant she was now working in, was extremely fortunate to have her devoted and able services. I believe she left the session surprised that she had been able to be so expressive with her anger towards me while also feeling validated of her self-worth.

Despite her psychological discomfort, G wanted to continue to not smoke. Together, we then explored several nonsmoking coping options that would be comfortable for her and practicable given her circumstances and resources. Also, to prepare G for termination, I pointed out that the time limitations of our 12-week program and suggested that she begin to work through these issues with the help of her regular therapist. G said she wanted to do that.

About 6 weeks after her quit day, as the active treatment period was coming to an end, G's emotional downturn had progressed to a severe depression. One week later, she was given a prescription for Zoloft.

Postcessation and Follow-Up

For some cases, counseling that takes place over 8 to 12 weeks with concomitant pharmacotherapy followed by booster sessions every few months may be adequate for maintaining long-term abstinence. However, I have also seen many instances when smoking cessation patients seek more frequent and more lasting clinical support after the cessation-related counseling has terminated. Duing the last 3 months, visits may occur less frequently, for example, once a month. Often, the patient's anticipation of seeing the therapist in another 4 weeks is a forceful motivation for not smoking again.

Between the last treatment visit and a scheduled Month 3 follow-up meeting, I saw G once and spoke to her by telephone twice. The first phone call came 2 weeks after the last treatment session. She wanted to see me because she felt very depressed. When I did see her, her face was drawn, her shoulders hunched, and her speech was slow and without lilt. She was clearly in a major depressive episode; still, she was committed to continuing not to smoke and she was also hopeful that with more time on Zoloft she would feel better. I encouraged her hopeful attitude, although, seeing her crestfallen manner at that time, I found it difficult to be certain of a positive outcome regarding the nicotine abstinence. G proffered more bad and good news. She had quit her job because she had felt that she would return to smoking if she had stayed. Encouraged by our discussions during the treatment sessions, she had begun to feel more comfortable about accepting the financial support her boyfriend had reassuringly offered. The second phone call came four weeks later. The depression had lifted. G had gone back to waitressing as a means of support for the meanwhile but she had also gone to a vocational appraisal program. It was for this new ability to consider a different career path which began during her smoking cessation treatment that she felt most grateful. She also reported that she felt closer than ever to her boyfriend.

The study protocol involved three other contacts over a period of 12 months after the end of the active treatment. By the 3-month follow-up which occurred through a telephone call, she was still taking Zoloft, and Buspar had been added to her regimen. At the time of the phone call, her mood was good. She had continued not to smoke, had begun a new job, and was engaged to be married.

An Epilougue

G called me again, on her own initiative. It had been exactly 3 years since she had stopped smoking. She wanted to thank me and to report on her progress. She was not smoking and was no longer using Zoloft or Buspar. She was now married, had completed a graduate degree, and was working as a professional in her field. And although there were times when she thought she would have really enjoyed a cigarette, she had not smoked since her quit day.

Although it seemed the psychological treatment had helped G stop smoking, what it did not prevent was the onset of a depressive episode. It may be the case that psychological counseling alone may not prevent the emergence of severe depression after smoking cessation among certain vulnerable smokers. Nevertheless, I believe that the treatment helped G to overcome what might have been a defeatist reaction to the depression. She actively sought the antidepressant medication and was hopeful that with its help she would feel better.

Other Cases

Space limitation permits only one detailed "Ms. G" story. However, I have worked with many more long-term abstainers, each case with its history of psychic struggle and unfolding of alternating negative and positive emotions brought on by nicotine withdrawal and, I believe, the psychological counseling. There was M, who denied a history of MDD but recalled extreme feelings of depression during a previous quit attempt. She smoked again at that time and within a day the symptoms disappeared. During the first 2 weeks after quitting, M called me every day, once from a plane to a business meeting in California. She talked alternately about her feelings of pride at having stopped smoking and the lost sense of self as she had become an ideal "corporate wife" to a prominent industry captain. In the course of dealing with postcessation emotions without the benefit of nicotine, she was confronted by old feelings of self-denigration and low self-esteem as her sense of self had disappeared in a high-profile marriage. However, stopping smoking, a goal she had small hopes of ever being able to reach, had brought about expressions of admiration from many friends and colleagues, and her own self-congratulation. With her new-found strength, as she stopped smoking and continued to do so, she broke out to gain prominence on her own merit in her own career.

It is difficult for me to ever forget Mrs. Z, a formally mannered grandmother of a toddler who began the way to her independence from smoking when she was able to accept and tolerate that she was capable of angry feelings, even toward her grandson, whom she wanted to hit as he fussed so on one evening of babysitting him. The craving to smoke that she experienced during that occasion provided the material that enabled us to examine how smoking had served to inhibit her forbidden anger. During one postquit session, as I verbalized the acceptability of that anger and enjoined her during one of the sessions to experience the anger and to accept herself for it, I witnessed, within moments, Z's physical posture change from one of taut rigidity to a soft relaxation and relief. In future sessions, she reported feeling generally less tense, and less troubled by cravings to smoke.

From the account of Ms. G's treatment, and the limited ones of 2 other cases described here, we can reiterate some of the principles and techniques that seem to characterize the essence of a psychotherapy for these emotionally vulnerable smokers. These include the promotion of the therapeutic alliance, encouragement of the patient's self-expression, and the therapist's interpretation of those self-expressions. Also important contributors to the change process were the educational sessions—which not only increased the patients' understanding of the disorder but in doing so enabled them to feel a sense of mastery over it. Related to this was a directive therapist style, which was necessary to counter the initial sense of helplessness that refractory smokers often come to treatment with. Moreover, a highly individualized approach, guided by details derived from a personalized history taking, increased the patients' sense of self-worth and self-confidence about being able to remain abstinent. It is also useful to consider that in all of these cases, the smoking cessation therapy was time limited, with the longest having taken place over 12 weeks. Among the cases I described, only G was concurrently in psychotherapy. However, many of the other ex-smokers I have worked with either were in concurrent therapeutic relationships or began such relationships after their work with me had ended. For the former, it is likely that the ongoing therapeutic relationship provided important additional support; in the latter, where patients began psychotherapy after the smoking cessation counseling, the changes it brought about (increased self-understanding, emotional awareness, and openness to the experience of negative feelings) required continued therapeutic attention.

To sum up, I have described a form of short-term insight-oriented psychological therapy for the treatment of nicotine dependence when the addiction to smoking is sustained by an inability to manage negative emotions. The focus of this approach is the recognition and acceptance of, and adaptive coping with emotional distress when the individual's wish to avoid painful mood states does battle with the emergence of such unwanted feelings. The therapist fosters the therapeutic alliance to encourage the patient's expression and experience of negative affect and to motivate the adoption of cognitive and behavior changes that dissipate the need to self-medicate by smoking.

REFERENCES

American Psychiatric Association. (1987). *Diagnostic and statistical manual of mental disorders* (3rd ed., rev.). Washington, DC: American Psychiatric Association.

Anda, R. F., Williamson, D. F., Escobedo, L. G., Mast, E. E., Giovino, G. A., & Remington, P. L. (1990). Depression and the dynamics of smoking. *JAMA, 264*, 1541–1545.

Balfour, D. J. K. (1982). The effects of nicotine on brain neurotransmitter systems. *Pharmacology and Therapeutics, 16,* 269–282.

Breslau, N., Kilbey, M., & Andreski, P. (1991). Nicotine dependence, major depression, and anxiety in young adults. *Archives of General Psychiatry, 458,* 1069–1071.

Breslau, N., Peterson, E., Schultz, L., Andreski, P., & Chilcoat, H. (1996). Are smokers with alcohol disorders less likely to quit? *American Journal of Public Health, 86,* 985–990.

Carmody, T. P. (1989). Affect regulation, nicotine addiction, and smoking cessation. *Journal of Psychoactive Drugs, 21,* 331–342.

Corrigall, W. A. (1991). Understanding brain mechanisms in nicotine reinforcement. *British Journal of Addiction, 86,* 507–510.

Covey, L. S., & Glassman, A. H. (1991). A meta-analysis of double-blind placebo-controlled trials of clonidine for smoking cessation. *British Journal of Addiction, 86,* 991–998.

Covey, L. S., Glassman, A. H., & Stetner, F. (1990). Depresssion and depressive symptoms in smoking cessation. *Comprehensive Psychiatry, 31,* 350–354.

Covey, L. S., Hughes, D. C., Glassman, A. H., Blazer, D. G., & George, L. K. (1994). Ever-smoking, quitting, and psychiatric disorders: Evidence from the Durham, North Carolina, Epidemiologic Catchment Area. *Tobacco Control, 3,* 222–227.

Covey, L. S., Struening, E. L., Larino, M., Glassman, A. H., Ferry, L. H., & Saunders, B. (1997, June). *Is there more to nicotine dependence than the DSM-IV criteria?* Paper presented at the 3rd Annual Meeting of the Society for Research on Nicotine and Tobacco, Nashville, TN.

Covey, L. S., & Tam, D. (1990). Depressive mood, the single-parent home, and adolescent cigarette smoking. *American Journal of Public Health, 80,* 1330–1333.

Fergusson, D. M., Lynskey, M. T., & Horwood, L. F. (1996). Comorbidity between depressive disorders and nicotine dependence in a cohort of 16-year olds. *Archives of General Psychiatry, 53,* 1043–1047.

Fiore, M. C., Novotny, T. E., Pierce, J. P., Giovino, G. A., Hatziandreu, E. J., Newcomb, P. A., Surawicz, T. S., & Davis, R. M. (1990). Methods used to quit smoking in the United States. Do cessation programs help? *JAMA, 263,* 2760–2765.

Glassman, A. H. (1993). Cigarette smoking: Implications for psychiatric illness. *American Journal of Psychiatry, 150,* 546–563.

Glassman, A. H., Helzer, J. E., Covey, L. S., Cottler, L. B., Stetner, F., Tipp, J. E., & Johnson, J. (1990). Smoking, smoking cessation, and major depression. *JAMA, 264,* 1546–1549.

Glassman, A. H., Stetner, F., Walsh, B. T., Raizman, P. S., Fleiss, J. L., Cooper, T. B., & Covey, L. S. (1988). Heavy smokers, smoking cessation, and clonidine. *JAMA, 259,* 2863–2866.

Hall, S. M., Munoz, R. F., & Reus, V. I. (1994). Cognitive-behavioral intervention increases abstinence rates for depressive-history smokers. *Journal of Consulting and Clinical Psychology, 62,* 141–146.

Hall, S. M., Munoz, R. F., Reus, V. I., Sees, K. L., Duncan, C., Humfleet, G. L., & Hartz, D. T. (1996). Mood management and nicotine gum in smoking treatment: A therapeutic contact and placebo-controlled study. *Journal of Consulting and Clinical Psychology, 64,* 1003–1009.

Henningfield, J. E. (1985). Abuse liability and pharmacodynamic characteristics of intravenous and inhaled nicotine. *Journal of Pharmacology and Experimental Therapeutics, 234,* 1–12.

Henningfield, J. E. (1995). Nicotine medications for smoking cessation. *New England Journal of Medicine, 333,* 1196–1203.

Hughes, J. R. (1994). Behavioral support programs for smoking cessation. *Modern Medicine, 62,* 22–27.

Hughes, J. R., Hatsukami, D. K., Mitchell, J. E., & Dahlgren, L. A. (1986). Prevalence of smoking among psychiatric outpatients. *American Journal of Psychiatry, 143,* 993–997.

Klerman, G. L., Weissman, M. M., Rounsaville, B. J., & Chevron, E. S. (1984). *Interpersonal psychotherapy of depression.* New York: Basic Books.

Lam, W., Sacks, H. S., Sze, P., & Chalmers, T. C. (1987). Meta-analysis of randomised controlled trials of nicotine gum. *Lancet, ii,* 27–30.

Leshner, A. I. (1997). Drug abuse and addiction treatment research. *Archives of General Psychiatry, 54,* 691–693.

Luborsky, L. (1984). *Principles of psychoanalytic psychotherapy. A manual for supportive-expressive treatment.* New York: Basic Books.

Patton, G. C., Hibbert, M., Rosier, M. J., Carlin, J. B., Caust, J., & Bowes, G. (1996). Is smoking associated with depression and anxiety in teenagers? *American Journal of Public Health, 86,* 225–230.

Pomerleau, C. S. (1997). Co-factors for smoking and evolutionary psychobiology. *Addiction, 92,* 397–408.

Schwartz, J. (1987). *Review and evaluation of smoking cessation methods: The United States and Canada, 1978–1985* (NIH Publication No. 87-2940). Bethesda, MD: U.S. Department of Health and Human Services.

Shiffman, S. M. (1986). Cluster analytic classification of smoking relapse episodes. *Addictive Behaviors, 11,* 295–307.

Shiffman, S. M. (1989). Tobacco "chippers": Individual differences in tobacco dependence. *Psychopharmacology, 97,* 535–538.

Thomas, C. L. (1993). *Taber's cyclopedic medical dictionary.* Philadelphia: Davis.

Tomkins, S. (1968). A modified model of smoking behavior. In E. F. Borgatta & R. R. Evans (Eds.), *Smoking, health, and behavior* (pp. 165–186). Chicago: Aldine.

U.S. Department of Health, Education, and Welfare. (1964). *Smoking and health: Report of the Advisory Committee to the Surgeon General of the Public Health Service* (PHS Publication No. 1103). Washington, DC: U.S. Government Printing Office.

U.S. Department of Health and Human Services. (1988). *The health consequences of smoking: Nicotine addiction. A report of the Surgeon General,* Publication No. (CDC) 88-8046. Rockville, MD.

Zelman, D. C., Brandon, T. H., Jorenby, D. E., & Baker, T. B. (1992). Measures of affect and nicotine dependence predict differential response to smoking cessation treatments. *Journal of Consulting Clinical Psychology, 60,* 943–952.

CHAPTER TEN

Group Psychotherapy for Hard-Core Smokers

Henry Spitz
Daniel F. Seidman
Columbia University

Treating hard-core smokers who are able to stop smoking but unable to stay off cigarettes poses one of the most challenging and vexing of clinical problems. The major focus of this chapter is a description of how a model psychotherapy group is used in treating this notoriously difficult clinical problem.

For the hard-core smoker, we recommend using a *relapse prevention group.* This psychotherapy model is targeted in a different way from short-term support groups designed to help people withdraw from cigarettes. In the latter approach, people who quit early are placed with people who cannot quit at all or not until the group ends. In contrast, a relapse prevention group is composed only of patients who have already quit, and focuses on the unique psychological benefits of a group as a tool to promote long-term abstinence. A major emphasis is on initial screening and preparation for the group. In our experience, introducing patients who are unable to stop smoking at all can be demoralizing or distracting to those who have stopped. Such individuals are dealing with different issues, are at a different stage of readiness to change,and can add a chaotic element to the group process, especially when they do poorly and drop out. As such, a demonstrated capacity to abstain for at least 24 hr is a key inclusion criterion.

As a general practice, group leaders need to exercise their gatekeeper function and to exclude those patients who, in their clinical judgment, are not ready to benefit from and will not help fulfill the goals of the group as a whole. Patients who want to quit but have not been able to stop smoking, may need to be referred for residential treatment (Hurt et al., 1992), or can be worked with individually to help them stop smoking and to prepare them for the type of relapse prevention group that we discuss in this chapter.

Feedback from a group of similarly addicted peers can be hard to dismiss or discount, without further self-appraisal. This is particularly the case when the feedback is similar to responses provided by the group leader. For some patients, hearing other smokers tell their stories may help break through a hard shell. For the hard-core smoker, staying off cigarettes often entails a difficult period of emotional readjustment. A group of peers who have "been there" can be a powerful model for identification and for alternative coping responses.

The literature on group treatment for smokers reveals long-term outcomes that are at least comparable to those found for individual treatments. Some studies also report superior end-of-treatment, 6-month, and 1-year results for group when compared with individual formats. Economic analysis also supports the use of intensive group counseling as the most cost-effective intervention for smokers (Cromwell, Bartosch, Fiore, Hasselblad, & Baker, 1997). This introduction briefly reviews general groups for smoking cessation, which offer treatment for quitting smoking as well as for relapse prevention, in contrast with the approach focused on relapse prevention presented in this chapter.

Schwartz (1987) provides an extensive review of group trials and methods and reports that group approaches are the mainstay of smoking cessation clinics. In his review of 46 widely disparate group trials, he reports a median quit rate of 27% with follow-ups that vary from 5 to 12 months.

Shewchuk et al. (1977), in an early paper on group treatment for heavy "hard-core" smokers, reported a superior end-of-treatment abstinence rate of 49% for group, compared to 38% for hypnosis, and 33% for individual counseling. At 1-year follow-up, only the success rate with group therapy showed superior results when compared to the success rate found in a non-treated sample. However, it should also be made clear that this study found *no* significant differences for group, 21%, hypnosis, 17%, and individual treatment, 19%, when they were compared with each other at 1 year. These authors summarize the smoking cessation and psychotherapy "treatment principles" employed in this study as:

1. Taking an individualized approach.
2. Adopting a "positive orientation."
3. Encouraging smokers to "assume responsibility" for their own behavior.
4. Promoting personal "contact and continuity" between therapist and patient.
5. Emphasizing "action" over "contemplation."
6. Focusing primarily on "obstacles to quitting," with secondary focus on quitting techniques.

7. Focusing on "maintenance" issues and follow-up contact.

A later research study by Hajek, Belcher, and Stapleton (1985) compared two group formats for smokers. These authors found significant advantages for what they call "group-oriented" groups (67% abstinent at end of treatment, 28% at 1-year follow-up) versus "therapist-oriented" groups (47% abstinent at end of treatment, 17% at 1-year follow-up). The treatment consisted of five 1-hr group sessions over a 4-week period. Group-oriented groups emphasize the autonomous development of group processes and resources such as:

1. Group pressure from social comparisons.
2. Group support from the sharing of mutual problems and the hopes of overcoming them.
3. Spontaneous group modeling of successful coping responses.

Therapist-oriented groups, in contrast, were defined in this study as emphasizing the educational (didactic) and motivational role of the group leaders.

A more recent report from Fiore et al. (1994) found superior outcomes for the group plus placebo patch (20.0%) versus the individual plus placebo patch (7.3%) counseling format at 6 months. (A confounding variable, though, is that the group sessions were 60 min and the individual sessions only 15 min.) The intensive group counseling employed in this study combined the elements of "skill training and group support." These authors concluded, based on the verbal reports of participants, that the social support of group sessions is most likely the active ingredient that produced greater abstinent rates for the group format. Finally, Hughes (1996), in a recent review of treatment efforts in nicotine dependence, presented an algorithm for smoking cessation in which he recommended group behavior therapy as a first-line psychological therapy.

Although some authors (Fiore et al., 1994) have suggested that social support is the active change agent in group treatments, in our view, group psychotherapy offers additional benefits, which it is the goal of this chapter to describe. These include: (a) the opportunity to learn a new repertoire of coping techniques firsthand from a group of peers; (b) a place for smokers to see their own psychological issues more clearly when expressed by others, and then to apply this learning to their own situations; and (c) an environment in which, because they share a common problem with others, smokers can feel less defensive and guarded and allow themselves to be more expressive about things that may seem "shameful" or "crazy."

The key initial tasks to start and maintain a relapse prevention group for treating nicotine addiction are (a) careful screening, diagnosis, and selection, and (b) preparation for the group experience.

GROUP SCREENING AND PREPARATION

Although the screening and evaluation elements discussed next are similar for individual and group treatments (except for obtaining a group history), the clinician considering referral for group has to review the first four elements in the context of the smoker's overall experience in groups throughout his or her life.

Screening and Evaluation

Screening involves five elements:

1. A health history.
2. A smoking history.
3. A substance abuse history.
4. A psychiatric history.
5. A group history.

A standard health questionnaire administered at the time of the first appointment accomplishes two important goals: it reveals smoking-related illnesses or symptoms (for both patients and their families), and it provides an opportunity to inquire about prior psychiatric treatments and illnesses (i.e., psychiatric comorbidity) such as depression, alcoholism and other substance abuse, anxiety disorders, or other psychiatric conditions.

A smoking history and tobacco use questionnaire, administered in the initial evaluation session, covers such areas as reasons to quit/reasons to smoke; length of time smoking and daily pattern of use; identification of relapse triggers; and history of nicotine withdrawal syndrome. In addition to data gathering, the initial interview accomplishes several clinical goals: (a) to develop a supportive therapeutic relationship and (b) to communicate to the patient an implicit message that specifically underlines the seriousness of the presenting problem of smoking. Taking a smoking history, in particular, provides the opportunity to observe the smoker's tendency to minimize, deny, or rationalize his or her addiction to tobacco use.

An initial evaluation for group psychotherapy focuses attention on smoking as a social or group activity. The extent of helpful social and clinical support, or lack thereof, in prior quit attempts and relapses is also assessed. An important goal in formulating an initial treatment plan is to uncover, and address with new strategies, problems not previously overcome in other quit attempts.

A brief evaluation is also made of alcohol/drug use (present and past) for the smoker, and of the smoker's psychiatric history and current mental status (Spitzer & Williams, 1996). These two elements, and their association with cigarette smoking, can provide further data to help formulate an effective initial treatment plan. It is sometimes important to inquire about any significant family psychiatric and substance abuse history as well. Associations between cigarette smoking, psychiatric disorders, and substance abuse, if prevalent in the smoker's family and social milieu, can present obstacles to the implementation of the treatment plan. Smokers coming in for cessation treatment may need an explanation of why psychiatric data (its absence or presence) is relevant to their current problem. A brief summary of findings concerning increased difficulties with cessation for smokers who have had a history of depression is usually sufficient (Glass, 1990).

The last element in a comprehensive screening for group is the group history, which explores the individual's past experiences in important groups such as the family, school, peers etc. The interpersonal "school" of evaluation for group therapy has produced a widely used set of criteria. It offers the therapist an evaluative framework for the question of when group is an appropriate option, as well as who the participants should be.

For example, it is essential from the interpersonal standpoint that the group therapist elicit a history of group function in much the same way that the sex therapist obtains a formal sexual history, or the internist takes a medical history. This is done by surveying the major areas of group function to date in the patient's life. Sequentially, these include the family of origin, early school history, peer-group relations in adolescence, work history, military experience, and social history, with particular focus on major emotional relationships.

The product of this investigation is a cross-sectional view of a person's ability or limitations in natural groups. From a pragmatic point of view, this may yield the most useful clinical data on an individual's potential for getting the most—or least—out of a group experience. Some examples follow that illustrate this premise: Patients with high levels of authority anxiety will reflect this in work histories characterized by conflict with superiors, in school situations through difficulties with teachers and administrators, and, of course, with parents.

On the other hand, patients with excessive peer anxiety stemming from disturbed sibling and/or peer-group relationships will show a corresponding historical pattern in dysfunctional relationships with their contemporaries. Because the group setting taps both peer (horizontal transference: member-to-member) and authority (vertical transference: member-to-leader) relationships, it offers a fruitful medium for resolving interpersonal conflicts involving both authority figures and peers.

The group history of an individual may reveal relationship problems of a chronic and specific nature. This information is helpful in two ways. If a prospective group member's style is one that is interpersonally destructive, as in sociopathy or impulse-control disorders, then the therapist is forewarned that including such a smoker could harm the group. It thus becomes data in the service of defining exclusion criteria. If, on the other hand, a pattern of disturbed interpersonal relationships of a more benign type is found, the patient can be placed in a group of specific composition, such as one in which those interpersonal problems can be readily reproduced and, it is hoped, resolved.

Such individual and personalized screening can usually be accomplished in the initial session, during which the therapist and the patient also formulate a treatment plan. Experience suggests that not more than 50% of the membership of any smoking cessation group should be composed of smokers with current symptoms of minor depression. The reason for this is that too many depressed people in a group can undermine the group's potential to instill hope, build confidence, and provide alternative models for coping and imitative behavior.

Readiness and Group Preparation

Preparation is crucial in starting a patient in a tobacco addiction group. Two criteria for "readiness" are:

1. A pretraining period of sustained abstinence of at least several weeks before beginning group.
2. Demonstrated capacity to achieve abstinence for a 24-hr period.

The latter, which is called a "prescribed abstinence period," is an important assessment tool. The 24-hr criterion is lenient, and may lead to more dropouts from the group. However, it also gives newly abstinent patients access to group support for relapse prevention earlier on in their treatment. It also serves to remind those group members with longer abstinence of their earlier struggle, thus reinforcing their ongoing commitment to finding fulfilling ways to live without nicotine.

In contrast, the first criterion—abstinence of several weeks—is more stringent. It will result in more potential group members being excluded from a group. However, it can also result in a higher level of long-term abstinence among the included group members. This criterion can also decrease anxiety and pressure on new members as they are already abstaining from smoking, and can increase group cohesion by minimizing the disruption due to dropouts by smoking group members.

What we advise in either case is to work individually with the patient to achieve abstinence and to give the patient a good picture of the group culture he or she will be joining. We find that this leads to a greater group cohesion and less rapid turnover in what can become a "drop in/drop out center," when active smoking addicts are freely entered into group.

Our group size is maintained at between five to nine members. More than nine members starts to feel impersonal, more like a quit smoking "class" than an intimate experience of confronting life's problems without nicotine. Less than five members severely limits the opportunities to develop the interpersonal group process.

Groups are run on an open-ended basis because it has been our experience that time-limited groups (such as 10 weeks) are unrealistic for many severely addicted patients. Group membership is also "rolling": As older members prepare to leave, new members are initiated.

Notice of 24 hr is required for absences, or else payment is requested. Or, as an alternative, a flat monthly fee is charged. This is to minimize absences and promote group cohesion and participation. Groups meet for either 75 or 90 min per session on a weekly basis.

Pregroup Preparation Process

In the initial visit, and again in the first group session, the group "ground rules" are presented. They include:

- Regular and on-time attendance.
- Confidentiality—what's said in group stays in group.
- No smoking (and honesty about slips).

We also explain the purpose or goal of the group, which includes:

- Living without tobacco—that is, learning to cope with life's problems without smoking.
- Finding new forms of day-to-day fulfillment that will strengthen the ability to avoid relapse by positively promoting abstinence.

A pregroup preparation checklist (see Table 10.1) helps ensure that elements essential for the success of the group are covered in a standardized way with all prospective group members.

Strongly encouraging or even requiring attendance at a peer-led Nicotine Anonymous meeting as part of preparing for a group gives prospective members a sample of the group experience. They can then review their reactions with the clinician to help identify potential strengths and liabilities before beginning in a leader-led smoking cessation group.

GROUP DYNAMICS

Yalom (1985) described a condensed list of group properties that he termed *therapeutic factors*. It included:

TABLE 10.1
Pregroup Preparation Checklist

General purpose and goals of the group
Group composition and size
Role and activity level of the leader
Observers, audiotaping, or videotaping of sessions
Physical arrangement of therapy room
Time period of each session; duration of the group (long-term vs. time-limited)
Loss and addition of group members
Rules about attendance
Fees and billing procedures
Other coexisting treatment: drugs, hospitalization potential, other therapies (simultaneous individual therapy)
Contacts and/or socialization among members outside the group
Modifications of the group contract (e.g., individual scheduling problems)
Confidentiality
Questions and answers about group therapy (try to clarify myths, misconceptions about group, and elicit early resistances to group participation)
Anything unique about the patient's life situation that might intrude on his or her ability to join, remain in, or participate in the group.

Note. From Spitz and Rosecan (1987, p. 179). Reprinted with permission.

1. *Imparting information*: a didactic component that can be quite valuable when centered on a theme common to all group members. Common examples of this group type are smoking education groups that provide accurate physiological and psychological data about smoking, and groups of previously hospitalized psychiatric patients in which information about mental illness is exchanged.

2. *Instilling hope*: a factor especially important in treating depression, alcoholism, and marital problems. Group members benefit from seeing others who have dealt with or mastered similar problems.

3. *Universality* is the recognition by all group members that they share a common set of concerns. Universal feelings such as fear of illness or guilt about the impact of their smoking on family and friends are evident as early as the first group session. The realization that members share similar life struggles sets the stage for identifications among members and provides the basis for group cohesion and support. An example of universalization occurred in a first group meeting when a member sheepishly confessed to smoking three packs a day. Instead of the anticipated response of humiliation or chastisement, the members all responded, in turn, with admissions about the extent of their own use of cigarettes. The sense of relief that emerged following this go-around was clear in the initial member's comment, "Well, I guess we're all in the same boat." Universality can thus help to counter feelings of low self-esteem and interpersonal alienation.

4. *Altruism* is when members are genuinely concerned about the emotional and physical well-being of others in the group, and behave in ways that reflect these concerns. Advice giving about ways that have been helpful to an individual who has been successful in quitting can be passed along to a fellow group member. When the member incorporates the suggestion offered, the donor of the advice feels a sense of personal fulfillment in having been helpful to someone else. This sense of altruism enhances self-esteem and empathy in group members. Altruism is also a quality useful in interrupting patterns of preoccupation with oneself, as in depressive and obsessional states.

5. *Family reenactment*: an effect where the group is seen as a "second-chance family," which mobilizes many of the unresolved problems related to the family of origin, while offering an opportunity to experience alternative modes of adaptation through the group process.

6. *Developing socialization techniques*: There is a chance to experience relationships in a safe, controlled setting, coupled with the availability of "accurate interpersonal feedback" from the group membership. This is especially useful with psychotic patients whose reality-testing ability is often seriously impaired.

7. *Imitative behavior*: a group dynamic whereby members can experiment with qualities they observe in other members. This can provide a source of new input into the behavioral repertoire of the withdrawn schizoid member who would be unlikely to take such action in his or her relationships outside the group.

8. *Interpersonal learning*: a complex factor that, broadly defined, parallels in the group setting elements seen in individual therapy such as transference, motivation, and insight.

9. *Group cohesion*: A central part of the binding force in therapy groups, cohesion is the attraction of the group to its members. Cohesion sets the stage for "affective sharing and acceptance," and although not synonymous with comfort, cohesion is considered a necessary prerequisite for change in group therapy.

10. *Catharsis*: a process that facilitates the affective as well as the cognitive aspects of the therapeutic experience. Judicious mobilization of strong affect is valued by many group leaders when defenses of intellectualization, denial, and/or isolation of affect are prominent, as they commonly are with people who develop substance abuse problems.

GROUP DYNAMICS APPLIED TO SMOKING CESSATION

The stages of a smoking cessation group are similar to the maturation process found in other psychotherapy groups.

Stage 1: Basic Trust, Resistance and Coping

The initial stage involves trust issues around affiliation/cohesion, and is accomplished in the context of a structured behavioral treatment that is focused on abstinence from smoking. The group is homogeneous in that all members are smokers with some abstinence who have a wish to continue to abstain from smoking. As such, war stories (such as great smoking tales or romantically recalled stories about smoking) are seen as a resistance, whereas discussion of coping strategies to deal with urges and cravings and close calls are considered appropriate.

Specific interventions in the initial stage of a group are aimed at building peer group support and creating a safe therapeutic environment to facilitate trust and self-disclosure. Appropriate group leader feedback highlights resistance to behavior change, such as when group members engage in excessive negativity to cover over fears of making changes in their lives.

Similarly, problems with managing stress and/or interpersonal conflict have often been responded to in the past by repetitively lighting up a cigarette and smoking. Such passive coping, in contrast to active coping, can have negative psychological as well as medical consequences. It is helpful to point out early in group that there are two different kinds of coping (Kobasa, 1982; Maddi, 1990; Maddi & Kobasa, 1984).

One kind of coping engages people in life's problems, where they commit themselves to overcoming challenges and transform short-term stress into long-term growth. A second kind of coping, in contrast, involves relying on old ways of doing things, repeating old patterns of behavior out of fear and helplessness. The group leader can suggest to each group member, "At each crossroad on the road of stopping smoking ask yourself (and be honest!): Is this a forward way of coping or is this a backward way of coping?"

Group discussions can then focus on developing concrete strategies and coping skills to help the group members live life more fully without smoking. In this framework, tendencies to justify returning to smoking as a coping strategy can be challenged as rationalizing, minimizing, or denying the addiction problem without really offering the smoker a long-term way out of it.

Stage 2: Relapse Prevention Training and Clinical Management of Slips and Relapses

In practice, stage 2 overlaps with stage 1. Throughout the group experience, an important consideration for the group process as a whole is the clinical management of slips and relapses. The use of slips and relapses in a smoking cessation group is similar to the cognitive-behavioral approaches to relapse prevention described in other substance abuse groups (Marlatt & Gordon, 1985; Spitz & Rosecan, 1987; Washton, 1987).

In brief, assessing relapse potential is an ongoing group task, with any slips openly addressed in group. Slips or near-slips by individual group members become an opportunity for all group members to closely examine their smoking triggers and to aggressively explore new and realistic alternative coping strategies. Group members learn by mutual identification that *a slip need not be a fall.* The smoker can learn from the group to better use available tools and supports.

Stage 3: Solidifying Abstinence

As the initial phases of building group rapport and developing relapse prevention skills progress, they begin to overlap with a third phase, which continues the process of solidifying abstinence. This phase involves exploring personality issues.

Heavily addicted smokers are unlikely to give up smoking without *getting something in return.* Some examples from our groups of how patients instill hope by example include:

- Increased pride in their health or body through changes in diet and exercise.
- Increased self-esteem through changes in asserting their feelings and needs.
- New and fulfilling activities or goals such as making positive changes in work or in relationships.

In this third phase, such issues as coping with loneliness, loss (current and past), and anger become prominent. The group members provide each other with a model showing that difficult feelings can be expressed and tolerated, and are not too painful to discuss. Open discussion can also bring relief and lead to new ways of seeing problems and coping with them as well. The group leader's interventions at this phase serve to increase patients' self-knowledge, facilitate productive interpersonal conflict resolution, and focus on here-and-now living. (See also the section on development of emotional self-awareness in chap. 12 of this volume.)

Group Themes

Certain repetitive themes or psychological problems commonly emerge in the third phase of smoking cessation groups. The group leader can employ such themes in the work of the group, where appropriate. They include:

- Patients' difficulty labeling feelings beyond focusing on somatic concerns or cravings to smoke.
- Patients' tendency to avoid interpersonal conflicts and to "smoke down" or "push down" negative feelings, as a patient in our program described it.
- Patients' tendency to wait for life to begin. As one patient put it, "smoking keeps you company while you get through each day waiting for life to begin."

Stage 4: Approaching Termination

Finally, a fourth stage can be described as a mature smoking cessation group, where the emphasis is on patients'applying their greater self-knowledge to relapse prevention training so they can greatly reduce their tendency to undermine their abstinence (and self-esteem). The "rolling" group format helps the long-term members who are terminating take the measure of their growth, whereas the new members who are starting have the experience of successful role models.

Interventions at this stage focus on a review of progress and the course of treatment; reminders of basic principles of relapse prevention; and addressing a sense of loss and accomplishment with approaching termination.

Case History

The patient was a 58-year-old divorced mother of an adult, chronically ill daughter. She had lost another child in a boating accident. She herself was severely ill with heart disease, diabetes, and cancer, yet continued to smoke 2½ to 3 packs per day.

When the patient tried to stop smoking she became, as she described it, "a real nut, crazy," "frantic," and felt she was "going out of her mind." She was in no way prepared to enter a group experience in this state. She wondered if she was suicidal to smoke after a heart attack and open heart surgery, and could only conclude that she was an "insane addict."

Initially we worked in individual sessions on stopping smoking, and her cardiologist prescribed an antidepressant and a patch. She reported being able to achieve a period of abstinence without becoming "vicious" or depressed. Six weeks after she stopping smoking, the patient described continued frequent urges to smoke.

At this point she had enough abstinence, and was stable enough in her mood, and we suggested she participate in a smoking cessation relapse prevention group. She began group the following week.

The experience of being in a group of peers who shared her problem with smoking helped this patient to decrease her sense of isolation and to open up. Not feeling judged as a "crazy nut" as she felt judged by her family, friends, and doctors made her feel "safe" in the group. Her peers, who were also nicotine addicts, helped her to feel more understood and self-accepting, and to hear feedback in a less defensive way. She began to use the group as a forum to work on her tendency to avoid conflict and to smoke instead. She described situations of interpersonal conflict with others outside group, and sought the group's feedback to help her to cope with them.

Eventually, through her work in the group, the patient was better able to understand her own defensive and avoidant behavior in interpersonal relationships. Another theme for her, and for many smokers in our experience, concerned the tendency to overextend physically and emotionally, which can result in increased medical problems and increased cravings to smoke. This patient was also able to use the group to work on her need to "not be all things to all people."

After 6 months in group the patient felt more secure in her abstinence from smoking and was more respectful of her personal limits and her need to live within them. This coincided with decreased cravings to smoke. She was less frustrated, helpless, and guilty in her relationships, and her behavior more reflected her need to be able to take care of herself emotionally as well as medically. She had stopped being overly available for others' needs (both in the group and outside the group) and was less resentful of others and less guilty about her own limitations.

This case serves as an illustration of how a relapse prevention group can decrease the isolation felt by many nicotine addicts as they struggle with their addiction and how such a group can help overcome interpersonal problems that may interfere with a smoker's capacity to stay off cigarettes in the long term.

We now describe how a psychotherapy group for relapse prevention compares with, and can work together with, other group formats, such as self-help groups. We also give a brief outline for making appropriate group referrals based on the initial screening and evaluation interview.

SMOKING CESSATION GROUP TREATMENT FORMATS

Formats to achieve the goal of staying off cigarettes can vary. Often, more than one format is appropriate, combining, for example, a psychotherapy group of the type we have described, along with a Nicotine Anonymous or another self-help group. Examples of group formats for smoking cessation are:

- Nicotine Anonymous/self-help
- Behavioral skills training

- Psychotherapy
- Hypnosis/health education

These formats can be complementary, not competing, and can work together to enrich the experience of the patient (see Table 10.2). For example, in self-help groups, leadership is peer based and the group seeks to promote mutual affirmation and immediate positive feedback among its members. In psychotherapy groups, on the other hand, leadership is provided by a professional with formal psychological training who works to balance group cohesion and mutual identification with the skillful use of group pressure and confrontation. In a psychotherapy group, differences as well as similiarities among group members are examined over time, as is the group interaction itself.

Referral to Group Formats

When psychiatric conditions and psychological disorders are present, a psychotherapy model of a smoking cessation group may be most appropriate. When there is a need for additional structure and support, referral to Nicotine Anonymous (a 12-step program based on the principles of Alcoholics Anonymous) may also be important. When other primary substance abuse problems, such as drugs/alcohol, are also present, appropriate referrals can be

TABLE 10.2
Addiction Group Formats

	Self-Help Group	*Psychotherapy Group*
Size	Large (size often unlimited)	Small (8–15 members)
Leadership	1. Peer leader or recovered addict	1. Mental health professional with or without recovered user.
	2. Leadership is earned status over time	2. Self-appointed leadership
	3. Implicit hierarchical leadership structure	3. Formal hierarchical leadership structure
Membership participation	Voluntary	Voluntary and involuntary (e.g., employer-referred)
Group governed	Self-governing	Leader governed
Content	1. Environmental factors, no examination of group interaction	1. Examination of intragroup behavior and extragroup factors
	2. Emphasis on similarities among members	2. Emphasis on differentiation among members over time
	3. "Here and now" focus	3. "Here and now" plus historical focus

(Continued)

TABLE 10.2
(Continued)

	Self-Help Group	*Psychotherapy Group*
Screening interview	None	Always
Group processes	Universalization, empathy, affective sharing, education, public statement of problem (self-disclosure), mutual affirmation, morale building, catharsis, immediate positive feedback, high degrees of persuasiveness	Cohesion, mutual identification, confrontation, education, catharis, use of group pressure re abstinence, and retention of group membership
Outside socialization	1. Encouraged strongly	1. Cautious re extragroup contact
	2. Construction of social network is actively sought	2. Intermember networking is optional
Goals	1. Positive goal setting, behaviorally oriented	1. Ambitious goals: abstinence plus individual personality issues
	2. Focus on the group as a whole and the similarities among members	2. Individual as well as group focus
Leader activity	1. Educator/role model catalyst for learning	1. Responsible for therapeutic group experience
	2. Less member-to-leader distance	2. More member-to-leader distance
Use of interpretation or psychodynamic techniques	No	Yes
Confidentiality	Anonymity preserved	Strongly emphasized
Sponsorship program	Yes (usually same sex)	No
Deselection	1. Member may leave group at their own choosing	1. Predetermined minimal term of commitment to group membership
	2. Members may avoid self-disclosure or discussion of any subject	2. Avoidance of discussion seen as "resistance"
Involvement in other groups/ programs	Yes	Yes—eclectic models No—psychodynamic models
Time factors	Unlimited group participation possible over years	Often time-limited experiences
Frequency of meetings	Active encouragement of daily participation	Meets less frequently (often once or twice weekly)

Note. From Spitz and Rosecan (1987, p. 162–163). Reprinted with permission.

made to self-help programs such as Alcoholics Anonymous or Cocaine Anonymous, as well as to a substance abuse group treatment program.

In cases where psychiatric/psychological and substance abuse factors are not at issue, but where the smoker scores high on a nicotine dependence scale, a behavioral skills training format may be optimal. Finally, in cases without the presence of cigarette-related illness or psychiatric/psychological and substance abuse problems, and where the smoker also scores low on a nicotine dependence scale, a brief behavioral management intervention, hypnosis group, or a health education class can also lead to a successful outcome.

SUMMARY

Comprehensive assessment and appropriate group formats will be increasingly crucial in successfully treating medically ill and other severely addicted smokers. Focusing on group preparation and following consistent group rules for "hard-core" smokers can make all the difference between a successful or unsuccessful long-term outcome in treating nicotine dependence.

A plan/program has been outlined that addresses addiction as a medical illness, assesses smokers' readiness, or lack thereof, to change, assesses individual and interpersonal function, looks for coexisting psychiatric problems, and thereby aims at greater patient specificity in treatment planning for smoking cessation. Several themes common to smokers' groups and suggested modes of intervention are outlined.

REFERENCES

Cromwell, J., Bartosch, W. J., Fiore, M., Hasselblad, V., & Baker, T. B. (1997). Cost-effectiveness of the Clinical Practice Recommendations in the AHCPR Guideline for Smoking Cessation. *JAMA, 278*(21), 1759–1766.

Fiore, M. C., Kenford, S. L., Jorenby, D., Wetter, D., Smith, S., & Baker, T. (1994). Two studies of the clinical effectiveness of the nicotine patch with different counseling treatments. *Chest, 105*, pp. 524–533, Number 2.

Glass, R. (1990). Blue mood, blackened lungs: Depression and smoking. *JAMA, 264*(12), 1583–1584.

Hajek, P., Belcher, M., & Stapleton, J. (1985). Enhancing the impact of groups: An evaluation of two group formats for smokers. *British Journal of Clinical Psychology, 24*, 289–294.

Hughes, J. R. (1996). An overview of nicotine use disorders for alcohol/drug abuse clinicians. *American Journal on Addictions, 5*(3), 262–274.

Hurt, R. D., Dale, L. C., McClain, F. L., Eberman, K. M., Offord, K. P., Bruce, B. K., & Lauger, G. (1992). A comprehensive model for the treatment of nicotine dependence in a medical setting. *Medical Clinics of North America, 76*, pp. 495–514.

Kobasa, S. C. (1982). The hardy personality: Toward a social psychology of stress and health. In G. S. Saunders & J. Suls (Eds.), *Social psychology of health and illness* (pp. 3–32). Hillsdale, NJ: Lawrence Erlbaum Associates.

Maddi, S. R. (1990). Issues and Interventions in Stress Mastery. In H. S. Friedman (Ed.), *Personality and disease* (pp. 121–154). New York: John Wiley and Sons.

Maddi, S. R., & Kobasa, S. C. (1984). *The hardy executive: Health under stress.* Homewood, IL: Dow Jones-Irwin.

Marlatt, G. A., & Gordon, J. R. (Eds.). (1985). *Relapse prevention: Maintenance strategies in the treatment of addictive behaviors.* New York: Guilford.

Schwartz, L. (1987). *Review and evaluation of smoking cessation methods: The United States and Canada, 1978–1985* (NIH Publication No. 87-2940). U.S. Department of Health and Human Services, Public Health Service, National Cancer Institute, Bethesda, MD.

Shewchuk, L., Dubren, R., Burton, D., Forman, M., Clark, R., & Jaffin, A. (1977). Preliminary observations on an intervention program for heavy smokers. *International Journal of the Addictions, 12*(2–3), 323–336.

Spitz, H., & Rosecan, J. (1987). *Cocaine abuse: New directions in treatment and research.* New York: Brunner/Mazel.

Spitzer, R., & Williams, J. (1996). *Patient problem questionnaire: Self report version of Prime M.D.* New York: State Psychiatric Institute Biometrics Research.

Washton, A. (1987). Outpatient treatment of cocaine abuse. In A. Washton & M. S. Gold (Eds.), *Cocaine: A clinician's handbook* (pp. 106–117). New York: Guilford Press.

Yalom, I. D. (1985). *The theory and practice of group psychotherapy* (3rd ed.). New York: Basic Books.

CHAPTER ELEVEN

Stopping Smoking: A Study on the Nature of Resistance and the Use of Hypnosis

Donald Douglas
Lenox Hill Hospital, New York

> The human condition is so wretched that while bending his every action to pander to his passions man never ceases groaning against their tyranny. He can neither accept their violence nor the violence he must do himself in order to shake off their yoke. Not only the passions but also their antidotes fill him with disgust, and he cannot be reconciled either to the discomfort of his disease or to the trouble of a cure. (de la Rochefoucauld, 1665/1986, p. 107)

Since smoking cessation was first widely recognized as a health measure in the 1960s, many psychological methods have claimed brief success. Cognitive, behavioral, conditioning, educational, persuasive and other techniques are being used, but none can be certified as consistently highly effective. As is so often the case, proliferation of methods occurs when none have worked very well. It is surely most significant that even the 12-Step Program so widely used for addictive substance abuse has offered little for smoking. It would appear that the very nature of smoking and of resistance to recovery from it has eluded us as much as have effective means of treatment. To this we must add that in our present state of knowledge even the most complete statistical comparison will not reveal the operative factors in release of the smoking addiction. Therefore, what follows is neither an extensive survey nor specific recommendation on techniques of treatment for smoking addiction, but rather an intensive examination—perhaps from a somewhat heterodox viewpoint—of the smoking process itself. The scope of this study is to elucidate the general nature of the resistance phenomenon together with its special relationship to smoking and the use of hypnosis: a search for deeper insight into the human nature that creates such addiction and resistance.

Hypnosis is gaining a place of special interest in the management of a variety of medical and psychological problems. One aspect of its particular usefulness is its potential for bypassing, transforming, and resolving resistance—a potential that is just beginning to be presently understood and realized. Considering the massive resistance to stopping smoking, it is notable that there is no developing history of improved methods in using hypnosis in treating smoking addiction. There is a considerable literature representing many variations on basic methods that may use hypnosis, but no clearly developed and effective practice; a review is provided in the annotated bibliography.

What has been found by most who attempt to treat smoking addiction is first, the importance of attention to individual and specific patterns of habit and response, and second, that repeated rather than single visits are needed for best results.

There is, however, a baffling third characteristic of smokers in general, more poignant than the simple basics just noted: Smokers seem to divide into two groups—those who are readily successful and those who are not. What is this difference between those who stop on their own or who are easy to help and those who have great difficulty or who cannot seem to stop permanently or even stop at all—for whom no method seems to work? It is with this second group of smokers that our study of resistance begins.

COMFORT-SEEKING: THE FIRST RESISTANCE

Respiration, Retrovirus and Addiction

Undoubtedly there is an organic pathophysiological basis for addiction to smoking as for any other form of substance abuse. Perhaps most closely related are the satiety seeking of certain eating disorders—so like the fleeting comforts of "snacking" on cigarettes. The common complaint of weight gain after stopping cigarettes seems very likely due not only to lowering of metabolism but also to replacement of one form of "snacking" by another. But there is a difference: "Snacking" on cigarettes might be described as a fixation at the preoral or respiratory phase—the earliest of postuterine life. To explain this important point a little further: For most smokers, and addictive overeaters as well as other substance abusers, the life pattern is rather quickly and unnoticeably subordinated to craving and its relief—the real onset of the addiction—but each addiction has something special. With smoking it is anchoring at a level deeper and even more primordial than eating. Protecting the increase of craving, at first by nonchalance and denial, then by evasion and finally in despair, the smoker seems to repeatedly take refuge in what is essentially a corruption of the earliest life function: a respiratory phase more primitive, as noted earlier, and less accessible to consciousness than the classical developmental stages of psychoanalytic theory. But there is more than theory. Pitiably demonstrative of what we may call "respiratory regression" are those smokers who, while suffering greatly from the diseases caused by smoking, most notably emphysema, go on making themselves worse by more smoking—as if comfort or escape from discomfort could only be experienced through a corruption of the respiratory function. An important and clinically useful obverse example is the frequently observed falling away of smoking in those who persist in aerobic exercises.

But whether or not we accept this, there is something more and very difficult. What begins as comfort-seeking eventually brings so much harm in exchange for so little comfort and becomes so obdurate and inaccessible to average understanding, judgment, and volition as to require a far more sinister analogy: In the pitiless light of modern science, smoking is clearly revealed as the cause not only of malignant changes at the most basic cellular level, but also of corruption at the highest psychic levels also. Not only lungs but also brain, not only breathing but also mind, are locked into repetitive servitude to the addiction—in this respect precisely like a retrovirus, which proliferates by moving into the nuclear core, usurping normal genetic functions and so degrading the host's normal life process. The cell retains its apparent structure for some time but loses the meaning and value of its true function by becoming subordinate to a lower level of life. What happens to cells happens to mind. Whether the smoker denies it or not, smoking not only usurps homeostatic self-control, it also usurps even the willingness to return to normality because normality is displaced by becoming something else. In addiction and especially in smoking, the addiction becomes the normal.

Without warning, the addictive cycle has begun. Then, as with all addictions, smoking becomes subject to paradoxical habituation; that is, depletion of satisfaction leads to more, not to less smoking. As use increases, the complex detoxification systems begin to fail through overload, so that smoking becomes integral first to appetitive function's degraded hedonic tone and then to the degraded cellular biochemistry. The retrovirus of comfort-seeking has taken over.

THE VICIOUS CYCLE OF "STOP-SMOKE"

The Second Form of Resistance

Sooner or later the smoker decides to stop. This intention is remembered with every cigarette and with all the details of smoking. The wish to stop becomes conditioned to smoking and smoking conditioned to the wish to stop—perhaps by 100,000 repetitions, perhaps to two or three times that. Then when at last the intention to stop is fully awakened and put into firm resolution to make maximum effort, the smoker must deal with an urge to smoke now monstrously reinforced by the very same intention, the very same resolution, the very same effort. This conditioned resistance very naturally and unconsciously resurrects a resistance from the past: the adolescent rebellion that initiates so much of smoking—a rebellion into adult captivity. Such is the stop-smoke cycle, and it can deceive many people who attempt to stop on their own without realizing how they have been trapped. It can also deceive their therapist, and some important details in technique derive from understanding just this stop-smoke conditioned cycle.

And now, having described the role of conditioning for comfort-seeking and for the stop-smoke cycle, we can no longer avoid those factors of personality—of human nature—that result in the distinction that was emphasized at the outset: the difference between those who can quit, some even quite easily, and those who cannot. We need nothing less than new insight. For this we may turn to the great French philosopher whose words stand at the beginning of this chapter. More than 300 years ago François, duc de la Rochefoucauld, in his *Maxims* described human nature in many aspects, including much that today might be termed *resistance.* His term was *self love,* and his comments open the next section.

A RESPONSIBLE AND POWERLESS ENEMY IS SO MUCH FUN: THE THIRD RESISTANCE

"You Have to Stop Me But I Won't Let You"

> Self love is love of oneself and of all things in terms of oneself . . . finds a living everywhere, on everything or on nothing, thrives equally well on things or on their absence, even joins forces with its declared enemies and identifies itself with their tactics and, most remarkable of all, hates itself with them, plots for its own downfall and even works to bring about its own ruin . . . all it cares about is existing, and provided it can go on existing it is quite prepared to be its own enemy. Hence there is nothing to be surprised at if it sometimes throws in its lot with the most rigorous austerity and brazenly joins therewith for its own destruction, for the moment of its defeat on one side is that of its recovery on another. When you think it is giving up what it enjoys it is only calling a temporary halt or ringing the changes, and at the very time when it is vanquished and you think you are rid of it, back it comes, triumphant in its own undoing. (de la Rochefoucauld, 1665/1986, p. 112)

Is the outlook as bitter as these words of de la Rochefoucauld seem to imply? It must often seem so for those who cannot stop smoking and for others who want them to stop. Can the great philosopher's words be as useful as they are lucid? Can we in this century approach "self love" a little differently? Has anything useful been learned? The smoker who cannot stop surely needs it.

Smoking frequently begins at the time of adolesence, of rebellion and conformity, a time of tremendous reaction to the "enemy's" failing control. This rebellious resistance not only contributes to the stop-smoke cycle, as mentioned, but also in quite another way. Unlike other addictions that may begin early in life, smoking seems quite harmless until its later stages, and even the idea of stopping is resented as an attack on what is defended as "comfort . . . relaxation . . . enjoyment."

Consequently, the resistance to stopping smoking becomes an extended and transformed adolescent dream of defiance, now with adult empowerment—in short, just those special processes generally designated as the *borderline syndrome.* The smoker may seem well integrated in many respects and yet may be reduced by addiction to the ego splitting, defiance, passivity, sabotage, ambivalence, evasiveness, and to the paradoxical reaction to failure that are unmistakably typical of the borderline personality disorder. To repeat, whether the smoker admits it or not, the smoker does not simply require cigarettes to function normally. The real treasure of resistance is hidden. For example, consider how closely the following description applies to the smoker who seems almost to enjoy his repeated failures:

> The need to defeat oneself as a necessary price to pay in order to defeat an unconsciously hated and envied helping figure is another related type of self-destructive motivation. Self-destruction here serves the purpose of "triumphing" over the envied object. The more serious cases of negative therapeutic reaction are often part of this group of patients. Severe forms of negative therapeutic reaction are linked with such "triumph" over others, in this case, the therapist and his life-affirmative tendencies. (Kernberg, p. 126)

How perfectly this describes the smoker who "cannot stop" or "cannot stay off cigarettes," and how much it echoes self love in its many aspects, now perhaps more familiar as borderline process. What is most striking—despite differences due to the elegance of 17th-century French prose and the 20th-century emphasis on etiology and psychodynamics—what is most striking is the perennial commonality: the maintenance of attachments at all costs by means of what are now known as vengeful impulses, false self, splitting of ego, failure of individuation, and the other aspects of the borderline that may be reviewed in much detail in the modern literature and may be applied directly and with great precision to understanding the general problems of resistance and specifically the problems of resistance to stopping smoking (Masterson, 1981; Masterson & Costello, 1980). This is not to declare that smokers suffer more than average self love or that they have a borderline disorder, but rather that the treatment-resistant group acts out self love in various ways at the borderline level for intermittent periods when the addiction is confronted. Certainly it seems that enjoyment of failure—the borderline's delight in triumph over the enemy rendered powerless by responsibility—must be faced by every therapist who sees this most resistant group of patients. Whether or not we hypothesize that addictive biochemistry is the primary source, the result is the same. The relative innocence of the adolescent rebellion is very typically transformed by the smoking addiction into the complexities of borderline resistance for whom a responsible powerless enemy is virtually a necessity. And surely, although it must be omitted here, there is a great deal more to be said about the development of borderline resistance in a society that makes the caretaker an enemy, rendered powerless by responsibility.

METANOIA: THE ONLY TRUE RECOVERY

At just this point we may now introduce a profound life-changing process—the only true means of dissolving borderline negativity and resistance—the secret that enables and distinguishes those successful in recovery. This process is usually termed *metanoia*: that is, a capacity for central change, for turning about and changing at the center rather than a change in behavior or external attitude. Metanoia is a term taken from the religious and philosophical literature and is used to indicate a complete and profound change in the direction of willing intention. It can almost be thought of as a kind of rebirth, but particularly for the smoker metanoia means the generation of willingness to bear the discomfort of withdrawal and to overcome the duplicity of the stop-smoke conditioned cycle, and to do both with a clear, unified motivation: that is, to replace the old with a better, new way of life. Metanoia is the fundamental reorientation essential to recovery from any addiction. Without it the long collapse into the morass of borderline resistance reactions will certainly present inevitable and insurmountable challenge to any form of therapeutic intervention. Smokers who "cannot" stop, and indeed many addicted in other fields of substance abuse, cannot seem to achieve the necessary awakening and activation toward metanoia. For them hypnosis can play a unique role in developing comprehensive strategies for dissolving comfort-seeking, stop-smoke cycle, and borderline resistance as already described.

HYPNOSIS IN SMOKING CESSATION

A full review of the use of hypnosis in dealing with smoking addiction is impossible here. A bibliography has been appended; it covers the full range of the use of hypnosis since smoking became a problem. We can here initiate only some selective observations, as follows.

Effective trance work includes understanding hypnosis, understanding the problem, and understanding the individual. The greatest of these is understanding the individual, especially in the case of the failing smoker for whom the foregoing studies of resistance can be useful when applied to a thorough understanding of the individual history.

In many cases, at least partial reduction of the borderline resistance reaction can be initiated by emphatic explanation that is corrective for those who think hypnosis is all-powerful and is disarming for those who are preparing to resist the hypnosis. A variety of metaphors, examples, direct statements, and interchanges may be necessary, but whatever is needed must be done to transmit the basic essential concept: *Hypnosis can empower the smoker's decisions but cannot change or substitute for them.* This concept is so necessary that further treatment, especially trance work, should not proceed until the patient has achieved full understanding and acceptance. Occasionally it may be preferable to delay or postpone or even not proceed with treatment at all, for if control and responsibility are not unequivocally accepted by the smoker, there is little chance of permanent success. Many patients can quickly learn an impressive degree of trance depth and trance phenomena, but this is no guarantee of good therapeutic outcome; even with every precaution, many smokers seem "unable" to take over their own control and responsibility. It is from this group that most failures seem to come, but even some of these can be helped with emphasis on use of the patient's memories, successes, and failure patterns, that is, significant attitudes and beliefs related to smoking and to personal responsibility for recovery. For the therapist this means utilizing every means to avoid, reframe, bypass, diminish, dissociate, or even confront and directly resolve the patient's direct and indirect subversive reactions of the borderline type.

As an example of the process of combining several techniques, we can begin with a reframe similar to that used in neurolinguistic programming (NLP). NLP refers to psychological reprogramming methods developed from observation of the hypnotic and psychotherapeutic techniques of Milton H. Erickson (Rosen, 1982). A number of authors have described the origin and development of NLP together with various aspects of its techniques used in combination with other forms of psychotherapy (Grinder & Bandler, 1976). In the example of reframe herein described, the patient is first asked to contact that part of the unconscious mind responsible for the smoking habit, and further, the patient is asked to allow this part of the mind to accept communication and to answer in some symbolic, usually nonverbal, form, such as nodding head, finger motion, and so on. The next communication is the acceptance of new ways of giving the smoker enjoyment, relaxation, or comfort—"The good stuff but not the bad stuff"—that is, all that smoking ever did, and doing it better (Lankton & Lankton, 1983). Once this is acceptable and the acceptance is indicated, the smoker is asked to use his or her "tremendous creative capacities of the unconscious mind" to create one or two or three or more methods of enjoyment, relaxation and comfort and to communicate to that part of the mind responsible for smoking in the past and now willing to accept change. These are not simply changes to discomfort, to void, or to unsatisfied cravings. Rather, each wish to smoke is to be replaced by the positive image of personal enjoyment, good health, and individual triumph. There is a great deal more that can be added during this process of reframing and of redirecting rebellion and attacking the displaced borderline resistance patterns. Time distortion has been mentioned; it can be quite useful. Other sensory techniques can disperse, displace, change, and diminish the total craving experience; frequently personal or even idiosyncratic metaphors, similes, or images may be developed for the individual patient (Wallas, 1985). A number of standard suggestions can be given directly and indirectly during this process, but the patient's own ideas, of health and sickness and even secret fears and secret hopes, are usually much more effective.

The presentation of this material to the patient can be done directly in the usual hypnotic techniques; the currently increasing practice of using audiocassette tapes is potentially very useful, particularly because a number of voice combinations are thereby available. One way to use more than one voice is with a prerecorded tape playing simultaneously while the therapist adds another voice. The voices of friends, family, or the patient's own voice can be used individually, in series, in parallel, or in combinations. These methods need not be elaborate at all; they are merely a way of redirecting the patient's awareness and resistance, conscious and unconscious. It is very effective for two therapists to work with one patient or for two patients or a patient and relative or friend to work together. The two voices may alternate or simultaneously represent many forms of the patient's resistance, motivation, conceptions of smoking, health, outcome, and many of the other associations as presented. The essence of this group of techniques is reduction of resistance by the voice not consciously followed, because the patient cannot really hear and mobilize resistance for both voices simultaneously all of the time. The patient should use the tapes for home practice; one way is to use a tape for 30 to 60 min every day for 30 or 40 days or more. These tapes may be overplayed, that is, used again during the therapeutic session, at which time the therapist can verbally introduce new material not on the tape, and therefore the resistances can be organized in whatever specific forms are most effective for the individual patient.

Work with hypnosis may be enhanced by behavioral techniques in some cases. Changes can be prescribed in various habits and motor patterns and in the many associations to smoking, such as food, coffee, and others. All of this is taught in ordinary consciousness and in the trance work in order to create replacement of trigger situations, that is, the stimuli for comfort-seeking and for the stop-smoking cycle, by self-hypnotic relaxation and relief on cue. The continued home practice mentioned already is very helpful here.

Many behavioral variations have been suggested to break up the stop-smoke cycle and to quell or distract from craving. Differing results have been claimed, but in the present era, and lacking the personal power of Jay Haley (1984) or Milton H. Erickson (quoted in Rosen, 1982), the present writer prefers "good deals" to ordeals: that is, there must be an immediate and increasing reward of some kind—pride, relief, visualizations of success and good health, even ego comparisons with smokers if that will do it, enjoyment of food or anything else, understanding and overcoming the craving and "weakness," increased self-reliance and much more. It is here that the unconscious search for reframing resources and methods is so important.

SUMMARY AND CONCLUSION

This chapter describes the smoking addiction as acting at once like a tenacious regression to the earliest life function of respiration and as a sinister retrovirus taking over the life of the host: regressive and preemptive addictive processes that derive from comfort-seeking, locked in by the stop-smoke cycle and defended by the complexities of the borderline syndrome. Specific management of the major resistances has been outlined with particular emphasis on their resolution into the process of metanoia, that is, the turning about at center without which no lasting recovery from any substance abuse can be achieved.

Such achievement is no easy process. The role of hypnosis in stopping smoking remains puzzling and unsatisfactory, still asking the same vexing questions that opened this study: Why can hypnosis help one group and not another? Who recovers and who does not and why? In our current practice hypnosis very frequently can make the process of recovery easier for even the most fortunate and less often may provide enough extra insight, replacement of stimuli, control, and relaxation to release an otherwise doomed smoker, but what makes the difference? And do these differences obtain for other of our patients?

For answer we may allow the duc de la Rochefoucauld to complete this presentation. The passage is blunt and plain yet profound and subtle; it is the quiet voice of truth, so easily misunderstood, so usually trivialized and frequently lost, for it casts a clear light even beyond the maze of self love into the depths of all resistance:

> Of all our passions the least well understood by ourselves is laziness. It is the most violent and malignant of all, though its violence is imperceptible and its ravages exceedingly difficult to see. If we carefully examine its power we shall see that in every eventuality it takes over the mastery of our emotions, interests and pleasures. It is the *remora* (parasite fish) which has the strength to bring the mightiest ship to a stand-still, a calm that is more dangerous to

> important affairs than breakers in the fiercest tempest. The tranquility of laziness casts a secret spell over the soul that suddenly puts a stop to the most relentless pursuits and brings to naught the most unbreakable resolutions. In conclusion, this passion can best be described by saying that laziness is as it were a peaceful state of the soul that consoles it for every loss and is welcomed as a substitute for every good. (de la Rochefoucauld, 1665/1986, p. 123)

We may hope that this brief study of the nature of addiction and its resistance to treatment with special reference to hypnosis has demonstrated the similarity—even the identity—of resistance in addiction with the ever-elusive nature of resistance to life itself. In dealing with addictions it is essential to acknowledge this identity, but this does not mean we yet understand it. We have presented here a few aspects of the paradoxical, out-of-balance disparities in treating the untreatable, of working with known and unknown quite impartially, of hope and despair in collusion, of resistance sharing with recovery, of insight reflecting opacity, of the obvious illuminated by the mysterious—all this learning and much more is right before us in this most commonplace and ordinary problem: stopping smoking. Indeed, from all the technical details and observations we have discussed, there arises a kind of questioning wonder at the immensity that lies between those who can release themselves from the secret spell over the soul, whatever its form, and those who remain in the recurrent trance of past attachments that in some form enslaves most of humanity.

REFERENCES

de la Rochefoucauld, François duc. (1986). *Maxims.* New York: Penguin Books. (Original work published 1665)

Grinder, J., & Bandler, R. (1976). *The strucutre of magic.* Palo Alto, California: Science and Behaviour Books.

Haley, J. (1984). *Ordeal therapy.* San Francisco: Jossey-Bass.

Kernberg, O. (1975). *Borderline conditions and pathological narcissism.* New York: Jason Aronson.

Lankton, S. R., & Lankton, C. H. (1983). *The answer within.* New York: Brunner/Mazel.

Masterson, J. F. (1981). *The narcissistic and borderline disorders.* New York: Brunner/Mazel.

Masterson, J. F., & Costello, J. L. (1980). *From borderline adolescent to functionary adult.* New York: Brunner/Mazel.

Rosen, S. (1982). *My voice will go with you.* New York: Norton.

Wallas, L. (1985). *Stories for the third ear.* New York: Norton.

SUGGESTIONS FOR FURTHER READING

The foregoing article represents a considerable departure from orthodox views; consequently, the bibliography is necessarily limited. For the practitioner interested in further instruction and comparison, the following sources are appended.

American Society of Clinical Hypnosis. (1973). *A syllabus on hypnosis and a handbook of therapeutic suggestions.* Des Plaines, IL: Author. Seven authors describe their methods in a useful sampling of mainstream methods.

Hammond, D. C. (Ed.). (1990). *Handbook of hypnotic suggestions and metaphors.* New York: Norton. Fifteen articles by 17 authors on hypnosis with smoking and addictions. Well-known authorities on smoking alone and/or in relation to other addictions.

Hoogdain, C. A. L. (1985). *Classical trance induction in Ericksonian psychotherapy: Smoking control.* In J. K. Zweig (Ed.), *Ericksonian psychotherapy II: Clinical applications* (pp. 292–298). New York: Brunner/Mazel.

Kroger, W. S., & Fezler, W. D. (1976). Excessive smoking. In *Hypnosis and behavior modification: Imagery conditioning* (pp. 191–200). Philadelphia: J. B. Lippincott. A combined approach of considerable interest and value.

Zeig, J. K. (1982). *Ericksonian approaches to promote abstinence from cigarette smoking.* In J. K. Zeig (Ed.), *Ericksonian approaches to hypnosis and psychotherapy* (pp. 255–269). New York: Brunner/Mazel.

The last three references give a total of 36 further bibliographic sources.

CHAPTER TWELVE

A Comprehensive Psychological Approach to Preventing Relapse

Daniel F. Seidman
Columbia University

Lirio S. Covey
New York State Psychiatric Institute, and Columbia University

Quitting smoking and maintaining abstinence are very different problems. In working with cigarette smokers we have found that three kinds of therapeutic changes—behavioral, cognitive, and affective (emotional) self-awareness—are helpful in relapse prevention. Depending on the clinician's comprehensive assessment of the smoker, the treatment plan should consider all three kinds of therapeutic changes, the timing of implementing them, and how they can contribute to a successful treatment outcome.

This approach is designed to work in tandem with pharmacotherapies such as nicotine replacement therapy, or other nonnicotine medications, which advise patients of the importance of participating in behavioral interventions and counseling.

Such an approach is also consistent with recent consensus findings concerning the long-term relapse risks for smokers. The U.S. Agency for Health Care Policy and Research (AHCPR) Clinical Practice Guidelines for Smoking Cessation (U.S. Department of Health and Human Services, 1996) lists four common risks for relapse encountered by patients: (a) weight gain; (b) negative mood or depression; (c) prolonged withdrawal symptoms; and (d) lack of support for cessation. This chapter is primarily concerned with strategies to address negative mood as a relapse trigger, but it also addresses these other problems associated with relapse as part of a comprehensive approach to preventing relapse.

This three-part treatment approach, developed for the hard-core smoker, conceptualizes nicotine dependence as not exclusively physiological and behavioral. An additional, major aspect of treatment, which is particularly important for relapse prevention, addresses the emotional and psychological adjustment after stopping smoking. Developing emotional confidence and coping skills (i.e., resilience) strengthens the smoker against potential relapse brought on by emotional triggers.

THREE KINDS OF PSYCHOLOGICAL CHANGE: AN OVERVIEW

Psychological deconditioning from smoking addiction begins with *behavioral change.* This consists of learning specific coping skills to establish abstinence and then applying these skills to external triggers or situations associated with relapse. Behavioral intervention is initiated when the smoker is ready to change, take action, and stop smoking (Prochaska & DiClemente, 1983).

The second kind of psychological intervention is *cognitive,* and overlaps with behavioral skills training to promote cognitive–behavioral change. Cognitive interventions address the need to identify and label internal emotional states such as anger, depression, and anxiety, which can become automatic triggers to relapse. They also challenge maladaptive beliefs, attitudes, and thinking associated with relapse, and seek to provide alternative and more adaptive ways of viewing life's problems which otherwise can foster relapse.

The third kind of psychological intervention discussed in this chapter focuses on *affective (emotional) self-awareness.* This refers to the necessary increase in a hard-core smokers' capacity to experience uncomfortable feelings, and to the realization that they don't have to use cigarettes to make themselves feel better. Emotional discomfort can be from sources as diverse as a setback on the job or a life-long feeling of inadequacy. But whether the source of such negative feelings is situational and short-term, or a long-term character trait, it is important for smokers to understand how negative affect serves as a relapse trigger so they can cope with it better in the future.

In this chapter we describe these interventions for smoking addiction, and illustrate them with case histories and specific examples. We also present a theoretical model of relapse prevention in smoking cessation treatment, which is not intended to be a comprehensive literature review (see Brown & Emmons, 1991). The three kinds of therapeutic change that we recommend are now presented in greater detail.

BEHAVIOR CHANGE

The treatment goal of behavior change in all drug abuse therapy is to establish and maintain abstinence—to separate the patient from the substance he or she is abusing. To achieve the goal of abstinence from cigarette smoking in particular, the treatment plan includes (a) behavioral skills training and (b) appropriate levels of social support (U.S. Department of Health and Human Services, 1996).

What is behavioral change and how does it contribute to abstinence from smoking? The tradition of Alcoholics Anonymous advises avoiding conditioned triggers such as "people, places, and things" associated with drinking. A conditioned response is like that exhibited by Pavlov's dog. The dog salivates when it hears the bell because it associates that bell with food. If the bell were not associated with food, it would not trigger salivation. Likewise, the smoker begins to crave cigarettes in situations he or she associates with having a smoke. When the smoker quits, "people, places, and things" associated with having or wanting a smoke become like that bell. Instead of triggering salivation, however, certain people, places, and things trigger a craving to smoke. In addition to external triggers to relapse behaviors, which the smoker can sometimes avoid, there often occur internal, that is, emotional, triggers, such as anger, depression, anxiety, and so forth. These must be dealt with by employing techniques other than avoidance, which we take up later in this chapter.

In an excellent paper on preventing relapse, Shiffman and his colleagues (Shiffman, Read, Maltese, Rapkin, & Jarvik, 1985, p. 489) identified seven common "relapse precipitants." These triggers include meal time, alcohol consumption, food substitution (i.e., smoking instead of eating), social situations, boredom, negative affect, and positive affect. This is part of what can be an extensive list for any given smoker! So when we recommend avoiding conditioned triggers, a smoker may resist our clinical recommendations by saying, "If I can't eat, feel positive or negative emotions, or socialize, what is there to look forward to in life?"

Our answer is that the goal of behavioral skills training is not only to help the smoker avoid relapse but to also develop new and fulfilling alternative ways of coping with these triggers.

Although it is not always possible to avoid triggers (such as having an unexpected encounter with someone who is smoking), it is possible to learn to anticipate triggers and develop techniques to cope with them. When avoidance or escape from high-risk situations is not possible, smokers need to remember that cravings are time limited and to try to distract attention from the craving and delay acting on it (Shiffman et al., 1985). In fact, Shiffman and his colleagues emphasized that relapse is really an interacton between "situational cues" (triggers to smoking) and "deficient coping skills" (inadequate responses to a relapse crisis). A list of behavioral techniques to prepare for quitting and to cope with withdrawal from cigarettes is provided in Table 12.1.

Each person must identify his or her own personal triggers and develop coping strategies that will work individually. These triggers and appropriate coping responses will be as similar or diverse as smokers themselves. For

TABLE 12.1
Behavioral Techniques

Before you quit:

1. Change to a brand of cigarettes you don't like. Try menthols if you don't like them, or nonmenthols if you do.
2. Put your cigarettes in a different place every day. Make it difficult to get to them. Put matches/lighters in another place so you must expend a lot of energy to get to smoke.
3. When you want to smoke, make yourself take "time out" to do it. That is, if you are at your desk, make yourself go to the hall or bathroom to smoke, etc. At home, go into a different room where you don't usually smoke.
4. Use smoke-holding technique: take a puff of a cigarette and hold for 30 seconds. Notice the bad taste and focus on the negative sensations.
5. Throw away *all* cigarettes, ashtrays, lighters. Ideally, this should be done on the night before your "Quit Day."

After you quit:

6. Save old, dirty cigarette butts in a jar with a little water in it. When you feel the urge to smoke, smell the jar.
7. Use deep breathing to relax when you feel the urge to smoke.
8. Make a list of activities that tempt you most to smoke and try to avoid those situations (e.g., drinking alcohol or coffee).
9. Play with paper clips, rubberbands, marbles, knitting, etc., to occupy your hands.
10. Chew sugarless gum, mints, or ice cubes.
11. Sip water or juice frequently.
12. Keep a supply of low-calorie, high-crunch snacks on hand in case of hunger pangs. Unbuttered popcorn or cut-up raw vegetables are good choices.
13. To avoid smoking after meals, get up from the table and brush your teeth or go for a walk.
14. Brush your teeth frequently and use a mouthwash.
15. *Exercise.* When you feel like smoking do some physical activity or take a brisk walk until the urge passes. Also, institute a regular exercise regime: walking, swimming, calisthenics, jumping rope, playing tennis—this will both decrease your need to smoke and help keep your weight down.
16. When you are having a strong "craving attack," time how long it lasts.

Note. This list is issued with an introduction: "The following is a list of behaviors which others have found to be helpful in stopping smoking. The first four suggestions are meant to be used in the days leading up to 'Quit Day' to help you to become more prepared to stop smoking; the others are recommended for use after you have stopped. Study this list and use the techniques regularly. Some will be more effective than others for you—the important thing is to stick with them." This list was prepared for the Smoking Cessation Clinic at New York State Psychiatric Institute by Fay Stetner, MA, MPA.

example, one patient realized she always experienced severe craving when she closed her car door. As she talked about it, she became aware that the moment she closed the door she looked forward to turning on the ignition and lighting a cigarette. Just recognizing the steps leading to the behavior (itself a cognitive intervention) enabled her to lessen that conditioned connection between the car door slamming and the craving to smoke. When the smoker can see the connection between the trigger and the craving, she can then also begin to use cognitive strategies such as constructive self-talk or self-coping statements, discussed later in this chapter, to help change the deeply conditioned and automatic behavioral response of smoking.

Once patients repeatedly experience a trigger and successfully avoid the conditioned smoking response, the association between them begins to diminish and the craving subsides. Over time the cravings become weaker and further apart, although periodically the ex-smoker may experience a temporary surge in cravings to smoke. It is important at these times for the clinician to reassure the patient that (a) cravings to smoke are an expected part of smoking cessation and will pass in time, and (b) he or she does not need to smoke to make the cravings go away. In fact, nothing seems to stimulate the craving to smoke more than actually smoking a cigarette!

Another patient found herself craving a cigarette in her "smoke-free" office. She later found that smoke from a smoker next door was coming in through her window. When she realized this, she had to decide how to cope with it. With the help of her group, she role played how she would be assertive with her smoking coworker in the next-door office. Later, when back at her job, she successfully communicated to the co-worker her genuine need for a smoke-free workplace. Such behavioral assertiveness is an example of a "life skill" (see Botvin & Epstein, chap. 3, this volume) that promotes a more satisfactory emotional adjustment to smoke-free living.

A third patient went out for a late-night drink of alcohol with a good friend and long-time fellow smoker. When, after three drinks, the friend began to smoke, the trigger was overwhelming and the patient slipped. In discussing the slip with her doctor, she learned from this experience that two drinks (when she was with a smoker) was her limit at that time, and that she needed to be very honest with herself about possible trouble when making plans involving drinking alcohol with friends who smoke.

SOCIAL SUPPORT AND THE NICOTINE WITHDRAWAL SYNDROME

In addition to learning behavioral skills, the second major aspect of the behavioral treatment plan is social support. Abstinence from smoking creates a state of disequilibrium (the nicotine withdrawal syndrome) for which a readjustment is necessary. When withdrawal is prolonged, defined here as longer than 5 weeks, AHCPR guidelines recommend considering the extension of nicotine replacement therapy (U.S. Department of Health and Human Services, 1996). It is also worthwhile to consider how stress may be magnifying craving and other withdrawal symptoms and how stress management principles can be applied to help manage a prolonged withdrawal syndrome.

As emphasized in the AHCPR smoking cessation guidelines (U.S. Department of Health and Human Services, 1996), increased clinical support plays an important role in a successful treatment outcome. One way to increase appropriate levels of such support is for the clinician to recommend to patients that they seek new support structures, such as those provided by individual and group counseling or peer groups, including Smokers' (Nicotine) Anonymous. These kinds of social support help patients develop new behaviors to cope with nicotine withdrawal syndrome. They also provide an "external control" structure to counter the smoker's tendency to lose control and the consequent high rate of relapse in the early period after quitting smoking.

We refer to establishing external structures and controls because heavily addicted patients are still likely to crave a smoke after their quit day. Smokers coming for treatment commonly have mixed feelings about stopping. Early in treatment, they also have not yet developed dependable ways to cope with their desire to smoke. Helpful social support can include the wish of patients to please their doctors, or to make a good report at their weekly group meeting. In other words, an ongoing supportive emotional relationship can lend smokers the hope, strength, and tools to abstain from smoking, so that they can then begin to develop these things in themselves.

The role of the clinician in this kind of intervention is that of a teacher, a guide, or a trainer. The clinician, by being genuinely knowledgeable and helpful in practical ways, acts as a source of motivation and faithful support. The hard-core, addicted patient must change the drug-seeking (smoking) behavior first, and only then can develop an honest appraisal of his or her addictive behavior.

This is in contrast to the strategy in traditional psychotherapies of waiting to develop the inner conviction of self-understanding offered by a "neutral" or "nondirective" therapist, which precedes behavioral change (Keller, 1996). Clearly, in smoking cessation treatment, the therapist is on the side of abstinence from smoking. With addicts, the therapist has to say "do this because it works," or "do this on doctor's orders" or by doctor's "prescription." The therapist thus assumes an active role in prescribing behavior change and as a coach in implementing it. The neutral nondirective approach may be why traditional psychotherapy approaches for addiction so often fail.

The patient's task in behavior change is to be a student, open to new ideas and ways of doing things that may be more successful than efforts previously made on his or her own. In the initial stage of stopping smoking, smokers are still in the "trial and error" phase of learning about their addiction; they may or may not be doing the things they need to do to avoid smoking. Their progress may be uneven. And if their strategy is working, they may not understand or be able to repeat their successes (abstinence) or avoid their mistakes (slips or near slips). Behavioral skills training and increased social support help the smoker benefit from the therapist's knowledge and experience of what works. These two aspects of behavioral treatment work together to help smokers overcome their ambivalence, which may show up as poor compliance with treatment tasks and the agreed-on treatment plan.

But what if the trigger to smoke is not an external situation for which an appropriate behavioral response can be found? What happens if the trigger is internal, such as a negative or a positive emotion? This brings us to the second kind of intervention.

COGNITIVE CHANGE

The goal of cognitive treatment is to question maladaptive beliefs, and to reframe illogical attitudes and irrational assumptions that can lead to "defeatist reactions" and relapse (Marlatt & Gordon, 1985). The goal of this facet of treatment is also to address the need to recognize, identify, and label internal feeling states associated with relapse.

For example, many smokers say, "I can't enjoy a good meal without a cigarette." This is reminiscent of the alcoholic who says he or she can't imagine going to a wedding without ceremoniously toasting the bride and groom. Other smokers give such examples of unrealistic thinking as "when life gets tough I need just one cigarette or a drink to feel all right and to get me through." In this example, the reality is of course that the smoker won't just have one cigarette, any more than an alcoholic will have just one drink.

How does the clinician achieve the treatment goal of changing (decreasing) irrational thinking or "rationalizations" associated with smoking behavior? Cognitive treatment questions and challenges such maladaptive beliefs as "I'll just have one smoke," and helps patients recognize how they serve to rationalize their addiction. Patients have to be trained in "trial thinking," to imagine themselves in the future and to picture where they are really going: back to smoking heavily and losing self-esteem because of the resumption of their addictive behavior.

Cognitive Treatment and Conditioned Cravings

Conditioned craving is what happens after years of smoking with coffee or smoking when stressed, angry, or depressed. The coffee or the stress and other emotions become paired with the smoking. Once this conditioning takes place, each time a smoker drinks coffee or experiences stress, these become conditioned stimuli ("triggers") to crave a cigarette. Conditioned cravings can thus be triggered by something internal (a feeling) as well as by something external (a situation).

By labeling a smoker's feelings and helping them to distinguish these feelings from the craving to smoke, cognitive treatment helps lessen the conditioned connection between such internal emotional triggers and subsequent smoking behavior. It is also important for the clinician to help identify how many heavily addicted smokers focus on their bodily sensations and physical ailments but cannot as readily verbalize their experience of themselves in emotional terms (see discussion of alexithymia later in chapter).

Conditioned Cravings and Negative Affect

Conditioned cravings divert (often very effectively) smokers from uncomfortable feelings they may be experiencing. For example, a smoker may be very upset about something happening in his or her life, but all the smoker is conscious of is wanting to smoke. For many nicotine addicts, smoking cigarettes has become a way of managing moods and altering feelings. In fact, an extensive literature has developed on the subject of "affect regulation" and nicotine addiction—in other words, the use of smoking to relieve stress and cope with dysphoria and anxiety (see Carmody, 1989, for a review). Numerous studies also point to a large role for negative emotional states such as anxiety, anger, and depressed mood as relapse triggers. For example, a study by Shiffman (1986) found that negative affect is associated with about 7 out of 10 relapse episodes. Another study (Brandon, Tiffany, Obremski, & Baker, 1990) also found that negative affect preceded initial lapse to smoking in almost two out of every three subjects.

Patients become so used to calming down by smoking when they are anxious, or getting a boost by smoking when they are depressed, that they have a very real difficulty even identifying these feelings. Again, like the bell paired with the food in Pavlov's experiment, the emotions are paired with the craving: All the dog knows when he hears the bell is that food is coming; all the smoker knows when he or she feels negative affect is that he or she wants to smoke. By identifying these feelings, the clinician can help the smoker to cope with them in new ways (without smoking). One way to cope with negative affect is to develop self-coping phrases or statements to be repeated in difficult moments such as: "It's all right, I can get through this discomfort without smoking and still feel good about myself. This will be over soon."

In cognitive treatment the clinician doesn't seek to understand in depth (or encourage a fuller emotional experiencing of) the person's feelings that have been masked by smoking. Early in treatment and early in abstinence, the clinician seeks only to label the feelings, and to modify negative mood through a combination of behavioral and cognitive techniques or what have been called *mood management* or *affect regulation* strategies (Carmody, 1989; Hall, Munoz, Reus, & Sees, 1993). Although it may seem basic to label feelings, it is fascinating to observe that smokers who are sophisticated and successful in dealing with the world around them may have absolutely no idea what they are experiencing or feeling inside themselves. For the addicted smoker, beginning to identify feelings, instead of automatically acting on them by smoking, is the first step in lessening and ultimately breaking the connection between feelings and cravings. Put another way, labeling these feelings helps begin to break the link that causes feelings to function as an "internal trigger" to relapse.

In addition to the awareness of internal triggers, there are also certain cognitive attitudes that can precede a slip and need to be identified and monitored. Three common cognitive precipitants of relapse (Marlatt & Gordon, 1985; Washton, 1987) useful to reframe in cognitive relapse prevention training are:

- The tendency to romanticize smoking.
- The tendency to want to test control, to test the strength of abstinence by taking a puff or "just one smoke."
- The tendency, if there is a slip, to attribute it to a long-standing personal trait such as weakness or lack of willpower. This tendency is called *AVE*, or the abstinence violation effect.

The tendency to romanticize smoking can be viewed as the smoker's selective inattention to other aspects of their presenting problem. Often it helps to review the smoker's presenting complaint and personal reasons for quitting. The clinician can then remind the smoker that smoking addiction was a "package" with not only positive features, but negative consequences as well. Addicted smokers cannot have only one pleasurable smoke here and there, but will predictably fall back into their old pattern of addicted smoking that brought them to treatment in the first place.

The tendency to test control involves one of the most difficult lessons learned by people who become addicted to drugs: addiction means addicts can no longer use the substance casually or recreationally, can no longer control their drug use. Many people have to learn this lesson again and again through hard experience and painful repetition. Testing control is the painful process of trying to have "just one" cigarette, only to resume smoking addictively and compulsively again.

The abstinence violation effect is a theory, developed by Marlatt, about the importance of a smoker's cognitive assessment or appraisal of their behavior after a brief slip, and how this can contribute to a full-blown relapse back to smoking (Marlatt & Gordon, 1985). The smoker who blames herself or himself for being "weak" usually continues smoking. While berating oneself, one doesn't take a good look at, and change, what one is doing. As an alternative, by looking at what went wrong, and applying the lesson learned to promote behavior change and abstinence, the patient can achieve a more successful outcome. Typically, instead of "beating herself (or himself) up" for her mistake, the patient can then more productively examine how to better use relapse prevention skills and social supports in the future.

Another cognitive attitude associated with relapse that often needs to be addressed in smoking cessation treatment concerns the issue of weight gain. Empirical research indicates that 80–85% of smokers will gain weight after stopping smoking, with the rest maintaining their precessation weight (Klesges, 1995). Unfortunately, while average weight gains of under 10 pounds are most often cited to patients (U.S. Department of Health and Human Services, 1996), recent work suggests that weight gains averaging 10 pounds and more are quite common, and that 15–20% of smokers will gain over 30 pounds (Klesges, 1995).

The fashion of thinness in modern Western culture dominates the popular view of attractiveness. But like the asthetic ideal of foot binding in China, thinness comes at a heavy price for most women because this "ideal" of weight and shape can involve a deformation of their normal and healthy bodies. The cultural ideal of thinness collides head-on for most women with the biological realities of their lives (Wilfley & Rodin, 1995). The advertising of the cigarette industry has clearly understood this discrepancy, and smoking cigarettes has been presented as an answer to women's pervasive concerns over weight gain. It would be a mistake to underestimate clinically how often the discrepancy between "ideal" and "real" weight contributes to the negative emotions and feelings of low self-worth that promote relapse back to smoking.

The AHCPR guidelines (U.S. Department of Health and Human Services, 1996) recommend that smokers make changes to promote good nutrition and healthy exercise habits, but discourage smokers from dieting too strenuously after quitting. The approach is to help smokers accept some weight in the short term and to advise them to wait until later, when they are more confident, to reduce any unwanted weight gained postcessation. Research on pharmacotherapy with nicotine replacement suggests choosing the gum over the patch as a more successful weight control strategy. Gross, Stitzer, and Maldonado (1989) found that subjects using nicotine gum versus subjects on a placebo gum showed about half as much weight gain for as long as they continued to chew the gum. In contrast, Perkins (1994), in a review of controlled studies of the patch, reported it to have no effect as a tool for weight control.

Christopher Fairburn, a leading researcher on eating disorders, traced low self-worth in patients with bulimia nervosa to their tendency to engage in "black and white" thinking with "shape and weight" as the central criteria for perfection versus failure (1995). Importantly, Fairburn wrote that for bulimia nervosa, "the chances of relapse are directly related to the presence of continuing concerns about shape and weight" (1995, p. 345). Concerns about shape and weight, and the negative emotions they engender, are a major obstacle for smokers as well who are trying to stay off cigarettes.

Certain researchers (Perkins, 1994) have advocated, as do the AHCPR smoking cessation guidelines, that smokers learn to accept more weight as opposed to trying to lose it right away after quitting smoking. This is because concerns about weight gain, as well as strict dieting to prevent it, are associated with lower quit rates.

Cognitive treatment for smoking cessation addresses smokers' maladaptive cognitions about weight gain and smoking. As an example, one female smoker stated she would rather have cancer surgery again than gain 5 pounds. Cognitive approaches to help smokers include the use of self-monitoring records that help track smokers' cognitions (beliefs and assumptions) about gaining weight. In reviewing these records, clinician and patient follow the smoker's distressing train of thought about gaining weight and address four questions:

1. What is the evidence for the smoker's beliefs? What really is the practical effect of gaining weight?
2. Is there an "alternative explanation" or "conclusion" that contradicts the belief? How else can the person view the impact of weight gain (even if he or she doesn't believe it)?
3. If the distressing belief is accurate, what are the implications (socially and professionally)? Are no "fat" people successful? Are no thin people unhappy?
4. Finally, does the belief lead to adaptive and rational action (Vitousek, 1995)?

An important principle of cognitive-behavioral treatment is for patients to go on as usual and not avoid their normal activities based on weight gain. The ability to carry on with, and not alter, their lives can decrease the overvaluation of weight gain as a central concern. Two strategies recommended by Vitousek (1995) to modify beliefs about weight and food in patients with anorexia nervosa are (a) to identify discrepancies the patients may have in standards for others versus themselves, and (b) to set up agreed-on criteria to evaluate the realistic impact of weight gain in the person's life. Such criteria might be in the form of a prediction about how other people will respond to any weight gain. Clinically it may be important to explore how other aspects of the person's work and social behavior are undervalued in contrast to the importance placed on weight and ideal body shape. It can also be worth pointing out that in smoking for weight control, the smoker buys into a package, and may not like all it contains. This is because the package also contains addiction and loss of control, guilt about damaging health, loss of sexual attraction due to unhealthy-looking skin and wrinkles, bad breath, smelly clothes, and discolored teeth (see chap. 4, this volume). As desirable as being thin might be, smoking can be as unattractive—depicted forcefully in the antismoking poster proclaiming "Smoking is so glamorous" under a photograph of a very wrinkled, very unhealthy-looking woman.

The clinician's role in a cognitive intervention strategy for smoking cessation, as in the behavioral treatment described in the previous section, is to provide structured guidance with clear goals, and how they will be achieved. Although in behavioral skills training the clinician is more directive in recommending alternative coping skills, in cognitive therapy the clinician takes a more collaborative and questioning stance (Young, Beck, & Weinberger, 1993), leaving a role for self-discovery in patients' ways of viewing problems associated with their smoking addiction.

Limitations of Cognitive-Behavioral Treatment for Smoking Cessation

In smoking cessation treatment, new attitudes and behaviors that accompany quitting often bring new rewards, which gradually reinforce these changes over time. However, in our own clinical work we have repeatedly observed a finding, confirmed by research (Brandon et al., 1990; Carmody, 1989; Shiffman, 1986), that the occurrences of strong and uncomfortable (negative) affects such as stress, anxiety, and anger, as well as depressive states postcessation (Covey, Glassman, & Stetner, 1990), serve as powerful relapse triggers back to smoking. Even after a year of nonsmoking behavior, smokers sometimes report being overwhelmed by such strong emotions as anger or sadness, which can reactivate the prior maladaptive attitudes and behaviors associated with smoking.

Occasionally (see Brandon et al., 1990), the trigger to resume smoking is simply the occurrence or appearance of an affectless "neutral" cue, such as being in a place previously associated with smoking, like a certain restaurant. Sometimes the lapse can be preceded by positive affects as well (Brandon et al., 1990). However, given the prominence of negative affect as a conditioned relapse trigger, a successful strategy for long-term relapse prevention must, in our view, effectively address this complex psychological issue.

The first two kinds of therapeutic changes we have described—behavioral and cognitive—do not always effectively secure the "emotional change" important in the long-term maintenance of abstinence and relapse prevention. The third kind of therapeutic change we discuss is achieving emotional self-awareness, which is combined with the behavioral and cognitive approaches previously discussed. This change seeks to address the common finding that, for many patients who seek help for their smoking addiction, relapse continues to remain the most likely outcome of their treatment for smoking cessation.

AFFECTIVE (EMOTIONAL) SELF-AWARENESS

The goal of this aspect of therapeutic change is to increase and strengthen the smoker's capacity to tolerate and to experience feelings, especially negative feelings, rather than act on them as conditioned triggers to relapse. This capacity has been referred to by Krystal (1975; Krystal & Raskin, 1970) as *affect tolerance.* To achieve this goal the smoker must be encouraged to "live through" emotional discomfort such as stress, anxiety, anger, and sadness (negative affects) as an alternative to seeking short-term relief from cigarette smoking. By developing self-awareness into their internal states of pleasure and unpleasure (negative affect), smokers who have quit can also develop the capacity to know and fulfill, where possible, their genuine emotional needs without cigarettes. (For case histories and specific examples of this, see the final section of this chapter.)

Many times smokers will say, "I know how to handle that situation, but didn't realize how angry or anxious I was and what was happening until later, and by then I was already smoking." Often, the nicotine addict intellectually knows what to do, but can't always apply it. To prevent relapse behavior, emotional change needs to go beyond labeling and identifying, as well as modifying and managing, emotions that serve as conditioned triggers to smoke. The distinction being made here is between (a) being able to recognize and talk about feelings in a cognitive or intellectual way on the one hand, and (b) being able to experience, and to develop affect tolerance for, feelings that are uncovered by stopping smoking on the other hand.

Dahl, an emotion theorist and researcher, stated (1991, p. 134) that emotions "function as wishes and beliefs in an evolutionarily given . . . nonverbal feedback information system." Dahl divided emotions into two major classes. The *IT emotions*, such as love, anger, and fear, are directed to the outside world and are concerned with the consummation of emotional wishes and somatic appetites. *ME emotions* (such as elation, depression, or anxiety), in contrast, involve internal experiences of pleasure and unpleasure, and a corresponding belief, or information feedback system, about the fulfillment or nonfulfillment of important wishes and appetites. "Positive" ME emotions are experiences people want to repeat (positive reinforcement), and "negative" ME emotions are experiences people want to get rid of (negative reinforcement).

According to Dahl, the discomfort of negative ME emotions functions as a cognitive belief, for example, that "my wishes are not going well" (anxiety) or that "my wishes can't be satisfied" (depression). These beliefs, when embedded in developmentally learned *schemas* (Young et al., 1993), or *frames* (Dahl, 1988) or core conflictual relationship *themes* (Luborsky, 1984), are based on learning from repetitive early childhood experiences. These prototypical cognitive–affective structures become maladaptive characterological responses; in other words, the patient may not only have an incapacity for tolerating affect, but may also have developed over time characteristic ways of defending against it (see next section).

The dysfunctional beliefs attached to these early experiences are thought by these authors (Dahl, 1988; Luborsky, 1984; Young et al., 1993) to be more susceptible to change when patients also experience their emotions, which are related to these beliefs, in a powerful and immediate way in the "here and now" of the psychological treatment relationship. The basic principle here is that, with skillful psychological help to overcome their psychological defenses, the more deeply patients can experience their emotional beliefs, the more accessible the beliefs are to change. Such heightened emotional experiencing, in this view, is the active ingredient that can lead to the therapeutic alteration of ingrained automatic patterns of behaving, thinking, and feeling.

Psychological Defenses Against Negative Emotions

When such a lifelong schema or frame reproduces negative feelings such as anxiety or depression, the person will tend to inhibit or defend himself or herself. "Such defenses, if invoked, vary greatly in their effectiveness, particularly against the NEG ME emotion itself, often leading to auxiliary means, such as alcohol and other drugs, to get rid of the aversive quality of the NEG ME emotion" (Dahl, 1991, p. 136). "Smoking nicotine," as well as using alcohol and other drugs, are the auxiliary means, the chemical defenses, that are used to decrease negative emotional states.

Psychological defenses are ways to diminish negative ME emotions. They are not really "mechanisms" but more characteristic modes of dealing with unpleasure (negative affect) and are associated with specific behavioral coping styles (Plutchik, 1995). Further, although they are discussed as separate "defense mechanisms" in theory, in clinical practice they are not so differentiated, and share the common feature of inhibiting, in Dahl's terms, negative ME emotions. For purposes of discussion we review three different psychological defenses—denial, externalization, and rationalization—and how they illustrate common clinical examples with smokers.

Denial. The psychological defense against the negative ME emotions most familiar to the clinician working with smokers is called *denial*, with its associated coping response of *minimization*: "There isn't a problem because I'm not addicted. I can quit whenever I really want to." In this case the smoker is denying the addiction itself (his or her difficulty controlling smoking, and that any negative consequences are connected with smoking) and so doesn't have to feel bad about it because it's "no problem."

Denial can be defined as a defensive refusal to recognize an external reality, or a "restriction" in perception, in the face of a disagreable or painful impression from the outer world (Freud, 1966). Interestingly, in our clinic, when we have smokers keep a diary of their cigarette smoking, they are often genuinely surprised to find out how many cigarettes they are really smoking. Some of these smokers have underestimated or minimized their smoking as a way to deny to themselves the seriousness of their addictive behavior. Frequent examples among smokers of the avoidance associated with denial are "I don't want to discuss this anymore" or "stop nagging, let's talk about something else."

Externalization. A second psychological defense, which others (Kaufman, 1994; Vaillant, 1986, 1992, 1993) have encountered in substance abusers and called *projection*, we refer to as *externalization*, with its associated coping response of blaming other people. This involves assigning responsibility for problems and feelings, which lead to relapse, to other people. A common clinical example of externalization or blaming other people is, "Yes I smoke, but no one understands me. If you had to live with my husband you'd probably do something worse."

Addressing this defense can be particularly important in treating smokers who view their problems as external and outside themselves, and who then feel victimized and helpless in the face of their addiction. Accepting responsibility for their addiction (as well as for their own happiness) can be an important step in achieving long-term abstinence and relapse prevention.

Rationalization. Finally, the third psychological defense often employed by smokers is called intellectualization or *rationalization*. This defense overlaps with the two other defenses we have been discussing and helps to make them possible. Although the smoker's logic may not look good when examined carefully by an outside observer, it works well to facilitate the behavior of the addiction because it is very believable to the cigarette addict.

Rationalization can be defined as the reassuring self-justification of behavior or thought that might otherwise be unacceptable to a person (Vaillant, 1992). One of the most fascinating aspects of working with smokers is watching their often creative and plausible ways of explaining away any possible consequences of their addictive behavior. A smoker's prime rationalization, as previously discussed, is "I will only have this one cigarette, and one cigarette will not harm or addict me."

This rationalization serves to protect addicted smokers from the painful reality that they can no longer control their smoking and be recreational smokers. A second example raises the question of distinguishing, especially in teenagers, between the defense of rationalization and the need for more education about the addictive consequences of smoking cigarettes. As one intelligent young man explained, "I'll just smoke for a few years and stop. People who say they're addicted are just making excuses or want to smoke."

Denial, externalization, and rationalization present formidable barriers to implementing a cognitive–behavioral treatment plan. They also present a barrier to the maintenance of therapeutic gains, and hence actively preserve the momentum of the physiological and conditioned aspects of smoking behavior. To successfully apply new behavioral skills and cognitive self-knowledge, many smokers need the clinician to point out to them how such different forms of defensive behavior protect them from experiencing painful feelings. This can allow for a deeper, more experiential, affective self-awareness into negative ME emotions such as anxiety and depression.

In our clinical experience with smokers, achieving such emotional self-awareness requires the clinician to (a) address defensive patterns such as denial, (b) evoke negative ME emotions, and (c) examine and challenge the cognitive messages (such as that "things don't ever work out for me") that are embedded in developmentally determined psychic schemas or frames of mind. It is also crucial that these three aspects of developing emotional self-awareness occur in the context of a supportive therapeutic relationship.

Affective Self-Awareness and the Therapeutic Relationship

For the addicted smoker, the crisis of quitting smoking brings unpleasant and, at times, overwhelming emotions to the surface. A skilled clinician can help mobilize these emotions for the purpose of emotional change and adaptation. Just seeking and maintaining a helping or therapeutic relationship to quit smoking can also bring out hidden emotions, which, when examined, can promote deeper and lasting emotional changes helpful in relapse prevention.

The clinician's role in promoting emotional change is to take a nonjudgmental and accepting stance to encourage emotional expressiveness and nondefensive personal self-disclosure. The patient's task is to discuss his or her feelings as openly as possible without censoring them or prejudging their importance in the process of emotional therapeutic change. It is also the clinician's task to help evoke emotional expressiveness in the patient, as smokers often cannot do this on their own.

This incapacity to verbalize emotion has been termed *alexithymia* and has been found to have a high prevalence among substance abusers, who may also have a limited cognitive capacity to cope with their overwhelming negative affects (Taylor, Parker, & Bagby, 1990). According to Taylor et al. (1990), alexithymic patients also manifest "a tendency to focus on and amplify the somatic sensations accompanying emotional arousal." The clinician working with hard-core smokers often must seek to elicit and develop the capacity to verbalize feelings (and for affect tolerance) by validating and accepting the patient's emotional reactions and experiences.

Despite these clinical efforts, there are those people whose defensiveness and lack of "psychological-mindedness" and/or unwillingness to work in a reflective psychological treatment modality may defeat a clinician's best efforts. Sometimes pharmacological treatment can help to stabilize the upsetting emotions associated with stopping smoking. This can place an "emotional floor" under the patient so he or she can begin to work more productively on the psychological aspects of his or her smoking addiction.

CASE HISTORIES: DEVELOPING EMOTIONAL SELF-AWARENESS

"Smokescreen"—Dealing With Feelings

Barbara described herself as a fair boss who tried to be everyone's friend. When she stopped smoking she found herself incredibly angry and irritable, and withdrew to protect others from her lashing out. She had used smoking to calm and soothe herself for so long that she did not recognize emotional pain for what it was. Smoking had been such an effective anesthetic to numb feelings and to manipulate mood that without it she felt like one big "raw nerve." Although a woman of the world in many ways, when it came to her emotions, she needed to go back to basics. She had always hidden her feelings under an emotional and a literal "smokescreen." Seeming to be full of good cheer, with a mask of bravado and a polished exterior, she left her own needs unmet. Smoking helped her to maintain her unhappy compromise with life. Giving up smoking meant much more to this patient than losing a bad habit. It meant confronting an emotional style of adaptation that was no longer working for her.

Jessica had spent years going to smoking cessation programs, traveling all around the country. She would always make many friends and stop smoking. However, when she returned home to her usual life, she always slipped back into smoking. She focused all her energy on her problem with quitting smoking, and when she entered the quit smoking support group she seemed to come in on a cloud of smoke. She had such a smokescreen around her that no one in the group could get to know her or figure out her story.

When Jessica stopped smoking, however, it was as if she became a new person. She began to talk openly about her marital problems and her fears of taking charge and changing her life. Jessica's preoccupation with smoking had hidden from her and from others her problems with living. After she gave up her cigarettes, when the smoke cleared, she began to settle down to looking at herself. Without her smokescreen, Jessica began to learn to better deal with, and not escape from, her feelings about her life. As painful as this was for her at times, Jessica became more comfortable with tolerating (and verbalizing to herself) her feelings and thus better able to assert her genuine emotional interests. This has left her with an increased self-confidence and decreased feelings of helplessness, powerlessness, and resentment of being at the "mercy of" others. She was able to achieve a greater affective self-awareness and has been smoke free for several years.

"Smoking It Down"—Avoiding Confrontation

A third patient, Jack, became enraged with a coworker in an important meeting. In his session all he could articulate was an increasing feeling of discomfort about not smoking and a wish to smoke to feel better. After labeling his feelings he realized that he had "thrown in the towel" with his colleague and had not found an appropriate rejoinder to her negative, destructive comments. He was left with a smoldering resentment.

Jack's resentment was fueling his wish to smoke. After becoming more aware of his feelings and seeing his situation in a different way, he was able to change his behavior. He later made time for a private talk with his colleague. He expressed himself clearly and directly with his coworker, and when it was over he felt at peace with himself. By confronting his coworker and overcoming his emotional turmoil, he felt less helpless and resentful. Interestingly, he also experienced less of a need and craving to smoke.

SUMMARY

To overcome a cigarette addiction and to not relapse, many patients need to work at the art of "here and now" living. Instead of identifying and dealing with their own feelings, or confronting others with their own legitimate needs, many smokers are waiting for life to begin. These smokers are always looking forward to those moments when they are puffing on a cigarette or taking "time out" for a cigarette break.

When many smokers successfully quit they experience a new vitality and energy for living. They seem genuinely excited by a sense of newness and freedom. Whatever the reason for this "pink cloud," one thing seems clear: To sustain abstinence, people must perceive benefits from quitting smoking. They need to get something, not just have something taken away.

Although medical detox in nicotine withdrawal syndrome is about making it easier to give up cigarettes, psychological deconditioning involves making behavioral, cognitive, and emotional changes to support long-term abstinence. In other words, the psychology of quitting and not relapsing involves making adaptive changes that can help smokers feel and live more fully without their old ways of artificially manipulating the biology of pain and pleasure through their cigarettes.

ACKNOWLEDGMENTS

The authors thank Michael S. Porder, MD, Fay Stetner, MA, MPA, and Susan Crawford, MA, for their careful reading of, and contributions to, this chapter. We also thank Ethan E. Gorenstein, PhD, for reviewing cognitive–behavioral strategies for dealing with weight gain, and Michael S. Porder, MD, who suggested the term *affective self-awareness* and also reviewed in detail this part of the chapter.

REFERENCES

Brandon, T., Tiffany, S. T., Obremski, K., & Baker, T. (1990). Postcessation cigarette use: The process of relapse. *Addictive Behaviors, 15*, 105–114.

Brown, R. A., & Emmons, K. M. (1991). Behavioral treatment of cigarette dependence. In J. Cocores (Ed.), *The clinical management of nicotine dependence* (pp. 97–118). New York: Springer-Verlag.

Carmody, T. P. (1989). Affect regulation, nicotine addiction, and smoking cessation. *Journal of Psychoactive Drugs, 21*, 331–342.

Covey, L. S., Glassman, A. H., & Stetner, F. (1990). Depression and depressive symptoms in smoking cessation. *Comprehensive Psychiatry, 31*, 350–354.

Dahl, H. (1991). The key to understanding change: Emotions as appetitive wishes and beliefs about their fulfillment. In J. Safran & L. Greenberg (Eds.), *Emotion, psychotherapy & change* (pp. 130–165). New York: Guilford Press.

Dahl, H. (1988). Frames of mind. In H. Dahl, H. Kachele, & H. Thoma (Eds.), *Psychoanalytic process research strategies* (pp. 51–66). New York: Springer-Verlag.

Fairburn, C. (1995). Short-term psychological treatments for bulimia nervosa. In K. Brownell & C. Fairburn (Eds.), *Eating disorders and obesity, a comprehensive handbook* (pp. 344–348). New York: Guilford Press.

Freud, A. (1966). *The ego and the mechanisms of defense.* New York: International Universities Press.

Gross, J., Stitzer, M. L., & Maldonado, J. (1989). Nicotine replacement: Effects on postcessation weight gain. *Journal of Consulting and Clinical Psychology, 57*(1), 87–92.

Hall, S. M., Munoz, R., Reus, V., & Sees, K. (1993). Nicotine, negative affect, and depression. *Journal of Consulting and Clinical Psychology, 61*(5), 761–767.

Kaufman, E. (1994). *Psychotherapy of addicted persons.* New York: Guilford Press.

Keller, D. (1996). Exploration in the service of relapse prevention: A psychoanalytic contribution to substance abuse treatment. In F. Rotgers, D. Keller, & J. Morgenstern (Eds.), *Treating substance abuse, theory and technique* (pp. 84–116). New York: Guilford Press.

Klesges, R. C. (1995). Cigarette smoking and body weight. In K. Brownell & C. Fairburn (Eds.), *Eating disorders and obesity, a comprehensive handbook* (pp. 61–64). New York: Guilford Press.

Krystal, H. (1975). Affect tolerance. In *The annual of psychoanalysis, a publication of the Chicago Institute for Psychoanalysis* (Vol. III, pp. 179–219). New York: International Universities Press.

Krystal, H., & Raskin, H. (1970). *Drug dependence.* Detroit, MI: Wayne State University Press.

Luborsky, L. (1984). *Principles of psychoanalytic psychotherapy. A manual for supportive-expressive treatment.* New York: Basic Books.

Marlatt, G. A., & Gordon, J. (Eds.). (1985). *Relapse prevention: Maintenance strategies in the treatment of addictive behaviors.* New York: Guilford Press.

Perkins, K. (1994). Issues in the prevention of weight gain after smoking cessation. *Annals of Behavioral Medicine, 16*(1), 46–52.

Prochaska, J., & DiClemente, C. C. (1983). Stages and Processes of self-change of smoking: Toward an integrative model of change. *Journal of Consulting and Clinical Psychology, 5,* 390–395.

Plutchik, R. (1995). A theory of ego defenses. In H. Conte & R. Plutchik (Eds.), *Ego defenses, theory and measurement* (pp. 13–37). New York: Wiley.

Shiffman, S. M. (1986). A cluster-analytic classification of smoking relapse episodes. *Addictive Behaviors, 11,* 295–307.

Shiffman, S. M., Read, L., Maltese, T., Rapkin, D., & Jarvik, M. E. (1985). Preventing relapse in ex-smokers: A self-management approach. In G. A. Marlatt & J. R. Gordon (Eds.), *Relapse prevention: Maintenance strategies in the treatment of addictive behaviors* (pp. 472–520). New York: Guilford Press.

Taylor, G., Parker, J., & Bagby, R. (1990). A preliminary investigation of alexithymia in men with psychoactive substance dependence. *American Journal of Psychiatry, 147,* 1128–1230.

U.S. Department of Health and Human Services. (1996). *Clinical practice guideline: Smoking cessation.* AHCPR Publication No. 96-0692. Rockville, MD: USDHHS.

Vaillant, G. (1986). Introduction. In G. Vaillant (Ed.), *Empirical studies of ego mechanisms of defense.* Washington, DC: American Psychiatric Press.

Vaillant, G. (1992). *Ego mechanisms of defense: A guide for clinicians and researchers.* Washington, DC: American Psychiatric Press.

Vaillant, G. (1993). *The wisdom of the ego.* Cambridge, MA: Harvard University Press.

Vitousek, K. (1995). Cognitive-behavioral therapy for anorexia nervosa. In K. Brownell & C. Fairburn (Eds.), *Eating disorders and obesity, a comprehensive handbook* (pp. 324–329). New York: Guilford Press.

Washton, A. (1987). Outpatient treatment of cocaine abuse. In A. Washton & M. S. Gold (Eds.), *Cocaine: A clinician's handbook* (pp. 106–117). New York: Guilford Press.

Wilfrey, D., & Rodin, J. (1995). Cultural influences on eating disorders. In K. Brownell & C. Fairburn (Eds.), *Eating disorders and obesity, a comprehensive handbook* (pp. 78–82). New York: Guilford Press.

Young, J., Beck, A., & Weinberger, A. (1993). Depression. In D. Barlow (Ed.), *Clinical handbook of psychological disorders: A step-by-step treatment manual* (2nd ed., pp. 240–277). New York: Guilford Press.

Part V

The Smoker and the Health Care System

CHAPTER THIRTEEN

Challenges and Techniques for the Treatment of Nicotine Dependence by Physicians and Dentists

Thomas J. Glynn
American Cancer Society

Marc W. Manley
National Cancer Institute

Sherry Mills
National Cancer Institute

Karen Gerlach
Robert Wood Johnson Foundation

Roselyn Epps
National Cancer Institute

The treatment of nicotine dependence remains a significant challenge to the medical community. Despite the wide acknowledgment of the key role physicans, dentists, and other health professionals need to play in reducing tobacco use (U.S. Department of Health and Human Services, 1994b), and the results of many clinical trials demonstrating that they can treat nicotine dependence successfully (U.S. Department of Health and Human Services, 1996), there remain a significant number of physicians, dentists, and their staffs who do not regularly provide treatment for what is the leading cause of preventable death in the United States (Lindsay et al., 1994).

BARRIERS TO THE TREATMENT OF NICOTINE DEPENDENCE IN MEDICAL PRACTICE

Before suggesting remedies for this dilemma, however, it is necessary to understand the reasons for the gap between the acknowledged importance of treating nicotine dependence and the relatively low rates of doing so in medical practice. More than a decade ago, a sample of family practice and primary care physicians were surveyed by Orleans and her colleagues to help understand why more of them were not treating patients for their nicotine dependence (Orleans, George, Houpt, & Brodie, 1985). Unfortunately, despite enormous advances in pharmacology, policy change, and positive clinical trial results, the reasons physicians cited for their low rates of treatment of nicotine dependence in the mid 1980s have changed very little in the ensuing decade.

As shown in Table 13.1, the primary reasons that physicians reported that they did not often treat nicotine dependence concerned inadequate training, lack of time, reimbursement issues, and beliefs both that patients would not be able to change their tobacco use behavior and that, even if delivered, treatments were ineffective. Significantly, in the same survey, patients themselves cited a number of barriers to receiving treatment for nicotine dependence. These included, as with the physicians, reimbursement issues, but also focused on ambivalence concerning the physician's role in treating nicotine dependence and the appropriateness of raising tobacco use as a health issue when most visits were not specifically related to the patient's tobacco use.

More recently, Wiggers and Sanson-Fisher (1994) employed Green and Kreuter's PRECEDE–PROCEED model (1991; Glanz & Rimer, 1996) to categorize the barriers that health professionals, and especially physicians, addressed in more general terms in the earlier Orleans et al. survey. They identified three constellations of factors that appear to impede the routine application of tobacco use cessation strategies by physicians.

Using Green and Kreuter's terminology, they referred to the first constellation as *predisposing factors*, which include practitioner knowledge about and

TABLE 13.1
Perceived Barriers to Treatment of Nicotine Dependence in Medical Practice

Physician
1. Lack of time
2. Lack of training
3. Lack of reimbursement
4. Belief that patients not able to change relevant behaviors
5. Belief that physician/dentist treatment of nicotine dependence ineffective
6. Belief that interventions by referral sources ineffective
Patient
1. Cost
2. Visiting physician/dentist for other purpose
3. Unaware of need for treatment of nicotine dependence
4. Unaware of physician/dentist role in treatment of nicotine dependence
5. Belief that physician/dentist role in treatment of nicotine dependence inappropriate

Note. Adapted from Orleans et al. (1985).

attitudes toward treatment of nicotine dependence and patient attitudes about receipt of such treatment. Their second constellation revolved around *enabling factors*, which include efficacy/effectiveness of tobacco use cessation interventions, availability of clinical guidelines, and practice organization conducive to providing treatment for nicotine dependence. Wiggers and Sanson-Fisher's final constellation was *reinforcing factors*, which referred to such issues as financial reimbursement, performance feedback, and peer support.

These are by no means insignificant issues—nor are they limited to physicians and their patients, because many of the same issues are raised when considering the role of dentists in treating nicotine dependence. Nevertheless, although each of these "factors" may impede the routine delivery of treatment for tobacco use, each is also an important and essential element in any strategy to incorporate such treatment in the practices of primary care physicians and dentists. Specific actions may be taken, in fact, to make these factors means of empowering rather than impeding progress toward the goal of routine treatment for nicotine dependence in primary care.

A summary of actions that can be taken to transform the predisposing, enabling, and reinforcing factors just discussed from impediments to means of empowering practice change and treatment of nicotine dependence is presented next, followed by a discussion of the importance of considering hard-to-reach, difficult-to-treat patients in any plan to increase the proportion of physicians and dentists who routinely provide treatment for nicotine dependence.

PROMOTING THE TREATMENT OF NICOTINE DEPENDENCE IN MEDICAL PRACTICE

There are a number of ways in which—through both individual and systemic change and commitment—the treatment of nicotine dependence can become routine in medical practice. Suggestions for doing so are included here within each of the Wiggers and Sanson-Fisher factors already discussed.

Predisposing Factors

These factors include practitioner knowledge about and attitudes toward treatment of nicotine dependence and patient attitudes about such treatment.

Concerning knowledge about treatment of nicotine dependence, the most telling issue may be the tobacco use status of physicians and dentists themselves. In the United States, tobacco use among these groups has become almost negligible (Nelson et al., 1994). This is important because it demonstrates practitioners' commitment to the importance of stopping tobacco use but, because they will likely never have undergone the difficulty of withdrawing from nicotine, it also may affect their attitudes about and ability to empathize with their patients' withdrawal symptoms and related problems. To help bring about this change in attitudes, practitioners will need to be trained, both in undergraduate medical/dental education and afterward, to recognize and understand the complexities of nicotine dependence and to help their patients through their decision to stop and subsequent withdrawal from nicotine.

As far as attitudes toward treatment of nicotine dependence are concerned, there seems now to be little question, on the part of both practitioners and patients, that this is a legitimate, necessary, and desired part of medical practice (e.g., Fiore & Baker, 1995; Orleans & Slade, 1993; Richmond, 1994). This is a very positive change that has occurred over the past decade, based on many factors including broad media attention to tobacco issues, widely publicized research findings linking tobacco use to an ever wider array of medical problems, and growing interest in preventive care as an accepted part of medical practice. This is especially true as managed care has expanded and, in some plans, begun to offer such services as cancer screening, nutrition counseling, and smoking cessation interventions. As accountability systems, such as the National Committee for Quality Assurance's HEDIS (Health Plan Employer Data & Information Set) performance measures (National Committee for Quality Assurance, 1996), become more common, we should also expect that provision of preventive services will also become more common and accepted as a minimum standard of care.

The effect of these changes in provider and patient behaviors and attitudes has been to make these predisposing factors less of an impediment to the routine delivery of nicotine treatment in primary care, but they have highlighted the need to address the behaviors and activities grouped under enabling factors.

Enabling Factors

These factors include the effectiveness of tobacco use cessation interventions, the availability of clinical guidelines, and medical practice organization conducive to providing routine treatment for nicotine dependence.

Substantial progress has been made in recent years in addressing these factors. As discussed later, primary care providers now have at their disposal both the information and the treatment techniques to help their patients stop using tobacco.

First, numerous clinical trials have demonstrated that physicians and dentists can effectively deliver treatment for nicotine dependence (e.g., U.S. Department of Health and Human Services, 1994b, 1996). An example of a successful treatment protocol is that developed by the National Cancer Institute (NCI), based on a series of clinical trials supported by the NCI in the late 1980s (Glynn & Manley, 1990).

The NCI protocol supports the notion that an effective smoking cessation intervention includes a brief physician intervention supported by office staff using simple procedures that ensure the efficient, systematic treatment of smoking patients at all office visits. The recommended intervention can be described as a self-help program that is encouraged, guided, and supported by physicians, nurses, and support staff.

It is important for both the physician and the patient to realize that smoking cessation is a process that takes place over time, and is not a single event of stopping. Because quitting smoking is a process, it is important for the physician and office staff to maintain continuity, provide a repeated and consistent message, and, most importantly, offer appropriate treatment at every visit.

The treatment of smokers is analogous to the treatment of patients with mild or moderate hypertension—screening is a continuing integral activity done routinely by the office staff at every visit, with physician treatment and follow-up of those identified as having the risk factor and requiring treatment.

The NCI-recommended intervention consists of the four As of clinical activities: Ask, Advise, Assist, Arrange. This intervention plan (Table 13.2) describes a general approach to smoking patients and can be used in almost any outpatient encounter. A typical intervention can be accomplished in a very short period of time, often 3 min or less. Each element of the intervention is described briefly next.

1. *Ask* about smoking at every clinic visit. A nurse or other staff member can easily ask patients "Do you smoke?" or "Are you still smoking?" at each visit, usually while measuring vital signs. Once it is known that a person smokes (or previously smoked), an identifier should be prominently placed on the chart to remind the physician and staff to discuss smoking at each visit.

2. *Advise* all smokers to stop. A clear statement of advice (e.g., "As your physician, I must advise you to stop smoking now") is essential. Many patients do not recall receiving this advice from their physician, so the statement must be easy to understand and memorable. Personalization of the message by referring to the patient's clinical condition, social roles, personal interests, or family history may add to the effectiveness of the advice. What motivates one person to stop smoking might not influence another person at all. Smokers are more motivated to stop if they have specific information about the effects of smoking on their life and the well-being of their family, as well as reinforcement of their personal reasons for stopping.

3. *Assist* the patient in stopping. When a patient is discussing stopping, his or her level of interest in stopping is usually evident. For patients who

TABLE 13.2
Synopsis for Physicians and Dentists:
How to Help Your Patients Stop Smoking

Ask about smoking at every opportunity.
1. "Do you smoke?"
2. "How much?"
3. "How soon after waking do you have your first cigarette?"
4. "Are you interested in stopping smoking?"
5. "Have you ever tried to stop before?" If so, "What happened?"

Advise all smokers to stop.
1. State your advice clearly, for example: "As your physician/dentist I must advise you to stop smoking now."
2. Personalize the message to quit. Refer to the patient's clinical condition, smoking history, family history, personal interests, or social roles.

Assist the patient in stopping.
1. Set a quit date. Help the patient pick a date within the next 4 weeks, acknowledging that no time is ideal.
2. Provide self-help materials. The smoking cessation coordinator or support staff member can review the materials with the patient if desired (call 1-800-4CANCER for NCI's Quit for Good materials).
3. Consider prescribing or recommending a pharmacologic product (e.g., transdermal patch, nicotine nasal spray, bupropion), especially for highly addicted patients (those who smoke one pack a day or more or who smoke their first cigarette with 30 min of waking).
4. Consider signing a stop-smoking contract with the patient.
5. If the patient is not willing to quit now: Provide motivating literature (call 1-800-4CANCER for NCI's Why Do You Smoke? Pamphlet). Ask again at the next visit.

Arrange follow-up visits.
1. Set a follow-up visit within 1 to 2 weeks after the quit date.
2. Have a member of the office staff call or write the patient within 7 days after the initial visit, reinforcing the decision to stop and reminding the patient of the quit date.
3. At the first follow-up visit, ask about the patient's smoking status to provide support and help prevent relapse. Relapse is common; if it happens, encourage the patient to try again immediately.
4. Set a second follow-up visit in 1 to 2 months. For patients who have relapsed, discuss the circumstances of the relapse and other special concerns.

Note. Adapted from Glynn and Manley (1990) and Mecklenburg et al. (1991).

do not want to stop, nagging is rarely of benefit. Physicians must accept the patient's decision, make sure that the patient is making an informed decision, and attempt to maintain the patient's trust and confidence so that smoking can be discussed at future visits.

For patients who express a sincere desire to stop smoking (70% or more of smokers), the physician should help them to pick a specific date for this action. There is evidence that patients who set a "quit date" are more likely to make a serious attempt to stop. This date should be soon (generally within 4 weeks), but not immediately, giving the patient the necessary time to prepare to stop.

Once a patient has selected a specific date to stop, information must be provided so that he or she can prepare for that date. For patients who can read, this is easily done by providing them with a self-help brochure. Effective brochures provide the patient with necessary information about smoking cessation (e.g., symptoms and time course of withdrawal, tips about stopping, good reasons for stopping, answers to common questions). These materials can be obtained from a variety of sources (e.g., American Cancer Society, American Lung Association, National Cancer Institute). Physicians new to the topic of smoking cessation can quickly add to their own knowledge by reading one of these brochures. Office staff can emphasize that the physician wants this material to be read, review the material with the patient, and answer any questions. The patient can then leave the office with a concrete plan for stopping, including a quit date, and information about preparing for that date and successfully stopping.

A number of pharmacologic agents are now available, and approved for use in the treatment of nicotine dependence by the Food and Drug Administration, that have proven useful as adjuncts to smoking cessation advice and counseling. Some of these agents are only available through physician prescription (nicotine nasal spray, bupropion), and others (transdermal nicotine patch, nicotine polacrilex gum) are available over the counter. Physicians should consider prescribing or recommending these products to those patients who are more highly addicted to nicotine.

4. *Arrange* follow-up visits. When patients know their progress will be reviewed, their chances of successfully stopping are improved. This monitoring may include a letter or phone call from the office staff just before the quit date, reinforcing the decision to stop. In addition, clinical trials strongly suggest that a visit with the physician or staff soon after a patient has stopped smoking is extremely important to the patient's ability to to remain a nonsmoker. Merely scheduling the visit may help the patient by providing a short-term goal (e.g., 1 to 2 weeks) that appears more manageable than "forever."

Most relapse occurs in the first weeks after cessation, and a person who comes to the office after stopping smoking for 1 to 2 weeks has a much improved chance of remaining abstinent. Follow-up visits should include an assessment of the patient's progress, discussion of any problems encountered, and discussion of pharmacological therapy if it was prescribed or recommended.

It is important to set up a second follow-up visit with the physician or staff member in 1 to 2 months. Studies show that the quit rate improves as the number of follow-up visits increases (e.g., Wilson, Taylor, Gilbert, & Best, 1988). A space for chart notation provides an easy way to keep informed about the patient's current smoking status and allows continued follow-up and reinforcement to be done, both at specifically scheduled smoking visits and when the patient is seen for other problems.

Following a protocol such as this will prove useful but, importantly, physicians and dentists are also beginning to understand that, although treatment success rates remain relatively low for individual patients, in comparison to treatments for many common illnesses seen in primary care (Glynn & Manley, 1989), they can have a broad public health effect—reducing premature mortality by as much as 20% in the United States—if treatment of nicotine dependence is delivered routinely.

Second, although various clinical guidelines have been available for some time (e.g., Glynn & Manley, 1990; Russell, Wilson, & Taylor, 1979; Schwartz, 1987), a significant step forward was taken in 1996 with the publication of the U.S. Agency for Health Care Policy and Research (AHCPR) Clinical Practice Guideline for Smoking Cessation (U.S. Department of Health and Human Services, 1996). The importance of this guideline lies in the breadth of research, the strength of the evidence, and the consensus-style approach that was employed in its development. Its three primary audiences are primary care clinicians, tobacco cessation specialists, and health care administrators, insurers, and purchasers.

The guideline is consistent with previous guidelines and quite direct in providing advice to primary care clinicians and tobacco cessation specialists:

- Clinicians should ask about and record the tobacco-use status of every patient.
- All smokers should be offered cessation treatment at every office visit.
- Provide treatment even if it is as brief as 3 min, although more intensive treatment is more effective.
- Nicotine replacement therapy, social support, and skills training are the most effective treatment components.
- Schedule follow-up contacts to prevent relapse.

The guideline provides considerably more detail regarding effective treatment techniques. It also strongly supports training for clinicians to improve their cessation treatment skills. The guideline urges that this training be aimed at both clinicans in training and practicing clinicians. For clinicians in training, this could be accomplished by devloping a specific curriculum devoted to tobacco use cessation that would be a part of every medical and dental student's education. For practicing clinicians, training would occur routinely if questions on effective tobacco use cessation techniques were included in licensing and certification exams for all clinical disciplines and if specialty societies adopted a uniform standard of competence in tobacco use cessation treatment for all of their members.

The final enabling factor concerns development of a practice organization conducive to routinely providing tobacco use cessation treatment. Earlier guidelines have emphasized the importance of this issue, recommending, for example, that the office or facility be, without exception, entirely tobacco free; that a coordinator be assigned the task of ensuring that the office/facility tobacco use cessation program be carried out; that systems be established for the identification of all tobacco users; that services be provided for the often-overlooked medically ill smoking patient; and that a series of follow-up contacts be provided to assure success or deal with the problems of relapse. The guideline supports these recommendations and adds the recommendation that individual or group practices and health care systems ensure that clinicians have the knowledge and training to treat tobacco use and that sufficient cessation resources be available to do so.

Reinforcing Factors

These factors include such issues as reimbursement, performance feedback, and peer support.

The absence of reimbursement for treating nicotine dependence is one of the most frequently cited barriers to the provision of this service by clinicians (Henry, Ogle, & Snellman, 1987; Orleans et al., 1989). For this and other preventive and clinical services, however, reimbursement does not appear to be the most important factor in determining whether clinicians offer them to their patients. Economic factors do not, for example, explain the low performance of sigmoidoscopic examinations, which are relatively well compensated (McPhee & Schroeder, 1987). Nevertheless, there are data indicating that physicians perform target preventive services more often when such services are covered by medical insurance (Logsdon, Lazaro, & Meier, 1989; McPhee et al., 1989) and, more specific to tobacco use, there is also evidence suggesting that reimbursing physicians for providing treatment for nicotine dependence decreases tobacco use among their patients (Cox & McKenna, 1990; Hughes et al., 1991). Further, treatment of nicotine dependence is often concomitant with treatment of smoking-related illnesses and events such as emphysema and myocardial infarctions (MIs), and the treatment for nicotine dependence when associated with these conditions should be accorded equal status with primary prevention.

The AHCPR guideline strongly supports reimbursement of clinicans for providing tobacco use cessation services. Specifically, it reommends to health care administrators, insurers, and purchasers that they:

- Reimburse providers for smoking cessation inpatient consultation services.

- Include effective smoking cessation treatments (both pharmacotherapy and counseling) as part of the basic benefits package for all individual, group, and health maintenance organization (HMO) insurance packages.
- Include smoking cessation treatment as a reimbursable activity for fee-for-service providers.
- Inform fee-for-service clinicians that they will be reimbursed for using effective smoking cessation treatments with every patient who uses tobacco.
- Include smoking cessation intervention in the job description and performance evaluation of salaried clinicians.

By following these recommendations, it will be possible to make treatment for smoking cessation a routine and institutionalized preventive and clinical care service.

Although reimbursement is a significant reinforcing factor in the delivery of treatment for tobacco use cessation, feedback from peers and patients on the usefulness and effectiveness of treatment also provides incentive for its delivery. Such feedback can be automatically generated at specific intervals or in response to specific actions, or lack of action, on the part of an individual clinician or an entire group (McDonald, Hui, & Smith, 1984). Although results of studies in which feedback is used to increase preventive practices are mixed, it appears that successful feedback requires prompt delivery and practical, effective suggestions for change or action (Burack & Liang, 1987) and that computer-generated systems of performance evaluation and feedback may be the most useful (McDonald et al., 1984). A review of this area concluded that feedback from colleagues and patients and their support in providing preventive and clinical services are both reinforcing and predisposing to increases in the delivery of such services (Burack & Liang, 1987).

Although many of the predisposing, enabling, and reinforcing factors discussed can now be effectively addressed, even the most significant treatment advances will not have an effect on tobacco use prevalence and public health if they are not able to be delivered to those patients at greatest risk and among whom tobacco use prevalence rates remain high.

IDENTIFYING AND MEETING THE NEEDS OF HARD-TO-REACH, DIFFICULT-TO-TREAT TOBACCO USERS

Tobacco users, as a group, are difficult to treat. As noted throughout this volume, nicotine dependence—classified by the American Psychiatric Association as a psychoactive substance dependence disorder (APA, 1987)—is a complex physiological and psychological condition that requires considerable skill and commitment on the part of the provider, as well as strong motivation on the part of the patient, if treatment is to be successful. Treatment complexity may be increased when the tobacco user is also a member of a special population that, by its members' behavior, social circumstances, ethnic/racial background, or other identifying characteristic, may add to the difficulty any tobacco user encounters when trying to stop.

The most comprehensive statement to date on the treatment of nicotine dependence is, as discussed earlier, contained in the Agency for Health Care Policy Research Clinical Practice Guideline on Smoking Cessation (U.S. Department of Health and Human Services, 1996). The guideline takes particular notice of "special populations" that may need a more focused, tailored approach to the choice, delivery, and efficacy of treatment.

Special populations identified in the guideline include women, racial and ethnic minorities, pregnant smokers, hospitalized smokers, smokers with psychiatric comorbidity, smokeless tobacco users, and children and adolescents. Other groups of tobacco users not cited in the guideline but who have been identified elsewhere as hard to reach and/or difficult to treat include drug abusers (Hurt, Eberman, Slade, & Karan, 1993), alcohol abusers (Hughes, 1990; Hughes, 1995), the un- or underinsured (Freeman, 1991) and those with incomes near or below poverty level (McWhorter, Schatzkin, Horm, & Brown, 1989).

As may be expected in the assessment of a relatively new area of clinical inquiry such as the treatment of nicotine dependence, there is mixed evidence as to the value of specialized treatments for particular populations of tobacco users. As summarized in the guideline and related research, the following describes recommendations to date:

Women. The same smoking cessation treatments appear to be effective for both men and women. Therefore, until additional evidence suggests otherwise, the same treatments can be used for both sexes, when other factors are equal (e.g., Manley, Epps, & Glynn, 1995).

Racial and Ethnic Minorities. Members of racial and ethnic minorities may be provided treatment modalities found effective among majority populations, but, wherever possible, these treatments should be modified or tailored to be appropriate for the ethnic or racial populations with which they are used (Glynn, Boyd, & Gruman, 1990). Data are sparse on the most effective treatments for racial and ethnic minorities; an upcoming U.S. Surgeon General's report on smoking and health plans to address this issue.

Pregnant Smokers. A quintessential example of the "teachable moment," pregnant smokers should be strongly encouraged to stop throughout their pregnancy, for their own health and the health of the fetus. Pregnant smokers may try to hide their tobacco use, making them difficult to treat, but the evidence to date demonstrates that intensive treatments should be offered, and minimal interventions used only if the more intensive treatments are not feasible (Mullen, Ramirez, & Groff, 1994).

Hospitalized Smokers. Because tobacco use can interfere with recovery and cause recurrences, all smokers who are hospitalized should have their tobacco use status documented at admission and discharge, should be assisted with quitting during hospitalization, and should be provided with advice and assistance on how to remain abstinent after discharge (Hurt, Lauger, & Offord, 1992; Stevens, Glasgow, Hollis, Lichtenstein, & Vogt, 1993).

Smokers With Psychiatric Comorbidity. There is a growing literature and body of clinical experience that suggests a strong interaction between tobacco use and psychiatric symptoms (Glassman, 1993; Glassman et al., 1993). Therefore, although not essential, it may be helpful to assess for psychiatric comorbidity prior to smoking cessation treatment. Such assessment may prepare the clinician for an increased posibility of tobacco use relapse or for worsening of the comorbid condition in response to nicotine withdrawal.

Smokeless Tobacco Users. There is little research on the effectiveness of treatments for smokeless tobacco use cessation. The current recommendation, therefore, is that clinicians should treat smokeless tobacco users with the same cessation interventions that are effective with smokers, until further evidence becomes available (Severson, 1993).

Children and Adolescents. As with smokeless tobacco use, there is little research on the most effective methods to treat youthful smokers. Therefore, the current recommendation for clinicians, when dealing with an under-18 smoker, is to consider using the same cessation interventions which have proven effective with adults (U.S. Department of Health and Human Services, 1994a). The most important message from clinicans for children and youth and their parents, of course, remains one of abstaining from any tobacco use and following previous guidelines for preventive action (U.S. Department of Health and Human Services, 1994b; Lynch & Bonnie, 1994).

Drug- and Alcohol-Abusing Smokers. In the absence of a significant body of clinical research about treating nicotine dependence in the context of drug and/or alcohol abuse, it appears that, once a smoking patient is screened for such use, standard treatment for smoking cessation may be used with these populations, given several caveats. These caveats include first determining the patient's interest in stopping smoking at all, the patient's interest in treating the drug/alcohol problem first or at the same time as the nicotine dependence, and closely monitoring the patient's recovery to ensure that smoking cessation does not threaten to trigger a relapse to drug/alcohol use (Hughes, 1993).

Underinsured, Low-Income Smokers. Tobacco use, although spread through all strata of our society, is becoming increasingly concentrated among the stratum with the lowest income. This group is also, and not surprisingly, likely to be among the 20–25% of the U.S. population that is uninsured or seriously underinsured, thus preventing its members from reaping the benefits of the treatment advances just outlined (Freeman, 1991). This group presents the greatest challenge to clinicians—because its members are large in number, because they are hard to reach due to their lack of access to the preventive and clinical care that should come with insurance coverage, and because they are difficult to treat due to what often may be only mild interest in cessation, their strong dependence on nicotine, and their inability to regularly purchase the nicotine replacement products that can aid in the cessation process.

Identifying and then reaching and effectively treating the special populations just discussed will remain for some time a significant challenge for clinicians involved in tobacco use cessation. As the most obvious barriers to doing so fall—such as research resulting in new, targeted treatments, changing attitudes about the importance of tobacco use cessation, and increasing the breadth of insurance coverage for preventive services—the goal of a tobacco-free society will be more readily achieved.

CONCLUSIONS

Significant and often sweeping changes have occurred over the past decade that have greatly increased the ability of clinicians, especially physicians and dentists, to effectively treat their patients who use tobacco. These changes include more widely held and negative attitudes toward tobacco use, an increased acceptance of the role of the clinician in treating nicotine dependence, availability of clinical trial evidence demonstrating that clinicians can effectively treat nicotine dependence, the approval of several pharmacological agents that can increase the effectiveness of clinician treatment for nicotine dependence, the development of practice models that can make the delivery of smoking cessation treatment (and other preventive services) easier and more cost-effective, and the development of a consensus practice guideline that provides specific details to clinicians for use in their treatment of patients who use tobacco.

Nevertheless, numerous other changes, advances, and actions are needed if we expect clinicians to be able to routinely provide effective treatment for all of their tobacco using patients. These include practical training in the treatment of nicotine dependence at both the undergraduate medical level and for practicing clinicians, and novel means of reaching and treating the special populations who remain at greatest risk for premature death and illness from their tobacco use. A national commitment will be required to support the research and policy change necessary to reach these goals.

Physicians, dentists, and tobacco use cessation specialists remain on the front line in the treatment of nicotine dependence. They now have specific guidelines for provision of that treatment, pharmacologic agents to increase the effectiveness of the treatment they provide, and greater patient desire to receive treatment for their nicotine dependence. The next steps involve universal training for proper treatment delivery, reimbursement for clinicians' efforts to do so, and provision of insurance coverage for those tobacco users most in need. We have made progress in moving toward a tobacco-free society, and taking these next steps in making it easier for clinicians to deliver effective treatment for nicotine dependence, and for patients to receive it, will bring us even closer.

REFERENCES

American Psychiatric Association. (1987). *Diagnostic and statistical manual of mental disorders* (3rd ed.). Chicago: Author.

Burack, R. C., & Liang, J. (1987). The early detection of cancer in the primary care setting: Factors associated with the acceptance and completion of recommended procedures. *Preventive Medicine, 16,* 739–751.

Cox, J. L., & McKenna, J. P. (1990). Nicotine gum: Does providing it free in a smoking cessation program alter success rates? *Journal of Family Practice, 31*(3), 278–280.

Fiore, M. C., & Baker, T. B. (1995). Smoking cessation treatment and the good doctor club [editorial]. *American Journal of Public Health, 85*(2), 161–163.

Freeman, H. (1991). Race, poverty, and cancer. *Journal of the National Cancer Institute, 83,* 526–527.

Glanz, K., & Rimar, B. K. (1996). *Theory at a glance: A guide for health promotion practice.* NIH Publication No. 95–3896. Bethesda, MD: National Institute of Health.

Glassman, A. H. (1993). Cigarette smoking: Implication for psychiatric illness. *American Journal of Psychiatry, 150,* 546–553.

Glassman, A. H., Covey, L. S., Dalack, G. W., Stetner, F., Rivelli, S. K., Fleiss, J., & Cooper, T. B. (1993). Smoking cessation, clonidine, and vulnerability to nicotine among dependent smokers. *Clinical Pharmacology Therapy, 54,* 670–679.

Glynn, T. J., Boyd, G. M., & Gruman, J. C. (1990). Essential elements of self-help/minimal intervention strategies for smoking cessation. *Health Education Quarterly, 17,* 329–345.

Glynn, T. J., & Manley, M. W. (1989). Physician, cancer control and the treatment of nicotine dependence: Defining success. *Health Education Research, 4,* 479–487.

Glynn, T. J., & Manley, M. W. (1990). *How to help your patients stop smoking: A National Cancer Institute manual for physicians* (NIH Publ. No. 90-3064). Bethesda, MD: U.S. Department of Health and Human Services, Public Health Service, National Institutes of Health, National Cancer Institute.

Green, L. W., & Kreuter, M. W. (1991). *Health promotion planning: An educational and environmental approach* (2nd ed.). Mountain View, CA: Mayfield.

Henry, R. C., Ogle, K. S., & Snellman, L. A. (1987). Preventive medicine: Physician practices, beliefs, and perceived barriers for implementation. *Family Medicine, 19*(2), 110–113.

Hughes, J. R. (1990). Treating smokers with current or past alcohol dependence. *American Journal of Health Behavior, 20,* 286–290.

Hughes, J. R. (1993). Treatment of smoking cessation in smokers with past alcohol/drug problems. *Journal of Substance Abuse Treatment, 10,* 181–187.

Hughes, J. R. (1995). Treatment implications and outcome. In J. Fertig, A. Abrams, O. Pomerleau, & L. Sobell (Eds.), *Alcohol and tobacco: From basic science to policy,* NIAA Monograph No. 30, pp. 171–185. Rockville, MD: National Institute of Alcohol Abuse & Alcoholism.

Hughes, J. R., Wadland, W. C., Fenwick, J. W., Lewis J., & Bickel, W. K. (1991). Effect of cost on the self-administration and efficacy of nicotine gum: A preliminary study. *Preventive Medicine, 20,* 186–196.

Hurt, R. D., Lauger, G. G., Offord, K. P., Bruce, B. K., & Dale, L. C. (1992). An integrated approach to the treatment of nicotine dependence in a medical center setting. *Clinical Proceedings, 67,* 823–828.

Hurt, R. D., Lauger, G. G., Offord, K. P., Bruce, B. K., Dale, L. C., McClain, F. L., & Eberman, K. M. (1992). An integrated approach to the treatment of nicotine dependence in a medical center setting: Description of the initial experience. *Journal of General Internal Medicine, 7,* 114–116.

Hurt, R. D., Eberman, K. M., Slade, J., & Karan, L. (1993). Treating nicotine addiction in patients with other addictive disorders. In C. T. Orleans & J. Slade (Eds.), *Nicotine addiction: Principles and management* (pp. 310–326). New York: Oxford University Press.

Lindsay, E. A., Ocuene, J. K., Hymowitz, N., Giffen, C., Berger, L., & Pomrehn, P. (1994). Physicians and smoking cessation: A survey of office procedures and practices in the Community Intervention trial for Smoking Cessation. *Archives of Family Medicine, 4,* 341–348.

Logsdon, D. N., Lazaro, C. M., & Meier, R. V. (1989). The feasibility of behavioral risk reduction in primary care. *American Journal Preventive Medicine, 5,* 249–256.

Lynch, B. S., & Bonnie, R. J. (1994). *Growing up tobacco free: Preventing nicotine addiction in children and youths.* Washington, DC: National Academy Press.

Manley, M. W., Epps, R. P., & Glynn, T. J. (1995). Smoking cessation. In V. L. Seltzer & W. H. Pearse (Eds.), *Women's primary health care: Office practice and procedures* (pp. 95–100). New York: McGraw-Hill.

McDonald, C. J., Hui, S., & Smith, D. M. (1984). Reminders to physicians from an introspective computer medical record system: A two-year randomized trial. *Annals of Internal Medicine, 100,* 130–138.

McPhee, S. J., Bird, J. A., Jenkins, C. N. H., & Fordham, D. (1989). Promoting cancer screening: A randomized, controlled trial of three interventions. *Archives of Internal Medicine, 149,* 1866–1872.

McWhorter, W. P., Schatzkin, A. G., Horm, J. W., & Brown, C. C. (1988). Contribution of socioeconomic status to Black/White differences in cancer incidence. *Cancer, 63,* 982–987.

Mecklenburg, R. E., Christen, A. G., Gerbert, B., Gift, H. C., Glynn, T. J., Jones, R. B., Lindsay, E., Manley, M. W., & Severson, H. (1991). *How to help your patients stop using tobacco: A National Cancer Institute Manual for the oral health team.* Bethesda, MD: National Institutes of Health.

Mullen, P. D., Ramirez, G., & Groff, J. Y. (1994). A meta-analysis of randomized trials of prenatal smoking cessation interventions. *American Journal of Obstetrics and Gynecology, 171,* 1328–1334.

National Committee for Quality Assurance. (1996). *Health plan employer data & information set.* Washington, DC: Author.

Nelson, D. E., Emont, S. L., Brackbill, R. M., Cameron, L. L., Peddicord, J., & Fiore, M. C. (1994). Cigarette smoking prevalence by occupation in the United States. *Journal of Medicine, 36*(5), 516–525.

Orleans, C. T., George, L. K., Houpt, J. L., & Brodie, K. H. (1985). Health promotion in primary care: A survey of US family practitioners. *Preventive Medicine, 14*, 636–647.

Orleans, C. T., Shoenbach, V. J., Salmon, M. A., Strecher, V. J., Kalsbeek, W., Quade, D., Brooks, E. F., Konrad, T. R., Blackmon, C., & Watts, C. D. (1989). A survey of smoking and quitting patterns among black Americans. *American Journal of Public Health, 79*, 176–181.

Orleans, C. T., & Slade, J. (Eds.). (1993). *Nicotine addiction: Principles and management.* New York: Oxford University Press.

Richmond, R. (Ed.). (1994). *Interventions for smokers: An international perspective.* Baltimore, MD: Williams & Wilkins.

Russell, M. A. H., Wilson, C., & Taylor, C. (1979). The effect of general practitioners' advice against smoking. *British Medical Journal, 2*, 231–235.

Schwartz, J. (1987). *Review and evaluation of smoking cessation methods: The United States and Canada: 1978–1985* (NIH Publication No. 87-2940). Bethesda, MD: U.S. Department of Health and Human Services, Public Health Service, National Institutes of Health.

Severson, H. H. (1993). Smokeless tobacco: Risks, epidemiology, and cessation. In C. T. Orleans & J. Slade (Eds.), *Nicotine addiction: Principles and management* (pp. 262–278). New York Oxford University Press.

Stevens, V. J., Glasgow, R. E., Hollis, J. F., Lichtenstein, E., & Vogt, T. M. (1993). A smoking-cessation intervention for hospital patients. *Medical Care, 31*(1), 65–72.

U.S. Department of Health and Human Services. (1994a). *Preventing tobacco use among young people: A report of the Surgeon General.* Atlanta, GA: Centers for Disease Control and Prevention.

U.S. Department of Health and Human Services. (1994b). *Tobacco and the clinician: Interventions for medical and dental practice* (NIH Publication No. 94-3693). Bethesda, MD: Author.

U.S. Department of Health and Human Services. (1996). *Clinical practice guideline: Smoking cessation* (AHCPR Publication No. 96-0692). Rockville, MD: Author.

Wiggers, J. H., & Sanson-Fisher, R. (1994). General practitioners as agents of health risk behavior change: Opportunities for behavioral science in patient smoking cessation. *Behaviour Change, 11*(3), 167–176.

Wilson, D. M., Taylor, D. W., Gilbert, J. R., & Best, J. A. (1988). Randomized trial of a family physician intervention for smoking cessation. *JAMA, 260*, 1570–1574.

CHAPTER FOURTEEN

The Role of the Dental Profession in Tobacco Cessation

Lynn M. Tepper
Daniel F. Seidman
Columbia University

It is well known by both the public and the health care professions that smoking tobacco causes lung cancer, pulmonary disease, and other serious conditions that ultimately reduce one's quality of life. Diseases of the oral cavity, such as leukoplakia, oral cancer, and periodontal diseases, are also associated with tobacco use; although this fact is less often recognized by the general public as well as practicing physicians, it can provide a valuable opportunity for intervention by the dental profession throughout the life cycle. One approach for prevention recommended by the National Cancer Institute is for dentists to advise youth not to start using tobacco, and to advise those in their care to quit (Moss, Allen, Giovino, & Mills, 1992). Advice from health professionals has been shown to be a powerful influence on patient decisions to stop or not begin using tobacco in the first place. The dental profession is in a unique position to influence the population because dentists and dental hygienists regularly see patients who are younger and healthier than primary care physicians and other health professionals.

The Mouth Is the Window to the Body. Tobacco-induced changes in the mouth can provide an excellent teachable moment in younger as well as older persons to encourage them to stop using tobacco. If changes associated with smoking can be readily shown by holding a mirror to the patient's mouth, these changes can then help focus the patient on the impact of smoking, which goes unseen and undetected throughout the rest of their body. Tobacco-induced changes in the mouth are often overlooked by primary care physicians, who tend to focus on routine medical examinations that often do not include the oral cavity. This may stem from their limited training in this area or from the assumption that their patients already receive regular dental care.

Recent initiatives in dental education have created new competencies for the dentist. Dental education in the last 20 years has expanded to include a more comprehensive knowledge of the behavioral, clinical, and basic biomedical sciences. Dentists as an important part of the health care team are expected to enhance and promote the total health of patients through oral health management. Behavioral skills, now considered a critical element in the practice of dentistry, can also help the dentist to address tobacco addiction when identified in their practice. A discussion about the present and future personal risks of tobacco's effects on thousands of other individuals does not mean as much to the patient as showing what is happening to the patient at the present moment, while a "captive audience" in their dental chair. Although dentists may occasionally refer patients to dental specialists for appropriate treatment, in the past they have not necessarily been prompted by training to make appropriate referrals to tobacco cessation specialists, or to offer their patients brief motivational tobacco cessation counseling when these conditions are diagnosed. This chapter discusses appropriate treatment protocols to help dentists provide brief interventions to their patients and refer them when necessary.

TOBACCO-INDUCED CHANGES IN THE MOUTH

Tobacco-induced changes in the mouth are readily apparent to the dentist who is trained to detect both undesirable cosmetic and potentially life-threatening oral conditions that are the result of tobacco use. Tobacco use results in numerous oral conditions.

The risk for particular oral diseases and conditions varies with the particular type of tobacco used and the form in which it is used, such as chewing tobacco, cigarettes, pipes, cigars, or snuff. The frequency and duration of the use of the tobacco product also contributes to the pattern and the severity of clinical presentation (U.S. Department of Health and Human Services, 1992). We divide tobacco-induced conditions into two categories, life-threatening and non-life-threatening, and recommend appropriate treatment protocols.

Life-Threatening Oral Changes

Oral Cancer. This condition involves lesions of the oral cavity, including the soft tissue linings of cheeks and lips, the tongue, the floor of the mouth, the gums, and the bony structure of the maxilla and the mandible. Although the number of smokers has diminished since the 1960's, the remaining smokers appear to be the heavier users, and therefore the effects on the mouth among this group may be even greater than the typical effects noted in the past. Although smoking tobacco is clearly associated with the development of oral squamous-cell carcinoma, about 9 out of 10 current smokers reported that they had not been screened for oral cancer in a 1992 study (Martin, Bouquot, Wingo, & Heath, 1997). The proportion of smokers (80%) among patients with oral cancer is two to three times greater than that in the general population (Neville, Damm, Allen, & Bouquot, 1995). The risk for a second primary cancer of the upper aerodigestive tract is two to six times greater for treated patients with oral cancer who continue to smoke than for those that stop smoking after diagnosis (Blott, 1988).

Smokeless tobacco users in Western cultures are at a similar risk compared with cigarette smokers for oral cancer. The use of smokeless tobacco has been shown to increase a chronic user's risk for oral cancer by a factor of four (Mattson & Winn, 1989). Various studies have suggested that the incidence of oral cancer among smokers varies from 2 to 18 times that of never smokers, with a median fourfold increased risk (U.S. Department of Health and Human Services, 1990). Regular use of alcohol increases the risk for oral cancer considerably, as smoking and alcohol work synergistically (Choi & Kahyo, 1991). The diagnosis of oral cancer, considered the most serious of oral conditions, should prompt the dentist to make an appropriate referral to a psychologist or psychiatrist specializing in tobacco cessation.

Leukoplakia. Leukoplakia is a white patch or plaque on the oral mucosa that cannot be wiped off and that cannot be classified clinically or pathologically as any other disease. It occurs six times more frequently in smokers than in nonsmokers, and may be regarded as a precancer. Although there are other factors, tobacco use is the most identifiable. Since this is also a very serious condition, appropriate referral to tobacco cessation experts is essential.

Referral Strategies. Studies have shown that referring smokers for help can result in a very low rate of follow-through (Lichtenstein & Hollis, 1992). When it comes to seeking treatment, smokers can be avoidant and resistant. In a study of three general population samples, approximately 40% of smokers are not thinking about stopping—that is, they are in the precontemplation stage. (Velicer et al., 1995). Approximately another 40% are ambivalent about quitting, and about 20% intend to quit in the near future (within a few months). Another way to look at the precontemplation group, especially when already seriously ill, is that they are in psychological denial and do not want to acknowledge their own negative feelings about being addicted. The clinician must recognize and respect the patient's wishes and psychological defenses.

Strategies for a patient who does not want to stop include providing written material to read and discuss at the next visit. Showing changes in the oral cavity that are induced by smoking, especially in very ill patients, can also help counter patients' denial and rationalization about their addiction to tobacco. The dentist can also suggest that although these changes are visible, other smoking-induced changes throughout the body may go undetected. Another important strategy for already ill patients is to suggest that they go for "just one visit" to a specialist or specialty clinic, which may be less frightening to them. Once they go for a visit, they may overcome at least some of the great fear that many smokers have about seeking help for this problem. It is usually good to give them a specific name, to know the clinician or clinic and be able to recommend it with a measure of confidence. It is important to avoid scare tactics, as this practice is more likely to produce anger and guilt in patients than to help them change deeply ingrained behaviors. Another strategy is to encourage patients to talk about their ambivalent feelings about smoking, the good as well as the bad. The dentist then supports the part of the patient that wishes not to be a smoker. The dentist can employ such statements as, "we now have tools available, both medical and psychological, to help you stop smoking," and "it's really not just a matter of being weak or strong when you are addicted to a drug." These referral strategies can also be employed when treating a patient with the non-life-threatening conditions described next, if the clinician has neither the time nor the inclination to provide the patient with structured psychological support.

Non-Life-Threatening Oral Conditions

The following conditions present more esthetic but less medically serious problems for users of tobacco products. When patients present with these conditions, the dentist may choose to treat their nicotine dependence by using brief, motivational interventions.

Snuff Dipper's Pouch. Snuff dipper's pouch is a white or white–red adherent lesion that is found in many smokeless tobacco users. Some oral pathologists classify it as a form of leukoplakia, and others classify it separately, referring to it as tobacco pouch keratosis (Neville et al., 1995). Most of these lesions will regress and some will disappear when the use of smokeless tobacco is discontinued (U.S. Department of Health and Human Services, 1986). Inflamatory conditions take time to regress after tobacco use ceases. Significantly, habit cessation almost always leads to a normal mucosal appearance withn 1 to 2 weeks (Neville et al., 1995).

Smoker's Palate. Also known as nicotinic stomatitis, this appears as a diffuse palatal keratosis with chronic inflammation of the palatal salivary glands. It is most often seen in pipe and cigar smokers. Nicotinic stomatitis does not appear to have a significant precancerous potential as compared with the palatal lesions produced by reverse smoking (the burning end is held in the mouth) as practiced in some regions such as the Caribbean and India (Reddy et al., 1974). This condition is completely reversible, as the palate returns to normal after 1 to 2 weeks of tobacco cessation (Neville et al., 1995).

Smokers Melanosis. Also called gingival melanosis, this is a melanin pigmentation that may occur in the attached gingiva of about 5–10% of smokers. This is more of an aesthetic problem than a life-threatening condition (Hedin, 1986). Cessation of smoking results in a gradual disappearance of the areas of related oral pigmentation conditions over a 3-year period (Neville et al., 1995).

Smoker's Lip. This is a burn from smoking unfiltered cigarettes down to the very end. It may occur when smoking under the influence of alcohol, drugs, or when the smoker is heavily sedated (Berry & Landwerlen, 1973).

Tooth Loss. Tooth loss is more common among tobacco users than nonusers in any age and gender cohort. In one study, tobacco users had 67% greater tooth loss than nonusers (Alquist, Bengtsson, Hollender, Lapidus, & Osterberg, 1989).

Tobacco Stains. Tobacco stains can penetrate into enamel and restorative materials, creating brown to yellow darkening of teeth, discoloration of nonmetallic restorations, and dark outlining around restoration margins (Christin, McDonald, & Klein, 1988). This condition can be most aesthetically displeasing and distracting, but is reversible after cessation either with regular oral phrophlaxis or crown bleaching.

Tooth Abrasion. This may result from extensive use of a pipe producing notches or wear patterns on the biting edge of teeth where the stem is habitually positioned (Christen et al., 1988). Discontinuation of pipe use stops abrasion, and cosmetic dentistry can restore worn surfaces.

Periodontal Disease. This includes all diseases and adverse conditions related to the supporting structures of the teeth. Destructive periodontitis in one study was 2½ to 3 times greater among smokers than nonsmokers at all ages and among both sexes (Bergstrom, 1986). Smokers have noticeably increased levels of pocketing, gum recession, bone loss, loss of attachment, and dental calculus and are more likely to be affected by acute necrotizing and ulcerative gingivitis (Palmer, 1987). Smoking impairs periodontal healing, but smoking cessation has been found to restore the normal periodontal healing response (Grossi et al., 1997).

Other Tobacco-Associated Oral Conditions

The following conditions are not necessarily primarily caused by tobacco use, but cigarette smoking is implicated in their etiology.

Gingival Bleeding. Gingival bleeding is less common in smokers than nonsmokers with similar hygiene practices. Impaired gingival bleeding may delay recognition of symptoms that would signal the development of periodontal disease (Kowolik & Nishet, 1983).

Dental Calculus. Calculus buildup is more common and extensive among smokers than nonsmokers (U.S. Department of Health and Human Services, 1992). Build-up slows down with discontinued use of tobacco.

Halitosis. Halitosis (bad breath) is one of the most commonly recognized noxious conditions associated with tobacco use. It usually regresses with discontinued tobacco use. There have been several conditions that have been discussed in the literature for which evidence of causal or closely related association with tobacco use is less strong, for which further investigation is recommended. These conditions include dental caries, dental plaque, lichen planus, oral clefts, reduced salivary flow, and diminished taste and smell.

These tobacco-induced, tobacco-related, and tobacco-aggravated oral conditions are certainly cause for concern, as they reflect the deleterious effect that tobacco use is having on the rest of the patient's body, which cannot be identified as graphically on examination as the oral cavity. Dentists should be able to recognize all common tobacco-related conditions so that the conditions can be discussed with or shown to patients as incentives to patients to discontinue their use of tobacco. "The mouth as the window to the body" concept places the dentist in an especially good position to promote tobacco cessation, and the opportunity must be seized!

INTEGRATION OF SMOKING CESSATION INTO DENTAL PRACTICE

The practice of dentistry emphasizes the key ingredients for tobacco cessation. The rationale for integrating smoking cessation is that the dentist is the public health practitioner who promotes prevention in oral health. Addressing smoking cessation fits well into this tradition in dentistry. The extremely addictive nature of nicotine prevents most people from quitting for good. People need to know that nicotine is found in all forms of tobacco, is highly addictive, can harm them, and can rob them of relationships and experiences that are important to them. More than 80% of tobacco-using dental patients want to stop (World Health Organization, 1980). Understanding that nicotine addiction holds together a chain of complex psychological and social factors that support its use is essential for the dentist as well as the patient to recognize and to understand. Some people can stop on their own, but many more need encouragement and guidance. Hard-core smokers need to be identified and referred for comprehensive treatment appropriate to the severity of their addictive illness.

A multifaceted approach is often the most effective approach. Helping patients to quit for good requires attention to their psychological and social dependence on nicotine in addition to the consideration of using pharmacotherapy such as a nicotine replacement product (gum, patch, spray or inhaler) to relieve the physical dependence until the craving subsides (see also treatment-related chapters of this volume).

Tobacco cessation courses are not common in dental education, but an increasing number of dental schools are including smoking cessation training in their curricula. For example, Columbia University School of Dental and Oral Surgery began required training in tobacco cessation in 1996, and offers a tobacco cessation clinic, staffed by attending psychologists, psychiatrists, dentists, and oral surgeons, for all patients at the medical center. Continuing education in dentistry should provide dental practitioners with tobacco cessation training to apply brief, motivational interventions for appropriate patients. It is also important to advise practitioners to identify appropriately trained specialists in treating hard-core smokers, such as psychologists and psychiatrists in their communities to whom they can make referrals. Together they can coordinate care for their more seriously ill patients in a team effort.

The Effectiveness of the Oral Health Team for Helping Smokers

Recent National Cancer Institute research has shown that the oral health team can be extremely effective in helping patients stop using tobacco. Studies have been done in private practice, dental schools, hospitals, and community health settings that show that brief interventions using a systematic approach to helping patients are the most effective (U.S. Department of Health and Human Services, 1992). Clinical research has shown that the oral health team can double, triple, or quadruple patient cessation rates by routinely using simple, brief intervention services. If 75% of oral health teams routinely helped patients and about 28 patients per team would stop, nearly

3 million additional ex-users would be added to the population each year (World Health Organization, 1980). A small but routine effort over years would help hundreds of patients in each practice. It is important for the oral health team to treat tobacco use prevention and cessation as a brief, routine activity during every office visit. It is also important to reinforce abstinence both in children and youth and in already addicted smokers who have quit.

Four steps recommended for brief, structured tobacco cessation intervention are described in more detail by Glynn and colleagues in chapter 13 of this volume. They are: asking the patient about tobacco use when they arrive for their first appointment each year; advising the patient to stop using tobacco by making such statements as, "As your dentist I am concerned about your oral and general health. I advise you to stop using tobacco"; assisting the patient in stopping by using a brief motivational intervention or referring to a tobacco cessation specialist when serious illness is diagnosed; and arranging patient follow-up services using the clinic recall system on a weekly, then monthly basis to reinforce success or assisting in establishing a new quit date. Clinical studies show that all four components, used routinely, result in much higher patient quit rates than if only two or three are used (U.S. Department of Health and Human Services, 1993).

The Dentist–Patient Relationship

From a behavioral health perspective, patient adherence with health recommendations involves the development of behavior that promotes optimal oral health through the identification and elimination of maladaptive behavior (smoking) and the implementation of positive behaviors (stopping smoking). Strategies can be used to help patients adhere to preventive and treatment regimens. Dental education now supports the notion that the patient is expected to share the responsibility for his or her own health, and a dentist–patient relationship that is both positive and supportive promotes that concept. Dentists' recommendations are most likely to be implemented by their patients if they (a) provide relevant information for developing appropriate health beliefs and attitudes, and (b) are active in helping their patients develop effective self-management strategies. The range of intervention is vast, from teaching basic oral hygiene habits such as flossing techniques, to helping the patient eliminate health habits that are life-threatening, such as tobacco use. Communication skills that promote behavior change include using language that is tailored to suit the individual patient, such as avoiding medical jargon that often results in lack of comprehension, repeating the message to enhance recall, allowing the patient time for formulating questions, allowing sufficient time for questions, thereby avoiding misunderstandings caused by not checking for comprehension, and providing key pieces of information early in the presentation, rather than tacking them onto the end of a clinical session (Geboy, 1986). Written information such as pamphlets, articles, and instruction sheets have the advantage of allowing the patient to process the material at his or her own pace, and emphasizing the importance of the information. Evidence clearly suggests that if the dentist is able to communicate sensitivity and caring, cooperation can be increased (Hornsby, Denneen, & Heid, 1985). The effective use of language, both verbal and nonverbal, not only insures that information is conveyed, but it is an instrument for emotional and attitudinal expression that can be used to influence patient behavior (Tepper, 1996). Providing effective feedback and supportive language will encourage patients to practice health behaviors that the dentist has recommended. The ability to listen effectively is perhaps the most undervalued of all communication skills, but is an essential component of a dentist's interpersonal skills. It assists in the establishment of rapport, and facilitates the acquisition of information about the patient and his health practices. The patient is more likely to develop trust and a cooperative attitude (Geboy, 1986).

SUMMARY

The process of stopping tobacco use takes time. Successful intervention is converting a contented user into a person who believes he or she should stop. Successful intervention is converting a dream of stopping some day to a decision to stop on a specific date. Successful intervention is helping a person through the quitting process, especially during the first critical weeks. People progressing through these steps need reinforcing messages in many environments. The dental office is one of many environments that can support these characteristics of successful smoking cessation practice, and influence patients and the public to avoid and discontinue the use of tobacco.

REFERENCES

Ahlquist, M., Bengtsson, C., Hollender, L., Lapidus, L., & Osterberg, T. (1989). Smoking habits and tooth loss in Swedish women. *Community Dentistry and Oral Epidemiology, 17,* 144–147.

Bergstrom, J. (1986). *Cigarette smoking as a risk factor of using smokeless tobacco* (NIH Publication No. 86-2874, pp. 123–131). Bethesda, MD: National Institutes of Health.

Berry, H. H., & Landwerlen, J. R. (1973). Cigarette smoker's lip lesion in psychiatric patients. *Journal of the American Dental Association, 86*(3), 657–662.

Blott, W. J. (1988). Smoking and drinking in relation to oral and pharyngeal cancer. *Cancer Research, 48,* 3282–3287.

Choi, J. K., & Kahyo, H. (1991). The effect of cigarette smoking and alcohol consumption on the etiology of cancer of the oral cavity, pharynx, and larynx. *International Journal of Epidemiology, 20,* 878–885.

Christin, A. G., McDonald, J. L., & Klein, J. A. (1988). A smoking cessation program for the dental office. *Indiana University School of Dentistry.*

Geboy, M. J. (1986). *Communication and behavior management in dentistry.* Baltimore, MD: Williams & Wilkins.

Grossi, S. G., Zambon, J. J., Machtei, E. E., Schifferle, R., Andreana, S., Genco, R. J., Cummins, D., & Harrap, G. (1997). The effects of smoking and smoking cessation on healing after mechanical periodontal therapy. *Journal of the American Dental Association, 128,* 599–607.

Hedin, C. A. (1986). Smoker's melanosis. *Academy Regia Odontologica, 51,* 62.

Hornsby, J. L., Denneen, L. J., & Heid, D. W. (1985). Interpersonal communication skills development: A model for dentistry. *Journal of Dental Education, 39,* 728–732.

Kowolik, M. J., & Nisbet, T. (1983). Smoking and acute ulcerative gingivitis. *British Dental Journal, 154,* 241–242.

Lichtenstein, E., & Hollis, J. F. (1992). Patient referral to a smoking cessation program: Who follows through? *Journal of Family Practice, 34*(6), 739–744.

Martin, L. M., Bouquot, J. E., Wingo, P. A., & Heath, C. W., Jr. (1997). Cancer prevention in the dental practice: Oral cancer screening and tobacco cessation advice. *Journal of Public Health Dentistry, 56,* 336–340.

Mattson, M. E., & Winn, D. M. (1989). Smokeless tobacco: Association with increased cancer risk. *NCI Monograph, 8,* 13–16.

Moss, A. J., Allen, K. F., Giovino, G. A., & Mills, S. L. (1992). Recent trends in adolescent smoking, smoking uptake correlates, and expectations about the future. *Advances in Data, Vital Health Statistics,* December 2, 221.

Neville, B. W., Damm, D. D., Allen, C. M., & Bouquot, J. E. (1995). *Oral and maxillofacial pathology.* Philadelphia: W. B. Saunders.

Palmer, R. M. (1987, November). Tobacco smoking and oral health. *Health Education Authority.* Occasional Paper No. 6.

Reddy, C. R. M. M., Raju, M. V. S, Sundareshwar, B., Ram Murthy, B., Sastry, P., & Narasinham, V. (1974). Palatal epithelial changes in reverse smokers having carcinoma of hard palate. *Indian Journal of Medical Research, 62,* 195–198.

Tepper, L. M. (1996). *Introduction to the patient.* New York: Columbia University Press.

U.S. Department of Health and Human Services. (1986). *The health consequences of using smokeless tobacco* (NIH Publication No. 86-2874, p. 112). Bethesda, MD: Author.

U.S. Department of Health and Human Services. (1990). *The health benefits of smoking cessation* (DHHS Publication No. CDC 90-8416, pp. 147–152). Rockville, MD: Author.

U.S. Department of Health and Human Services, National Institutes of Health, National Cancer Institute. (1992). *Tobacco effects in the mouth* (NIH Publication No. 92-3330, pp. 5–13). Rockville, MD: Author.

U.S. Department of Health and Human Services, Public Health Service, National Institutes of Health. (1993). *How to help your patients be tobacco-free* (NIH Publication No. 93-3161, p. 118). Bethesda, MD: Author.

Velicer, W. F., Fava, J. L., Prochaska, J. O., Abrams, D. B., Emmons, K. M., & Pierce, J. P. (1995). Distribution of smokers by stage in three representative samples. *Preventive Medicine, 24,* 401–411.

World Health Organization. (1980). Guide to epidemiology and diagnosis of the oral mucosal diseases and conditions. *Community Dentistry and Oral Epidemiology, 8,* 1–26.

CHAPTER FIFTEEN

Afterword: The Public Health Perspective: Have Hard-Core Smokers Been Written Off?

Cheryl Healton
Columbia School of Public Health

The preceding chapters set forth the treatment approaches for the hard-core smoker with particular attention to special populations, comorbidities, and areas of current debate (e.g., the role and effectiveness of nicotine replacement therapy). These recommendations for clinicians and indeed for smokers themselves must be accompanied by public policy decisions that will determine access to and shape health care reimbursement for smoking cessation programs, support treatment research to improve cessation effectiveness, and define the most effective secondary preventive interventions for former and current smokers. All of these public health decisions require special consideration for chronic hard-core smokers.

At the present time approximately one in four Americans smoke. Though in the years since the 1964 U.S. Surgeon General's report on smoking the proportion who smoke has fallen from 40% in 1965 to 27% today, the rate of cessation has leveled off, and many of the remaining smokers have a long-term addiction to nicotine (Janofsky, 1993). The U.S. Public Health Service has embraced the laudable goal for the year 2000 of reducing by 7% to 15% the percentage of Americans age 20 and older who smoke (U.S. Department of Health and Human Services, 1990). In its final report, the Advisory Committee on Tobacco Policy and Public Health (Kessler and Koop, Co-chairs) proposed a minimum reduction in children and adolescent smoking of 65% during the next decade (Kessler & Koop, 1997). The important public health goals embodied in these two recommendations, however, can only be achieved through a combination of primary and secondary prevention approaches (i.e., sharply reducing the number who start smoking and the number of those who successfully quit).

Herein lies the national public policy challenge: to maintain and strengthen efforts to reduce smoking initiation, but at the same time, aggressively pursue strategies to reduce the number of individuals who actually smoke, especially the chronic hard-core smokers. Ironically, the effort to successfully treat the long-term smoker may be hampered by the culture of contempt toward smokers that has evolved in the last two decades. Although successfully fueling the growth in public and workplace prohibitions and possibly contributing to the reduced uptake of smoking, these cultural changes may also have undermined efforts to expand research for cessation and other treatment for chronic hard-core smokers. Simply put, the villainization of smoking and smokers may be coming back to haunt us, as an absent political will to treat a "lifestyle" illness.

It is against this background of the special challenges of the hard-core smokers and the barriers to their successful treatment that we must examine the critical questions that go to the heart of our commitment to the health of the hard-core smoker:

1. Are we prepared to use health insurance plans to subsidize the smoking cessation efforts of the 80% of smokers who want to quit? Are we as a society willing to support repeated unsuccessful attempts to quit? Are we willing to dedicate substantially more resources to develop better, more efficient and effective smoking cessation programs directed at a variety of populations, as well as underwrite their broad dissemination through health plans?
2. Have we amassed and applied a sufficient current body of knowledge concerning the efficacy of secondary screening (most notably chest x-rays, stress tests, other radiological screening) to facilitate early intervention for morbidities common in current and former heavy smokers (e.g., lung cancer and coronary artery disease)?

SMOKING CESSATION: DEMAND, EFFICACY, AND AVAILABILITY

Approximately 80% of smokers express a desire to quit smoking and a substantial number have attempted to quit. In addition to the consumer-induced demand, increasing yet still insufficient numbers of clinicians and provider organizations are referring patients to cessation services or developing their own cessation programs (i.e., health maintenance organization [HMO] based programs, programs designed for hospital inpatients). Despite this laudable trend, existing cessation programs, even those in which interventions are substantial, have only marginal long-term success rates, and some studies have found self-help to be of equal efficiency when compared with formal programs (Fortmann & Killen, 1995). The addition of nicotine replacement therapy appears to have boosted the quit rates, particularly when combined with support groups (Lando, Pirie, Roski, McGovern, & Schmid, 1996). However, for some populations (e.g., heavy chronic smokers) and when used alone, its success is equivocal (Cepeda-Benito, 1993). An intervention designed by Mayo Clinic researchers for inpatients who had smoking-related nonfatal illnesses and agreed to a 2-week residential cessation program achieved a biologically verified abstention rate of 29% at 1-year follow-up, suggesting that in the arena of smoking cessation more may be more (Hurt et al., 1992). Kottke and his colleagues (Kottke, Battista, DeFriese, & Brekke, 1988) found that the number of intervention modalities used in a cessation program was positively associated with successful cessation, and an analysis of the cost-effectiveness of the clinical practice recommendations of the Agency for Health Care Policy and Research (AHCPR) concluded that "the more intensive the cessation intervention the lower the cost per year of life saved" (Cromwell, Bartosch, Fiore, Hasselblad, & Baker, 1997).

There are a number of explanations for the relatively modest success of most cessation programs, including:

1. The failure to properly assess the smoker and tailor the program to the smoker's particular circumstance (i.e., level of motivation, level of nicotine dependence, and presence of psychiatric conditions).

2. The cohort of adults who still are smoking, particularly those who have been addicted for decades, are now a highly selected population, many of whom have comorbidities such as drug abuse and depression. Also, the most highly addicted are probably the least likely to have successfully quit in the past, thus producing a hybrid group who are most treatment resistant (i.e., the least addicted have long since quit; they are among the 15% reduction in adult smokers from 1965 to 1997).

3. The programs themselves, particularly the broadly disseminated ones, are mostly modest with regard to the intensity of the intervention. A plethora of programs labeled as "brief one-minute interventions" for physicians to apply in their practice have achieved only modest success. Imagine the probable success of a similarly labeled program for the chronic heroin abuser. This is not a far-fetched analogy if one stops to consider the known addictiveness of nicotine and the nature of the population who have not yet been able to quit.

4. Patients have difficulty accessing programs because they have no insurance coverage or although insured, their plan does not cover smoking cessation treatment including reimbursement for nicotine replacement products. Some plans cover only first quit attempts, a particularly irrational policy because virtually all successful quitters had prior unsuccessful attempts.

What explains the low prevalence of high-quality and accessible smoking cessation programs? One reason is the absence of reimbursement incentives by insurers and employers for clinicians and patients, which probably explains much of the shortfall in referrals and treatment uptake. However, probably the most important factor is the misguided belief among the public (three out of four of whom never smoked or are former smokers) that it is relatively easy to quit. This widespread belief does not create fertile soil for the propagation of more and higher quality smoking cessation efforts. Moreover, it may fuel overt hostility toward the smoker, which manifests itself in the form of employer discrimination against smokers (i.e., not hiring them), fiscal penalties for life and health insurance, and truncated treatment and research budgets in the areas of smoking cessation and the treatment of conditions more common among current and former smokers (e.g., emphysema, lung cancer). Like AIDS, smoking has been broadly labeled as a lifestyle choice, despite the long-standing consensus concerning the highly addictive nature of nicotine.

The economic consequences of substantially increasing the proportion of Americans who can successfully quit smoking would be considerable. These benefits should be included in the calculus of deciding how great will be our investment in smoking cessation efforts. These advantages include reduced morbidity and mortality from smoking-related causes, both directly among the smoker, and indirectly among those exposed to secondhand smoke. They also include substantial indirect benefits such as reduction in household fires, one in four of which are attributed to smoking. As Lichtenstein and Glasgow noted in their discussion of the cost-effectiveness of smoking cessation efforts among those with smoking-related illnesses, "quitting smoking is cheaper than another MI [myocardial infarction]" (1992). In an analysis limited to evaluation of health care costs alone, Barendregt and colleagues (1997) concluded that health care costs would be higher overall (by 7% among men and 4% among women) if universal smoking cessation were achieved (the study country was the Netherlands). However, if quality of adjusted life years were used to assess smoking cessation instead, this would show that universal smoking cessation (and for that matter all points along the continuum toward it) results in substantial benefits by increasing the life expectancy of successful quitters.

Smoking can also be viewed as socially contagious; thus, increasing the numbers who successfully quit could reduce the numbers who start, and improve the self-efficacy among those who see others succeed in their attempt to quit. The average cost of highly successful (i.e., 20–30% smoke free at 1 year) smoking cessation programs should probably fall somewhere between the current low-tech physician pep talk with and without nicotine replacement, and the highly intensive Mayo Clinic 2-week inpatient model with intensive follow-up services. It is not unreasonable to expect to pay

$2,000 on multiple occasions to achieve successful cessation in a chronic long-term smoker. These funds would support physician and nonphysician counseling, nicotine replacement therapy and other drugs as needed, the organization and conduct of support groups. In some instances residentially based nicotine withdrawal/detoxification may be crucial. If, on average, each smoker "consumed" $10,000 attempting to successfully quit, the costs amortized over all insured (both public and private) over the collective life spans would be modest indeed. Cromwell and colleagues (1997) calculated the cost of universal implementation in the United States of the AHCPR clinical practice guidelines to be $6.3 billion per year or $32 per capita to yield 1.7 million new quitters. Such a macro-scale effort would reap far greater economic benefits if it could contribute to our actually achieving our year 2010 smoking objectives—now, just a gleam in the eye of the Secretary of Health and Human Services.

SECONDARY PREVENTION IN THE CURRENT AND FORMER SMOKER

A debate is igniting concerning the efficacy of the annual chest x-ray to screen and more effectively treat current and former smokers for early lung cancer. The essence of this debate contends that the large-scale prospective clinical trials that led to the abandonment of the annual chest x-ray routine screenings may have falsely concluded that chest x-ray provides no added value due to a flawed outcome measure. Also, one of the four large-scale studies was designed to test sputum cytologic study and x-ray combined and thus was not able to address the efficacy of chest x-ray specifically. The authors concluded that for the period 1980–1994, 31,540 lives could have been saved in the United States using routine chest x-rays of current and former heavy smokers, if their thesis is correct (Strauss, Gleason, & Sugarbaker, 1995). It also is noteworthy that none of the population-based evaluations of the efficacy of chest x-ray included women as subjects—despite the fact that lung cancer was then a growing cause of cancer death among women (and indeed, it is now the leading cause of cancer death). This is particularly unfortunate given the fact that a substantial proportion of women smoke and they are less successful in cessation attempts.

Here again it is clear that the villainization of the smoker may color the research and treatment landscape. Why haven't we conducted further studies to determine if more lives can be saved with detection and improved surgical and other treatment?

This raises yet another issue—the increased risk of cardiovascular disease among smokers, notably coronary artery disease (CAD) and cerebral vascular disease. The former is well documented to be underdiagnosed and undertreated among women (Blustein, Arons, & Shea, 1995; Wenger, Speroff, & Packard, 1993). Although Wenger and colleagues have concluded that "neither exercise testing nor any other simple test is of value for large-scale screening for coronary heart disease in truly asymptomatic patients (either men or women), even when coronary risk factors are present," those with early symptoms or abnormal electrocardiograms (EKGs) are probably plentiful among the population of chronic smokers. Given the rapid decline in myocardial infarction (MI) risk among women who quit smoking, virtually indistinguishable from those who never smoked within 3 years of cessation (Rosenberg, Palmer, & Shapiro, 1990), broader screening is probably warranted, as is further research for presymptomatic screening approaches. Given the fact that a medical crisis represents a teachable moment and that heart disease can be detected by stress tests and other screening and early treatment begun, should separate guidelines for screening exist for chronic heavy smokers? Might a warning about specific CAD findings have induced some to quit? Might pharmacological and other interventions save some lives? Might a national policy of more extensive disease screening among smokers send an important message and achieve a desired end: fewer smokers, less disease progression, and improved treatment outcome?

Even if future studies strongly support the reintroduction of the routine chest x-ray and expanded clinical preventive screening for cardiovascular disease, broadly disseminated uptake will be slow in this era of managed care and in light of the assumption by many that tobacco use is simply a "lifestyle choice."

Enlightened public policy designed to meet the nation's tobacco cessation goals should include markedly expanded tobacco cessation tailored to specific populations and supported by health care plans, ongoing research and clinical application of secondary prevention to decrease tobacco related morbidity and mortality, and adoption of the recommendations of the final report of the Advisory Committee on Tobacco Policy and Public Health. These recommendations can only be fully implemented through the combined forces of litigation against the tobacco industry and a mix of federal, state, and local legislation both to regulate the industry and to support research and treatment. Hopefully, public policy decisions will focus on treatments for the hard-core smoker as well as balance the need for primary prevention, cessation and treatment research, and adequate reimbursement for cessation programs, screening, and tertiary care.

REFERENCES

Barendregt, J. J., Bonneux, L., & van der Maas, P. J. (1997). *NEJM, 337*(15), 1052–1057.

Blustein, J., Arons, R., & Shea, S. (1995). Sequential events contributing to variations in cardiac revascularization rates. *Medical Care, 33*(8), 864–900.

Cepeda-Benito, A. (1993). Meta-analytical review of the efficacy of nicotine chewing gum in smoking treatment programs. *Journal of Consulting and Clinical Psychology, 61*(5), 822–830.

Cromwell, J., Bartosch, W. J., Fiore, M. C., Hasselblad, V., & Baker, T. B. (1997). Cost-effectiveness of the clinical practice recommendations in the AHCPR Guideline for Smoking Cessation. *JAMA, 278*(21), 1759–1766.

Fortman, S. P., & Killen, J. D. (1995). Nicotine gum and self-help behavioral treatment for smoking relapse prevention: Results from a trial using population-based recruitment. *Journal of Consulting Psychology, 63*(3), 460–468.

Hurt, R. D., Lowell, C. D., Offord, K. P., Bance, B. K., McClain, F. L., & Eberman, K. M. (1992). Inpatient treatment of severe nicotine dependence. *Mayo Clinic Proceedings, 67,* 823–828.

Janofsky, M. (1993, December 19). 25-Year decline of smoking seems to be slowing. *New York Times,* p. 1.

Kessler, D. A., & Koop, C. E. (1997, July). *Final Report of the Advisory Committee on Tobacco Policy and Public Health* (Unpublished Advisory Committee Report to Congress commissioned by a bipartisan group of Members of Congress).

Kottke, T. E., Battista, R. N., DeFriese, G. H., & Brekke, M. L. (1988). Attributes of successful smoking cessation interventions in medical practice, a meta-analysis of 39 controlled trials. *JAMA, 259*(19), 2883–2889.

Lando, H. A., Pirie, P. L., Roski, J., McGovern, P. G., & Schmid, L. A. (1996). Promoting abstinence among relapsed chronic smokers: The effect of telephone support. *American Journal of Public Health, 12,* 1786–1790.

Lichtenstein, E., & Glasgow, R. E. (1992). Smoking cessation: What have we learned over the past decade. *Journal of Consulting and Clinical Psychology, 50*(4), 518–527.

Rosenberg, L., Palmer, J. R., & Shapiro, S. (1990). *New England Journal of Medicine, 322*(4), 213–217.

Strauss, G. M., Gleason, R. E., & Sugarbaker, D. J. (1995). Chest x-ray screening improves outcome in lung cancer: A reappraisal of randomized trials on lung cancer screening. *Chest, 107,* 2705–2795.

U.S. Department of Health and Human Services. (1990). *Healthy people 2000: National health promotion and disease prevention objectives* (DHHS Publication No. [PHS] 91-50212, pp. 133–141). U.S. Government Printing Office, Washington, DC.

Wenger, N. K., Speroff, L., & Packard B. (1993). Cardiovascular health and disease in women. *New England Journal of Medicine, 329,* 247–256.

About the Contributors

David Adams, PhD, MPH was formerly Research Director of the Cabarrus Family Medicine Program. He is Assistant Clinical Professor, Department of Family Medicine and Public Health, James Quillen School of Medicine, East Tennessee State University, Johnson City, Tennessee.

Gilbert J. Botvin, PhD earned his doctorate from Columbia University in 1977 in both developmental and clinical psychology. After working for 3 years at the American Health Foundation, where he served as Director of Child Health Behavior research, he joined the faculty of Cornell University Medical College. He is currently a professor of Public Health and Psychiatry at Cornell University Medical College, Director of Cornell's Institute for Prevention Research, and an attending psychologist at the New York Hospital-Cornell Medical Center.

Neal R. Boyd, EdD, MSPH did graduate work in Health Behavior/Education and Behavioral Science at the University of Tennessee at Knoxville and the University of Alabama at Birmingham School of Public Health. He has been a faculty member and university administrator at the University of Southern Mississippi, a Research Fellow at the National Cancer Institute, and currently is the Associate Director of Tobacco Control Research at Fox Chase Cancer Center.

Joseph A. Califano, Jr. is founding Chairperson and President of the National Center on Addiction and Substance Abuse at Columbia University. He is Adjunct Professor of Public Health (Health Policy and Management) at Columbia University's Medical School (Department of Psychiatry) and School of Public Health, and a member of the Institute of Medicine of the National Academy of Sciences. In January 1977, Mr. Califano became Secretary of Health, Education, and Welfare. He served in that Cabinet post until August 1979.

Lirio S. Covey, PhD (Co-editor) is Associate Professor of Clinical Psychology (in Psychiatry), Columbia University, and Research Scientist, New York State Psychiatric Institute. Dr. Covey has treated several hundred addicted smokers as Co-Director of the Smoking Cessation Research Clinic at the Psychiatric Institute.

Donald B. Douglas, MD is a diplomate of the American Board of Psychiatry and Neurology and of the American Board of Medical Hypnosis. He is currently Associate in Neurology and in Psychiatry at Lenox Hill Hospital in New York City.

Michelle Drayton-Martin, RN, MPH was the founding Director of Healthy Start/NYC, and remained with the project through its demonstration phase (1991–1997). Ms. Drayton-Martin is presently with Communications, Inc. in New York City. She holds a Master's degree in Public Health, a Bachelors of Science in Nursing, and a Certificate in Executive Management of Not-for-Profits from Columbia University School of Business.

Thomas Eissenberg, PhD is Assistant Professor of Psychology, Virginia Commonwealth University. He received his PhD in Psychology from McMaster University in Ontario, Canada and his postdoctoral training in Human Behavioral Pharmacology from Johns Hopkins University.

Roselyn Epps, MD is a medical officer at the National Cancer Institute and helps develop strategies to train professionals in smoking prevention and cessation techniques. She serves as a national and international consultant. Formerly, she practiced medicine, served as D.C. Acting Public Health Commissioner and was a professor at Howard University College of Medicine.

Jennifer A. Epstein, PhD completed her degree in Social Personality Psychology at Columbia University. She is an Assistant Professor of Psychology in the Department of Public Health at Cornell University Medical College.

Karen K. Gerlach, PhD, MPH was a Cancer Prevention Fellow at the National Cancer Institute in Bethesda, Maryland when this chapter was written. Dr. Gerlach is currently an epidemiologist in the office on Smoking and Health at the Centers for Disease Control and Prevention in Atlanta, Georgia. She received her PhD in Microbiology and Immunology from Indiana University School of Medicine and her MPH degree from the Johns Hopkins University School of Hygiene and Public Health.

Alexander H. Glassman, MD is Chief of Clinical Psychopharmacology at the New York State Psychiatric Institute and Professor of Psychiatry at Columbia University. Dr. Glassman is an internationally recognized expert in the treatment of depression and a leading expert in psychiatric issues related to nicotine dependence research and treatment.

Thomas J. Glynn, PhD is Director, Cancer Science and Trends, American Cancer Society. He was formerly Chief of the Cancer Prevention and Control Research Branch at the National Cancer Institute (NCI). At NCI he directed the development of a national program of research aimed at reducing the incidence and prevalence of cancer, primarily through dietary change, tobacco use reduction, and adherence to cancer screening guidelines.

Cheryl Healton, Dr PH is Head of the Division of Sociomedical Sciences and Associate Dean at the Columbia University School of Public Health. She earned her Dr.PH from the Columbia School of Public Health. Prior to her appointment at the School of Public Health she was Assistant Vice President and Associate Dean of Columbia's College of Physicians & Surgeons.

Jack E. Henningfield, PhD is Associate Professor of Behavioral Biology, Johns Hopkins School of Medicine and Vice President, Research and Health Policy, Pinney Associates. Until August 1996, Dr. Henningfield was Chief of the Clinical Pharmacology Branch of the National Institute on Drug Abuse (NIDA). He currently serves as President (1998–1999) of the Society for Research on Nicotine and Tobacco.

J. Andrew Johnston, Pharm D received a BS in pharmacy from the University of South Carolina and a Doctor of Pharmacy at the University of Tennessee. Following specialty training in Psychopharmacy, he practiced at the Veterans Administration Hospital and the University of Tennessee in Memphis. For the past 15 years Dr. Johnston has been involved in developing psychotropic compounds at Glaxo Wellcome Inc. He is currently a Senior Clinical Program Head in CNS Clinical Research.

Marc W. Manley, MD, MPH is Chief of the Public Health Applications Branch in the Division of Cancer Prevention and Control of the National Cancer Institute. Dr. Manley directs a national program to train health professionals in effective smoking cessation techniques. Dr. Manley received his MD from the University of Washington in Seattle. He received an MPH and completed the Preventive Medicine Residency Program at the Johns Hopkins University.

Sherry Mills, MD, MPH received her undergraduate degree in Human Biology from Brown University, her medical school training at the University of Cincinnati, College of Medicine, and completed her residency in Internal Medicine at Providence Hospital, Washington, DC. Dr. Mills also received a Masters of Public Health degree from The Johns Hopkins School of Hygiene and Public Health, and completed a residency in preventive medicine. She is currently serving as a cancer control research scientist in the Prevention and Control Extramural Branch of the National Cancer Institute.

Naomi Rock Novak, MS formerly the Director of Public Directions and Resource Development for Healthy Start/NYC is now director of Public Relations, Community Outreach, and Volunteers for Saint Michael's Medical Center, Newark, NJ. She is also the president of Allegheny International Associates, a communications and marketing firm specializing in science, hi-tech, health, and medicine. Ms. Novak has a Master's in Journalism from Columbia

C. Tracy Orleans, PhD is a Senior Program Officer and Senior Researcher at the Robert Wood Johnson Foundation, where she has responsibility for numerous research-based tobacco control, substance abuse prevention, behavioral medicine, and chronic disease management projects. A clinical psychologist, she also serves as Adjunct Full Member of Fox Chase Cancer Center, Philadelphia, PA, and Adjunct Professor in the Department of Psychiatry at the University of Medicine and Dentistry of New Jersey.

Mark D. Robinson, MD is the Associate Director of the Cabarrus Family Medicine Residency Program and the founder and medical director of the Cabarrus Nicotine Dependence Center in Concord, North Carolina. Dr. Robinson is a Consulting Associate in the Department of Community and Family Medicine at Duke University.

Lorna Role, PhD was educated at Harvard, receiving a B.A. in Applied Mathematics in 1975 and her Ph.D. from the Medical Sciences division in Physiology in 1981. She was then appointed as an assistant professor at Columbia P&S in the Department of Cell Biology and Anatomy in the Center for Neurobiology in 1985 and granted tenure in 1992.

Jeffrey S. Rosecan, MD is an Assistant Clinical Professor of Psychiatry in the Department of Psychiatry, Columbia University. He is co-author of *Cocaine Abuse: New Directions in Treatment and Research*, and is founder of the Cocaine Abuse and Chemical Dependency Program, Columbia Presbyterian Medical Center.

Daniel F. Seidman, PhD (Co-editor) received his PhD in Clinical Psychology from Columbia University. He is Assistant Clinical Professor of Medical Psychology (in Psychiatry), Columbia University, College of Physicians and Surgeons. Dr. Seidman is Director of Smoking Cessation Services at the Behavioral Medicine Program of Columbia University.

Jill Shamban, MS received her Masters of Science in Health Policy and Management from the Harvard School of Public Health in 1989. She was formerly Program Manager for Healthy Start/NYC and is now the owner of Shamban Consulting which specializes in health and social services management and research.

Henry I. Spitz, MD is Clinical Professor of Psychiatry in the Department of Psychiatry of Columbia University, College of Physicians & Surgeons. He is also Director of Group Psychotherapy and Marital Therapy at New York State Psychiatric Institute and at the Columbia-Presbyterian Medical Center. He, along with Jeffrey Rosecan MD, is editor and contributor to the text: *Cocaine Abuse: New Directions in Treatment and Research.*

Maxine L. Stitzer, PhD is Professor of Psychiatry and Behavioral Sciences at John Hopkins University School of Medicine. She received her PhD in Psychology and training in Psychopharmacology from the University of Michigan. She has been president of the Division on Psychopharmacology and

Substance Abuse of the American Psychological Association, served on the AHCPR Smoking Cessation Guidelines panel, and on the Board of Directors of the College on Problems of Drug Dependence, and is a former president (1997–1998) of the Society for Research on Nicotine and Tobacco.

Lynn Tepper, PhD is Associate Clinical Professor and Director of the Behavioral Science Program at Columbia University School of Dental and Oral Surgery and School of Public Health. She is also Director of the Institute of Gerontology at Mercy College in Dobbs Ferry, NY, and is on the faculty of Long Island University where she teaches Health Psychology in the Department of Graduate Psychology and through the Internet.

Frances Trakis-Manners, MS, RD formerly the smoking cessation Coordinator for Healthy Start/NYC, is now a consultant to smoking cessation programs and coalitions committed to advocacy and education regarding the risks of smoking. She received her Masters of Science in Public Health Nutrition from Columbia University in 1978. Ms. Manners was instrumental in the development of the Healthy Start/NYC Smoking Cessation Program.

Author Index

C

D

E

F

G

I

J

K

L

T

Y

Z

Subject Index

D

E

F

G

H

I

L

M

N

O

P

Q

R

S

T

For Product Safety Concerns and Information please contact our EU representative GPSR@taylorandfrancis.com Taylor & Francis Verlag GmbH, Kaufingerstraße 24, 80331 München, Germany

Printed and bound by CPI Group (UK) Ltd, Croydon, CR0 4YY

08/06/2025

01896998-0013